The Effects of Mycotoxins on Human and Animal Health

The Effects of Mycotoxins on Human and Animal Health

A Special Focus on the Cellular and Molecular Mechanisms Responsible for Mycotoxin Toxicity

Editors

Daniela Eliza Marin
Ionelia Taranu

MDPI • Basel • Beijing • Wuhan • Barcelona • Belgrade • Manchester • Tokyo • Cluj • Tianjin

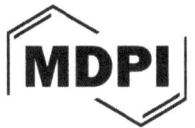

Editors
Daniela Eliza Marin
National Institut for Research and Development
for Biology and Animal Nutrition
Romania

Ionelia Taranu
National Institut for Research and Development
for Biology and Animal Nutrition
Romania

Editorial Office
MDPI
St. Alban-Anlage 66
4052 Basel, Switzerland

This is a reprint of articles from the Special Issue published online in the open access journal *Toxins* (ISSN 2072-6651) (available at: https://www.mdpi.com/journal/toxins/special_issues/Mycotoxins_Cellular_Molecular).

For citation purposes, cite each article independently as indicated on the article page online and as indicated below:

LastName, A.A.; LastName, B.B.; LastName, C.C. Article Title. *Journal Name* **Year**, *Volume Number*, Page Range.

ISBN 978-3-0365-3028-4 (Hbk)
ISBN 978-3-0365-3029-1 (PDF)

© 2022 by the authors. Articles in this book are Open Access and distributed under the Creative Commons Attribution (CC BY) license, which allows users to download, copy and build upon published articles, as long as the author and publisher are properly credited, which ensures maximum dissemination and a wider impact of our publications.

The book as a whole is distributed by MDPI under the terms and conditions of the Creative Commons license CC BY-NC-ND.

Contents

About the Editors vii

Preface to "The Effects of Mycotoxins on Human and Animal Health" ix

Daniela Eliza Marin, Cristina Valeria Bulgaru, Cristian Andrei Anghel, Gina Cecilia Pistol, Madalina Ioana Dore, Mihai Laurentiu Palade and Ionelia Taranu
Grape Seed Waste Counteracts Aflatoxin B1 Toxicity in Piglet Mesenteric Lymph Nodes
Reprinted from: *Toxins* **2020**, *12*, 800, doi:10.3390/toxins12120800 1

Roua Gabriela Popescu, Cristina Bulgaru, Arabela Untea, Mihaela Vlassa, Miuta Filip, Anca Hermenean, Daniela Marin, Ionelia Țăranu, Sergiu Emil Georgescu and Anca Dinischiotu
The Effectiveness of Dietary Byproduct Antioxidants on Induced CYP Genes Expression and Histological Alteration in Piglets Liver and Kidney Fed with Aflatoxin B1 and Ochratoxin A
Reprinted from: *Toxins* **2021**, *13*, 148, doi:10.3390/toxins13020148 15

Diana Herman and Peter Mantle
Rat Tumour Histopathology Associated with Experimental Chronic Dietary Exposure to Ochratoxin A in Prediction of the Mycotoxin's Risk for Human Cancers
Reprinted from: *Toxins* **2021**, *13*, 205, doi:10.3390/toxins13030205 37

Gerald Schwerdt, Michael Kopf and Michael Gekle
The Impact of the Nephrotoxin Ochratoxin A on Human Renal Cells Studied by a Novel Co-Culture Model Is Influenced by the Presence of Fibroblasts
Reprinted from: *Toxins* **2021**, *13*, 219, doi:10.3390/toxins13030219 47

Jinling Cui, Shutao Yin, Chong Zhao, Lihong Fan and Hongbo Hu
Combining Patulin with Cadmium Induces Enhanced Hepatotoxicity and Nephrotoxicity In Vitro and In Vivo
Reprinted from: *Toxins* **2021**, *13*, 221, doi:10.3390/toxins13030221 61

Cristina Valeria Bulgaru, Daniela Eliza Marin, Gina Cecilia Pistol and Ionelia Taranu
Zearalenone and the Immune Response
Reprinted from: *Toxins* **2021**, *13*, 248, doi:10.3390/toxins13040248 73

Chao Gu, Xiuge Gao, Dawei Guo, Jiacai Wang, Qinghua Wu, Eugenie Nepovimova, Wenda Wu and Kamil Kuca
Combined Effect of Deoxynivalenol (DON) and Porcine Circovirus Type 2 (Pcv2) on Inflammatory Cytokine mRNA Expression
Reprinted from: *Toxins* **2021**, *13*, 422, doi:10.3390/toxins13060422 93

Po-Yen Lee, Ching-Chih Liu, Shu-Chi Wang, Kai-Yin Chen, Tzu-Chieh Lin, Po-Len Liu, Chien-Chih Chiu, I-Chen Chen, Yu-Hung Lai, Wei-Chung Cheng, Wei-Ju Chung, Hsin-Chih Yeh, Chi-Han Huang, Chia-Cheng Su, Shu-Pin Huang and Chia-Yang Li
Mycotoxin Zearalenone Attenuates Innate Immune Responses and Suppresses NLRP3 Inflammasome Activation in LPS-Activated Macrophages
Reprinted from: *Toxins* **2021**, *13*, 593, doi:10.3390/toxins13090593 109

Roua Gabriela Popescu, Sorin Avramescu, Daniela Eliza Marin, Ionelia Țăranu, Sergiu Emil Georgescu and Anca Dinischiotu
The Reduction of the Combined Effects of Aflatoxin and Ochratoxin A in Piglet Livers and Kidneys by Dietary Antioxidants
Reprinted from: *Toxins* **2021**, *13*, 648, doi:10.3390/toxins13090648 125

About the Editors

Daniela Eliza Marin is Senior Researcher in the Laboratory of Animal Biology and Scientific Secretary of the National Institute for Research and Development in Biology and Animal Nutrition, Baloteşti, Romania. For more than 20 years, she has acquired expertise in mycotoxins and their effects on the animal health. She has coordinated two international projects and five national projects in toxicology and she was involved in more than 30 national and international projects as team member. She is a reviewer for more than 20 international journals and Academic Editor for the journals *Toxins* and *Romanian Biotechnology Letters*. Out of 120 published papers, more than 50 were published as the main author or co-author in peer-reviewed journals, mainly in Toxicology. She was Evaluator or Scientific Officer for different research agencies (UEFISCDI—Romania, National Science Centre—Polonia, Agence Universitaire de la Francophonie etc.).

Ionelia Taranu is a senior researcher at the National Research and Development Institute for Biology and Animal Nutrition (INCDBNA-IBNA), Balotesti, Romania. She is the head of Animal Biology Laboratory, IBNA, in which she coordinates a team of seven scientists and four technicians working on nutrition and immunology field. The research work of Dr. Ionelia TARANU is substantiated in 152 scientific publications (of which 71 are ISI), mainly dealing with the impact of feed quality (optimization of dietary composition) and feed security (feed contamination) on the performance, gastro-intestinal barrier and health of farm animals (immune response modulation to various dietary factors: novel feed, contaminants: mycotoxins, pre- and probiotics: bioactive compounds, fibers, bacteria, etc.). She is an independent evaluator expert (ID: EX2002B070822) for the EU Commission and invited expert of EFSA and other research agencies (UEFISCDI—Romania, ANCSI—Romania, Dutch Technology Foundation, National Science Centre-Polonia, FWO, Suisse).

Preface to "The Effects of Mycotoxins on Human and Animal Health"

Mycotoxins are secondary metabolites mainly synthesized by fungi belonging to the Aspergillus, Fusarium and Penicillium genera. The contamination of cereals and agricultural products by mycotoxins may lead to a variety of adverse health effects, ranging from acute to chronic toxicity, with serious health implications for both humans and animals. The toxic effects of mycotoxins are characterized by lesions in target organs such as the liver and kidneys and in the pulmonary, intestinal, immune and central nervous systems, which can vary according to the type of toxin, time of exposure, mycotoxin concentration, animal species, sex, etc. At the cellular level, many processes such as apoptosis, genotoxicity, oxidative stress and inflammation have been described as being responsible for the effects of mycotoxins.

Immune response is one of the most affected by the exposure to mycotoxins. Chronic or sub-chronic exposure to mycotoxins is responsible for impaired immunity, decreased resistance to disease, increase in the predisposition of animals to infections and, consequently, decreased productivity. However, the mode of action of mycotoxins on different effectors of the immune response and the molecular mechanisms involved need further research. Another subject of interest is related to the concomitant exposure of human and animals to mycotoxins and other food/feed contaminants such as viruses, bacteria, pesticides, heavy metals, etc., which can have additive or synergic toxic effects and thus can amplify the mycotoxins toxicity.

Mycotoxins represents an important threat for the global economy and there is a permanent need to find new solutions for the mitigation of the mycotoxin effects in human and animals. Among them, the nutritional solutions represent a more convenient approach due to their low toxicity and their high content in bioactive compounds that can improve the health of human and animals exposed to mycotoxins.

The present Special Issue aims to improve our knowledge concerning mycotoxin toxicity by investigating their mode of action and the molecular mechanisms involved at the level of organs involved in the metabolism and excretion (liver and kidney) as well as at the level of the immune response effectors. Additionally, the efficacy of some dietary byproduct antioxidants, such as mitigation agents, in improving the health of animals exposed to individual mycotoxins or combination of mycotoxins was investigated.

Daniela Eliza Marin, Ionelia Taranu
Editors

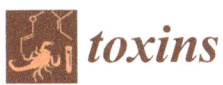

Article

Grape Seed Waste Counteracts Aflatoxin B1 Toxicity in Piglet Mesenteric Lymph Nodes

Daniela Eliza Marin *, Cristina Valeria Bulgaru, Cristian Andrei Anghel, Gina Cecilia Pistol, Madalina Ioana Dore, Mihai Laurentiu Palade and Ionelia Taranu

National Institute for Research and Development for Biology and Animal Nutrition, INCDBNA Balotesti, Calea Bucuresti nr 1, Balotesti, 077015 Ilfov, Romania; cristinavaleria11@yahoo.com (C.V.B.); andrei.anghel@ibna.ro (C.A.A.); gina.pistol@ibna.ro (G.C.P.); dore.madalina@ibna.ro (M.I.D.); mihai.palade@ibna.ro (M.L.P.); ionelia.taranu@ibna.ro (I.T.)
* Correspondence: daniela.marin@ibna.ro; Tel.: +40-213512082

Received: 13 November 2020; Accepted: 13 December 2020; Published: 15 December 2020

Abstract: Aflatoxin B1 (AFB1) is a mycotoxin that frequently contaminates cereals and cereal byproducts. This study investigates the effect of AFB1 on the mesenteric lymph nodes (MLNs) of piglets and evaluates if a diet containing grape seed meal (GSM) can counteract the negative effect of AFB1 on inflammation and oxidative stress. Twenty-four weaned piglets were fed the following diets: Control, AFB1 group (320 µg AFB1/kg feed), GSM group (8% GSM), and AFB1 + GSM group (8% GSM + 320 µg AFB1/kg feed) for 30 days. AFB1 has an important antioxidative effect by decreasing the activity of catalase (CAT), superoxide dismutase (SOD), and glutathione peroxidase (GPx) and total antioxidant status. As a result of the exposure to AFB1, an increase of MAP kinases, metalloproteinases, and cytokines, as effectors of an inflammatory response, were observed in the MLNs of intoxicated piglets. GSM induced a reduction of AFB1-induced oxidative stress by increasing the activity of GPx and SOD and by decreasing lipid peroxidation. GSM decreased the inflammatory markers increased by AFB1. These results represent an important and promising way to valorize this waste, which is rich in bioactive compounds, for decreasing AFB1 toxic effects in mesenteric lymph nodes.

Keywords: aflatoxin B1; grape seed meal; mesenteric lymph nodes; piglets

Key Contribution: Aflatoxin B1 induces inflammation and oxidative stress in mesenteric lymph nodes. In the mesenteric lymph nodes of AFB1-intoxicated piglets, grape seed meal can improve some markers of inflammation and oxidative stress.

1. Introduction

The gut is constantly exposed to potentially harmful contaminants from food or feed, such as mycotoxins [1]. Aflatoxin B1 is a mycotoxin produced by different species of fungi, especially *Aspergillus flavus* and *A. parasiticus* [2]. AFB1 is a potent carcinogen in humans and animals [3] and, for this reason, was classified in Group 1 of human carcinogens on the basis of toxicological data. Aflatoxins can contaminate different commodities such as cereals, nuts, dried fruits, and spices [4].

AFB1 is absorbed in the proximal part of the gut at high rates regardless of the species [5]. As the passage of the toxin across the intestinal barrier is very high, AFB1 can compromise the intestinal epithelium even before the absorption in the upper part of the gut. Indeed, it was shown that AFB1 induced inhibition of epithelial cell growth [6], an increase of apoptosis [6], and an increase of apoptotic markers (Bax and caspase-3) [7]. Additionally, AFB1 induced dysregulation of intestinal microbiota [8] and affected intestinal barrier function [9,10]. After absorption in the intestinal villi, the lipophilic compounds, such as AFB1, are first transported via the mesenteric lymphatic duct and then through the thoracic duct before entering the blood circulation [11]. Mesenteric lymph nodes (MSLs) are important for the proper functioning of the immune system of the gut, acting as filters for nutrients and microbial substances that enter through the lymph in the intestinal lamina propria [12]. MSLs are responsible for tolerance induction to food particles, but they also contribute to the prevention of the systemic inflammatory response that can result from the bypass of portal circulation [13].

AFB1 is a potent immunomodulator as the toxin has been shown to impair both the innate and acquired immune responses [14,15]. However, until now, little is known about the effect of AFB1 on gut immunity and, especially, mesenteric lymph nodes as local effectors of the immune response in the gut.

Grape seed meal (GSM) represents the residue left after grape seed oil extraction; this waste can be recycled in order to enrich the feed rations of farm animals [16,17]. GSM has a high content of bioactive compounds: polyunsaturated fatty acids (mainly linoleic acid, n-6), in addition to oleic acid (n-9), dietary fiber, phenolic acids, resveratrol, proanthocyanidins, and flavonoids [18,19]. In living organisms, the beneficial effects of bioactive plant compounds as counteracting agents for AFB1 toxicity have been investigated both in vivo and in vitro [20]. An in-vitro study performed on human hepatocytes has shown that an extract from palm kernel cake, rich in phenolics, has beneficial effects by upregulating the genes involved in the response to oxidative stress and downregulating the genes associated with inflammation and apoptosis in AFB1-exposed hepatocytes [21]. Additionally, in vivo studies have demonstrated that in rats, oxidized tea polyphenols can form a complex with AFB1 that leads to a decrease of AFB1 absorption and, implicitly, a reduction of its toxicity [22].

In particular, the bioactive compounds from grape seed were shown to have beneficial effects on intoxication with AFB1. In a recent study, the supplementation of an AFB1-contaminated diet with grape seed proanthocyanidin extract reduced AFB1 residue in the liver and significantly mitigated the negative effects caused by AFB1 in broiler chickens [23]. Through their alimentation, rich in cereals, especially maize, pigs are particularly exposed to mycotoxins. We have demonstrated that GSM addition into a diet contaminated with AFB1 ameliorates histological liver injuries, reduces the parameters associated with oxidative stress in piglets [24], and is able to change the microbiota composition already affected by AFB1 exposure [25]. The present study is a continuation of our previous studies and aims to investigate if AFB1 can affect mesenteric lymph nodes as the gate of toxic substances in intestinal lamina propria. Additionally, this study aims to evaluate if the administration of a diet containing grape seed meal can counteract the negative effects of AFB1 on inflammation and oxidative response.

2. Results

2.1. Effect of Grape Seed Meal and Aflatoxin B1 on Oxidative Damage in Mesenteric Lymph Nodes

AFB1 induces a significative decrease in the activity of the enzymes involved in the response to oxidative stress, with 27% for catalase (CAT; $p = 0.0248$), 22% for glutathione peroxidase (GPx; $p = 0.0034$), and 10.2% for superoxide dismutase (SOD; $p < 0.0001$), as compared with the control piglets (Figure 1). Additionally, exposure of piglets to 320 µg AFB1/kg feed, significantly decreased the total antioxidant status (−20.5%; $p = 0.0001$) associated with an increase of lipid peroxidation (+52.3%; $p = 0.0001$), as assessed by the TBARS method. When piglet diet included 8% of grape seed meal, no effect was observed on the activity of the enzymes involved in antioxidative defense, total antioxidant capacity (TAC), or lipid peroxidation. However, the concomitant administration of both grape seed meal and toxin resulted in a significant increase of GPx (by 119.3%; $p = 0.0048$), SOD (by 105.9%; $p = 0.0046$), and TAC (by 112%; $p = 0.0180$), as compared with the AFB1 group, while decreasing lipid peroxidation (by 12.3%; $p = 0.018$). GSM was not able to significantly increase CAT activity ($p = 0.331$, as compared with the AFB1 group).

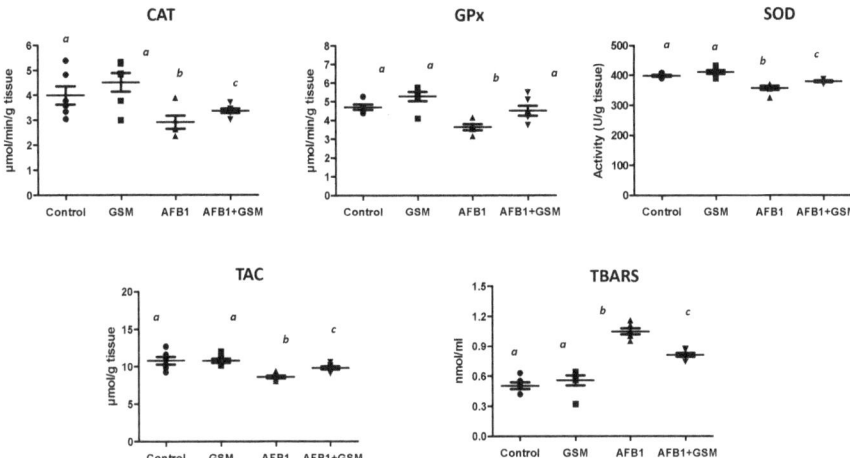

Figure 1. Effect of grape seed meal and AFB1 on oxidative damage in mesenteric lymph nodes. Data represent mean ± SD, n = 6. One-way ANOVA tests, followed by a Fisher's PSLD test, were used for statistical data analyses. [a–c] indicate statistically significant differences between treatments ($p < 0.05$).

2.2. Effect of Grape Seed Meal and Aflatoxin B1 on Inflammatory Cytokine Synthesis in Mesenteric Lymph Nodes

Piglets' exposure to AFB1 contaminated diet was responsible for a a significant increase in the synthesis of IL-1β ($p = 0.0068$), IL-8 ($p = 0.0010$), and for a tendency of increase in the synthesis of IL-6, IFN-γ, and TNF-α ($p > 0.05$; Figure 2).

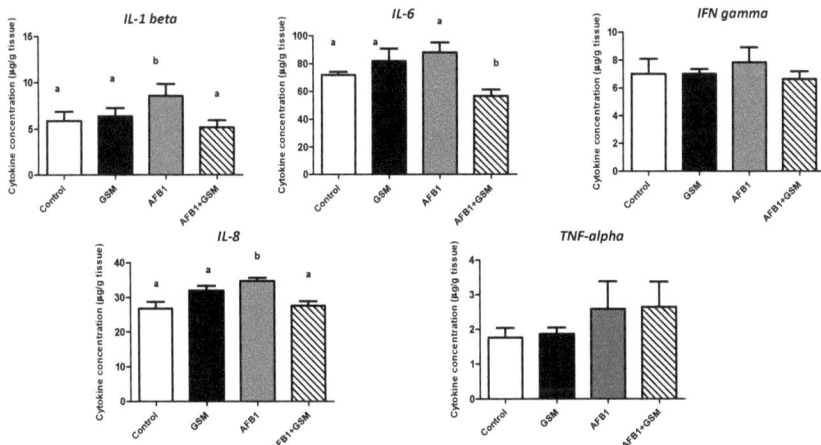

Figure 2. Effect of grape seed meal and AFB1 on inflammatory cytokine synthesis in mesenteric lymph nodes. Data represent means ± SD, n = 6. One-way ANOVA tests, followed by Fisher's PSLD test, were used for statistical data analyses. [a–c] indicate statistically significant differences between treatments ($p < 0.05$).

GSM diet did not affect the synthesis of inflammatory cytokines, the concentration of analyzed cytokines being very similar to the concentration measured in the mesenteric lymph nodes of the control group.

GSM administration to the piglets exposed to AFB1 (AFB1 + GSM diet) had an important anti-inflammatory effect, decreasing inflammatory cytokine synthesis towards the control level. Inclusion of GSM into the AFB1-contaminated diet (AFB1 + GSM group) was responsible for a decrease in the synthesis of IL-1β (8.57 ± 2.97 to 5.16 ± 1.75 μg/g tissue), IL-8 (34.7 ± 2.07 to 27.59 ± 3.07 μg/g tissue), IL-6 (81.9 ± 14.9 to 57.97 ± 9.88), and IFN-γ (8.13 ± 2.54 to 6.72 ± 1.47 μg/g tissue) towards the levels of the control group.

This decrease was significant for IL-1β ($p = 0.0009$), IL-6 ($p = 0.044$), and IL-8 ($p = 0.0018$) and not for IFN-γ ($p = 0.371$). GSM was not able to counteract the increase of TNF-α induced by the toxin ($p = 0.389$).

2.3. Effect of Grape Seed Meal and Aflatoxin B1 on Cell Signaling Pathways in Mesenteric Lymph Nodes

In order to validate the qPCR analysis and to demonstrate that GSM can restore the negative effects, such as inflammation and the oxidative response triggered by AFB1, we assessed by Western blot the expression of three proteins involved in NF-kB and Nrf2 signaling pathways: phospho-p38 MAPK, phospho-NF-kBp65, and Nrf2 (Figure 3A–C).

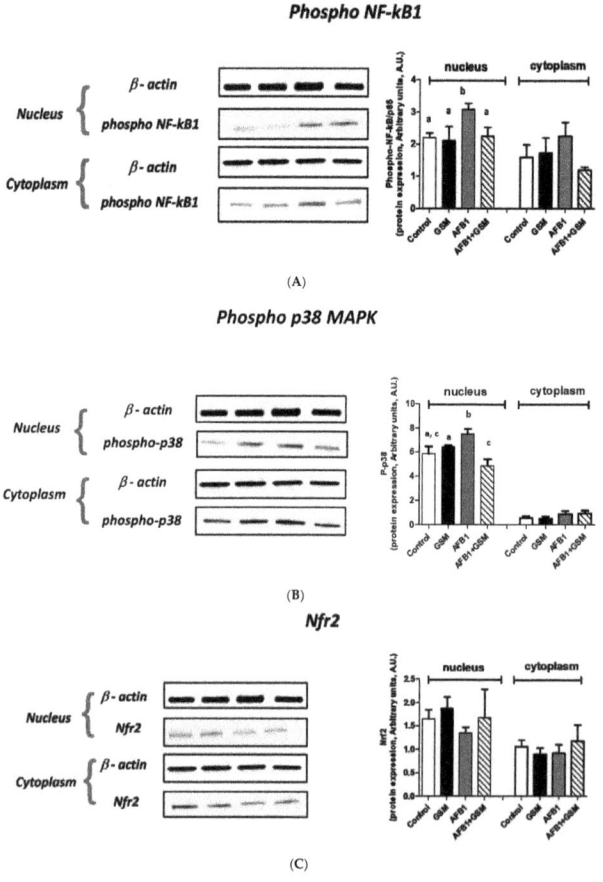

Figure 3. Effect of grape seed meal and aflatoxin B1 on cell signaling pathways in mesenteric lymph nodes: (**A**) phosphor-NF-kB1; (**B**) phosphor-p38 MAPK; (**C**) Nrf2. Data represent mean ± SD, $n = 6$. One-way ANOVA tests, followed by Fisher's PSLD test, were used for statistical data analyses. $^{a-c}$ indicate statistically significant differences between treatments ($p < 0.05$).

Feeding piglets with the diet contaminated with 320 µg AFB1/kg feed resulted in a significant nuclear increase in protein expression of both phosphorylated forms of NF-kBp65 ($p = 0.049$, Figure 3A) and p38 MAPK ($p = 0.028$, Figure 3B), while Nrf2 expression was not affected ($p = 0.55$, Figure 3C) in the AFB1 nuclear fraction when compared with control.

No significant alteration of the expression of these three proteins was noticed in the cytoplasm, although a slight increase of NF-kB expression in the AFB1 group was observed. As compared with the control, concomitant administration of both GSM and AFB1 resulted in a decrease of the expression of both phospho-p38 MAPK (4.86 ± 0.54 vs. 5.86 ± 0.59 A.U.) and phospho-NF-kBp65 (2.24 ± 0.28 vs. 2.19 ± 0.14 A.U.).

Additionally, the expression of Nrf2 increased toward the control level in the AFB1 + GSM group as compared with the control in both nucleus (1.64 ± 0.19 vs. 1.67 ± 0.69 A.U.) and cytoplasm (1.06 ± 0.11 vs. 1.17 ± 0.28 A.U.). The expression of the proteins involved in the inflammation signaling pathway decreased significantly in the AFB1 + GSM group as compared with the AFB1 group: −35% for phospho-p38 MAPK ($p = 0.0017$) and −27% for phospho-NF-kBp65 ($p = 0.05$), respectively.

2.4. Effect of Grape Seed Meal and Aflatoxin B1 on mRNA Gene Expression Involved in Inflammation

Exposure to AFB1-contaminated diet was responsible for a significant increase in the expression of the majority of the investigated genes. AFB1 contamination led to a highly significant increase in the expression of several proinflammatory markers: IL-8 ($p = 0.001$), IL-1β ($p = 0.023$), and IL-18 (0.07) (Table 1).

Looking at the gene expression encoding for signaling molecules with a key role in the inflammation pathway, a similar increase was observed for (i) transcription factors: c-Jun ($p = 0.013$), NF-kB p65 ($p = 0.004$), STAT3 ($p = 0.011$); (ii) MAP kinases: extracellular signal-regulated kinase ERK 1 ($p = 0.039$); (iii) metalloproteinase MMP2 ($p = 0.001$). When compared with the control diet, GSM alone had no effect on inflammatory markers or signaling molecules, with the exception of some genes, but resulted in a decrease in inflammatory response of the mesenteric lymph nodes, compared with the AFB1 group. In the AFB + GSM group, GSM was responsible for a significant decrease of the expression of ERK-1 ($p = 0.006$), c-Jun ($p = 0.028$), IL-18 ($p = 0.002$), and IFN-γ ($p = 0.002$), while the AFB1 × GSM effect for the other gene expressions was not significant ($p > 0.05$).

Table 1. Effect of the exposure of piglets to aflatoxin B1 and/or aflatoxin B1 + grape seed meal on selected gene expression in mesenteric lymph nodes.

Gene Expression	Control	GSM	AFB1	GSM + AFB1	p Value	
					AFB1 Effect	AFB1 × GSM Effect
ERK-1	1.0 ± 0.73	3.53 ± 0.63	34.6 ± 0.63	1.96 ± 0.73	0.039	0.006
c-JUN	1.0 ± 0.28	0.94 ± 0.35	6.83 ± 0.62	1.07 ± 0.13	0.013	0.028
p38 a	1.0 ± 0.68	0.86 ± 0.03	2.21 ± 0.64	0.47 ± 0.24	0.108	0.782
JNK1	1.0 ± 0.59	0.56 ± 0.48	2.53 ± 0.57	0.78 ± 0.15	0.211	0.543
JNK2	1.0 ± 0.28	0.62 ± 0.51	3.12 ± 0.69	0.73 ± 0.25	0.170	0.297
NF-kB p65	1.0 ± 0.36	0.80 ± 0.66	7.97 ± 0.42	1.57 ± 0.08	0.004	0.112
STAT 3	1.0 ± 0.84	1.25 ± 0.62	17.4 ± 0.71	2.93 ± 0.17	0.011	0.681
MMP 2	1.0 ± 0.45	0.75 ± 0.58	12.5 ± 0.66	2.34 ± 0.10	0.001	0.168
TNF α	1.0 ± 0.10	0.95± 0.05	7.75 ± 0.49	3.22 ± 0.07	0.187	0.107
IL-1 β	1.0 ± 0.15	0.76 ± 0.34	15.3 ± 0.71	0.66 ± 0.10	0.023	0.073
IL-8	1.0 ± 0.49	0.94 ± 0.05	17.5 ± 0.37	0.87 ± 0.46	0.001	0.168
IL-18	1.0 ± 0.28	0.96 ± 0.61	26.8 ± 0.22	0.35 ± 0.14	0.076	0.002
IFN γ	1.0 ± 0.25	1.68 ± 0.82	14.2 ± 0.29	0.37 ± 0.14	0.326	0.002

2.5. Correlations between Gene Expressions of Transcription Factors, MAP Kinases, Metalloproteinases, and Cytokines in Pigs Fed AFB1 and AFB1 + GSM Diets

In order to confirm the inflammatory effect of AFB1 and to better understand the mechanism involved in GSM action in counteracting the AFB1 effect, mathematical correlations were established between the expressions of transcription factors, MAP kinases, metalloproteinases, and cytokines in mesenteric lymph node samples derived from pigs fed AFB1 or AFB1 + GSM diets. As expected, the expression of all the inflammatory markers analyzed in the present paper was positively correlated (Figure 4).

	ERK-1	c-JUN	p38 α	JNK1	JNK2	NF-kB	STAT 3	MMP 2	TNF α	IL-1 β	IL-8	IL-18	IFN γ
ERK-1	1	0.929	0.541	0.832	0.789	0.927	0.512	0.871	0.666	0.317	0.651	0.873	0.577
c-JUN		1	0.571	0.84	0.887	0.951	0.647	0.923	0.694	0.285	0.628	0.836	0.654
p38 α			1	0.597	0.766	0.33	0.397	0.345	0.701	0.325	0.876	0.745	0.612
JNK1				1	0.904	0.808	0.311	0.72	0.468	0.337	0.531	0.7	0.414
JNK2					1	0.792	0.506	0.765	0.595	0.188	0.691	0.798	0.541
NF-kB						1	0.573	0.958	0.572	0.259	0.488	0.75	0.557
STAT 3							1	0.662	0.496	0.041	0.586	0.641	0.78
MMP 2								1	0.544	0.097	0.464	0.689	0.573
TNF α									1	0.606	0.834	0.894	0.85
IL-1 β										1	0.37	0.569	0.573
IL-8											1	0.864	0.787
IL-18												1	0.89
IFN γ													1

Figure 4. Gene expression correlations in lymph nodes of piglets exposed to AFB1 versus control.

Highly significant correlation was obtained between the expression of NF-kB, the key signaling molecule of the inflammation pathway, and the expression of (i) transcription factor c-Jun (R^2 = 0.95); (ii) MAPK signaling molecules: ERK1 (R^2 = 0.927), JNK1 (R^2 = 0.808), JNK2 (R^2 = 0.792); (iii) metalloproteinase MMP2 (R^2 = 0.958); (iv) inflammatory cytokine IL-18 (R^2 = 0.75). When mathematical correlations were performed between inflammatory gene expressions of lymph nodes derived from the AFB1 + GSM group and those of the AFB1 group (Figure 5), a highly significant correlation were observed between the expression of NF-kB and the expression of c-JUN (R^2 = 0.965), p38 (R^2 = 0.924), JNK 1 (R^2 = 0.828), JNK 2 (R^2 = 0.986), STAT 3 (R^2 = 0.982), MMP 2 (R^2 = 0.952), TNF-α (R^2 = 0.817), IL-8 (R^2 = 0.822), IL-18 (R^2 = 0.872), and IFN-γ (R^2 = 0.875), which clearly demonstrate the anti-inflammatory effect of GSM on the mesenteric lymph nodes of AFB1-intoxicated piglets.

	ERK-1	c-JUN	p38 α	JNK1	JNK2	NF-kB	STAT 3	MMP 2	TNF α	IL-1 β	IL-8	IL-18	IFN γ
ERK-1	1	0.727	0.704	0.616	0.672	0.745	0.695	0.795	0.89	0.55	0.38	0.764	0.748
c-JUN		1	0.87	0.799	0.863	0.965	0.953	0.936	0.786	0.417	0.81	0.876	0.824
p38 α			1	0.897	0.963	0.924	0.964	0.966	0.695	0.288	0.679	0.689	0.751
JNK1				1	0.937	0.828	0.87	0.829	0.576	0.38	0.59	0.672	0.702
JNK2					1	0.896	0.927	0.929	0.623	0.261	0.672	0.664	0.7
NF-kB						1	0.982	0.952	0.817	0.507	0.822	0.872	0.875
STAT 3							1	0.966	0.755	0.436	0.801	0.8	0.835
MMP 2								1	0.799	0.268	0.739	0.795	0.796
TNF α									1	0.529	0.615	0.876	0.907
IL-1 β										1	0.518	0.593	0.727
IL-8											1	0.774	0.776
IL-18												1	0.898
IFN γ													1

Figure 5. Gene expression correlations in lymph nodes of piglets exposed to AFB1+ GSM versus AFB1-exposed piglets.

3. Discussion

Mycotoxins are responsible for important decreases in productivity and health in the animal sector, and finding new solutions for the reduction of their toxic effects represent a continuous challenge for scientists. For some mycotoxins, such as aflatoxins, zearalenone, and ochratoxin, the use of high-affinity binders represents a promising solution as they can form stable complexes that cannot be adsorbed in the gut and are eliminated through feces, thus reducing the toxins' systemic absorption [26,27].

According to Commission Regulation (EC) no 386/2009, mycotoxin adsorbents, which are able to mitigate the toxins' effects through the reduction of intestinal absorption, were classified as a new functional group of feed additives. As stipulated in this regulation, the mycotoxin adsorbents should suppress or reduce the absorption, promote the excretion of mycotoxins and, at the same time, increase the quality of the feed, assuring the protection of public and animal health. At present, the use of mycotoxin adsorbents represents the best method for protecting animals against the harmful effects of contaminated feed [28,29].

From the mycotoxin adsorbents group, aluminosilicates are the most tested, but their use is limited due to their capacity to bind other molecules besides mycotoxins, such as vitamins and minerals that cannot be further absorbed in the gut [30]. Additionally, many binders have proven a high efficacy for mycotoxin adsorption using in-vitro abiotic systems, but these qualities were not confirmed by the in vivo studies [31].

Grape residues, as agroindustrial waste, are frequently discarded in open areas, representing a problem for the environment [32]. In order to avoid this, investigations have been done for their use for other purposes. Highlighting their chemical composition, rich in bioactive compounds, has led to their use as food/feed additives and pharmaceuticals [33]. For example, grape seed waste has been used in animal farm production in order to get functional foods, such as eggs or meat enriched in PUFAs or polyphenols [16,34].

The use of grape waste as binders of mycotoxins is of recent interest. Thus, the bioactive compounds from grape byproducts (grape pomace) were shown to efficiently adsorb AFB1 in abiotic systems [35]. Grape pomace was also efficient in reducing the urinary mycotoxin biomarker of AFB1 and zearalenone in an in-vivo trial, where piglets were fed a bolus contaminated with a mixture of mycotoxins (fumonisin B1, deoxynivalenol, zearalenone, AFB1, and ochratoxin A), through the reduction of gastrointestinal mycotoxin absorption [36].

As the information related to the effect of AFB1 on the lymphatic system and, in particular, the lymph nodes are scarce, the present study investigated the effect of AFB1 on the mesenteric lymph nodes of piglets after weaning. Additionally, we have investigated if a diet containing grape seed meal can counteract the negative effect of AFB1 on inflammation and oxidative response in piglets' MSL.

Many studies have shown that oxidative stress represents one of the causes for AFB1-induced toxicity, which leads to the generation of reactive oxygen species (ROS), resulting in lipid, protein, and DNA damage and, consequently, cell injury [37].

Oxidative stress plays a negative role in chronic inflammatory diseases [38], and our previous data indicate that oxidative stress and inflammation are tightly correlated in animals exposed to mycotoxins [39,40].

In the present study, our results have shown that AFB1 has an important antioxidative effect by decreasing the activity of principal enzymes involved in the response to oxidative stress (CAT, GPx, SOD) and total antioxidant status while increasing lipid peroxidation, as compared to oxidative stress parameters in the MSL of control piglets. As a result of the exposure to AFB1, an increase of transcription factors, MAP kinases as signaling molecules, and metalloproteinases and cytokines as effectors of inflammatory response were observed in the mesenteric lymph nodes of the intoxicated piglets. According to the most recent data, AFB1 has a rather biphasic effect on the immune response, with a stimulatory effect in the first phase, followed by a suppressive action in the second phase [41]. Immuno-stimulation induced by AFB1 increases the synthesis of inflammatory markers and free radicals, which lead to chronic inflammation and cancer [42,43]. Anti-inflammatory activities of plant bioactive compounds have been reported in acute and chronic inflammation in animal models [44,45], and recent data have shown that they can be used for counteracting the toxic effect of AFB1 [24,46,47]. Our previous results have shown that GSM addition into AFB1-contaminated diet induced the amelioration of liver injuries and decreased inflammation and oxidative stress in the liver of intoxicated piglets by decreasing the MAPKs and NF-κB signaling pathways overexpressed by the AFB1 diet [24].

Although the immune system represents one of AFB1's targets, few studies have investigated the potential beneficial role of bioactive compounds on the immune organs. For example, curcumin, a powerful plant antioxidant, decreases the weight of spleen and bursa of Fabricius, as well as the ratio of spleen/bursa, in broilers fed AFB1, towards similar values to the control group [48]. Additionally, in AFB1-intoxicated mice, lycopene, another plant bioactive compound, can alleviate AFB1-induced immunosuppression by increasing spleen weight, spleen coefficient, T-lymphocyte subsets, and IL-2, IFN-γ, and TNF-α gene expression in spleen [49]. Similarly, our results have shown that GSM was able to decrease proinflammatory cytokine gene expression and protein synthesis (IL-1β, IL-6, IL-8, IL-18, and IFN-γ), as well as the gene and protein expressions of important markers of signaling inflammation—ERK-1, c-Jun, phospho-p38 MAPK, phospho-NF-kBp65—as molecules involved in the NF-kB signaling pathway.

It was shown that phytocompounds can alleviate the immunosuppression induced by AFB1 in the spleen of mice through the inhibition of oxidative stress and mitochondria-mediated apoptosis [49]. Indeed, our results have shown that GSM induced a reduction of AFB1-induced oxidative stress by increasing the activity of enzymes involved in the response to oxidative stress (GPx and SOD) and decreasing lipid peroxidation.

The mechanism responsible for the beneficial effect of GSM in counteracting AFB1 toxicity is not clear. Recent studies have shown that grape pomace was able to efficiently bind AFB1, decreasing in this way the toxin's absorption and increasing its excretion [35,36]. Likewise, our in vitro studies, performed on a panel of eight agroindustrial wastes, have shown that GSM was the most efficient binder of AFB1; these results suggest that this waste has a high capacity to bind AFB1 (Palade et al., submitted). The decrease of the toxic effects of AFB1 in the MSL of the AFB1 + GSM group, observed in our study, can be related to the capacity of GSM to adsorb AFB1 and increase its elimination.

Some hypotheses concerning the GSM way of action can be formulated based on previous literature studies. The first one, related to the high cellulose content (37.8%) of GSM [24], has a great potential to adsorb AFB1 by electrostatic attractions and hydrogen bonding, resulting in the formation of a mycotoxin monolayer on its surface [48]. The second one is based on the ability of polyphenols to form a complex with AFB1 mycotoxins. In a recent study, Lu et al. (2017) demonstrated that polyphenols from fermented tea can reduce AFB1-induced liver injury as they bind the toxin in a complex (C-AFB1 complex) and, consequently, inhibit AFB1 absorption and increase toxin elimination through feces [22]. Another interesting hypothesis is that of Ali Rajput et al., who considered that the protective effects of the bioactive compound proanthocyanidin, from grape seed, may be due to AFB1 biotransformation in the gut, which leads to the reduction of AFB1 absorption [23]. However, more studies are necessary to elucidate the interaction between grape waste and AFB1.

4. Conclusions

In conclusion, our study demonstrates that before being transported via the mesenteric lymphatic duct and entering the blood circulation, AFB1 exerts proinflammatory and pro-oxidative effects in the mesenteric lymph nodes of intoxicated piglets. Grape seed meal, a waste product generated after oil extraction, has been shown to have the capacity to reduce the inflammation and oxidative stress triggered by AFB1. These results represent an important and promising way to valorize this waste, rich in bioactive compounds, for decreasing AFB1 toxic effects on mesenteric lymph nodes.

5. Materials and Methods

5.1. Animals and Dietary Treatments

Twenty-four crossbred weaned piglets (TOPIGS-40), 4 weeks old, were randomly assigned to the experimental groups and fed the following treatments for 30 days: Control (fed a maize-soybean diet), AFB1 group (diet contaminated with 320 μg AFB1/kg feed), GSM group (diet with 8% grape seed meal included), and AFB1 + GSM group (basal diet with 8% GSM and 320 μg AFB1/kg feed), as previously described by Taranu et al. [50]. Each experimental group was represented by 6 piglets (2 pens/treatment and 3 pigs/pen). Piglets had access ad libitum to water and feed during the experimental period.

The experimental protocol was approved on 5 February 2020 by the Ethical Committee (no. 52/2014 of INCDBNA Balotesti) and the animal handling was done in accordance with EU Council Directive 98/58/EC and Romanian Law 206/2004.

Animals were slaughtered at the end of the experiment by exsanguination, and samples of the mesenteric lymph nodes were taken on ice and stored at −80 °C until the assessment of the immune and stress oxidative parameters.

5.2. Composition of the Grape Seed Meal

Dried grape seed meal (GSM), resulted after oil extraction, was provided by S.C. OLEOMET-S.R.L., Bucharest, Romania. Analyses consisting of chemical composition (fat, protein, ash, fibers), total and specific polyphenol content, as well as polyunsaturated fatty acids (PUFA) and antioxidant capacity, were performed for GSM characterization, as already described by Taranu et al. [51].

5.3. Toxin

Pure AFB1 (FERMENTEC, Jerusalem, Israel) was used to contaminate both AFB1 and GSM + AFB1 diets. Briefly, 50 mg toxin was dissolved in dimethyl sulfoxide and mixed with the control diet in order to achieve a final AFB1 concentration of 320 µg/kg diet. The final AFB1 concentration was confirmed by ELISA and UPLC analysis (320 ± 10.9 µg AFB1/kg diet). In the control diet, the AFB1 concentration was 2.4 ± 0.15 µg/kg diet. The diets were analyzed for contamination by other mycotoxins (ochratoxin A, fumonisins, deoxynivalenol, zearalenone); the levels found were under the EU limits for pigs.

5.4. Determination of Total Antioxidant Status

A total antioxidant capacity (TAC) assay has already been described by Marin et al. [39]. The method consists of the measurement of the absorption of 2,20-azinobis-[3-ethylbenzothiazoline-6-sulfonic acid cation (ABTS+)] in samples of mesenteric lymph nodes, and the results are expressed as mmol TEAC (trolox equivalent antioxidant capacity)/g tissue.

5.5. TBARS Assessment

Thiobarbituric acid reactive substances (TBARS) were measured in samples of frozen mesenteric lymph nodes, as already described [39]. The results are expressed as nmol/mg protein.

5.6. Enzyme Activity Assessment

The activities of superoxide dismutase (SOD), catalase (CAT), and glutathione peroxidase (GPx) were measured using Cayman kits (Cayman Chemical, Ann Arbor, MI, USA), according to the instructions provided by the manufacturer [52]. A Tecan microplate reader (SunRise, Vienna, Austria) was used for the measurement of the absorbance.

5.7. Cytokine Measurement

Cytokine concentration was assessed in mesenteric lymph nodes, as already described by Marin et al. [39]. Briefly, the homogenates from 1 g of frozen sample for each animal, in buffer with complete protease inhibitor cocktail, were used for the analyses of cytokine content by ELISA. Bradford assay was used for the analyses of total protein content. Monoclonal antiporcine antibodies for IL-1beta, IL-6, IL-8, and TNF alpha were used as capture antibodies, and biotinylated antiporcine IL-1beta, IL-6, IL-8, and TNF alpha were used as secondary antibodies (R&D Systems; Minneapolis, MN, USA). Results were presented as micrograms of cytokine/g tissue.

5.8. Extraction of Total RNA and cDNA Synthesis

RNA extraction followed by cDNA synthesis was carried out as described by Pistol et al. [53]. Briefly, a Qiagen RNeasy midi kit (QIAGEN GmbH, Hilden, Germany) was used for the extraction of total RNA from frozen mesenteric lymph node samples and then treated with ribonuclease inhibitors and purified on columns of silica gel. Concentration and quality were analyzed using a Nanodrop ND-1000 (Thermo Fischer Scientific, Waltham, MA, USA), and integrity was analyzed using agarose gel electrophoresis. Then, 100 ng of total RNA samples were used for the generation of cDNA using an M-MuLV Reverse Transcriptase Kit (Thermo Fischer Scientific, Waltham, MA, USA). A GeneQuerry™ Pig cDNA Evaluation Kit (ScienCell, Carlsbad, CA, USA) was used for the assessment of the absence of contamination with genomic DNA and the successful reverse transcription of tRNA to cDNA and cDNA quality.

5.9. Detection of Inflammatory and Signalling Gene Expression by qPCR Array

Real-time PCR was used to evaluate the expression of transcription factors: c-Jun, nuclear factor NF-kappa-B p65 (NF-kB p65), and signal transducer and activator of transcription 3 (STAT3); MAP kinases: extracellular signal-regulated kinase (ERK 1), c-Jun N-terminal kinase (JNK 1, JNK2) and p38, and metalloproteinase MMP2; cytokines: tumor necrosis factor (TNF alpha), interleukin beta (IL-1 beta), interferon gamma (IFN gamma), interleukin 8 (IL-8), and interleukin 18 (IL-18), as already described by Marin et al. [40]. The sequence of gene-specific primer pairs and the conditions used for the reactions have already been published in our previous papers [54–56]. Duplicates were performed for each gene, and melting curves were used for the confirmation of the formation of single PCR products. For all primers, negative controls were used, consisting of qPCR mix except for cDNA. Two reference genes—beta-actin (ACTB) and hypoxanthine-guanine phosphoribosyl-transferase (HGPRT)—were used for the relative quantification of gene expression changes, and the results were expressed as fold change, as compared with the control group (Fc), using the $2^{(-\Delta\Delta CT)}$ method [57].

5.10. Western Blot Analysis

The protein expression level of three proteins involved in cell signaling—MAPK-p38, NF-kB phosphorylated form and Nrf2 (Nuclear factor erythroid 2-related factor 2)—were measured by Western blot. Cytoplasmic and nuclear fractions of tissue lysates were obtained using the protocol recommended by Thermo Fisher Scientific (Rockford, IL, USA NE-PER) for Nuclear and Cytoplasmic Extraction Reagent Kits, as described by Pistol et al. [53]. After assessment of protein concentration (Pierce BCA Protein Assay Kit, Thermo Fischer Scientific, Waltham, MA, USA), lymph nodes lysates, undiluted (cytoplasmic lysates) or $\frac{1}{2}$ diluted (nuclear lysates), were separated on a 10% SDS-PAGE and transferred onto a 0.45-µm nitrocellulose membrane. After being blocked overnight with 5% nonfat dry milk, the membrane was incubated after washing with primary antibodies from Cell Signaling Technology (Beverly, MA, USA) for phospho-MAPK-p38 (rabbit antiporcine phospho-MAPK-p38), phospho-NF-kB/p65 (rabbit antiporcine phospho-NF-kB p65), β-actin (rabbit antiporcine β-actin), and Nrf2 (rabbit polyclonal antibody; Abbexa, Cambridge, UK) for 2 h at room temperature. Then, the membranes were incubated with a horseradish-peroxidase-conjugated antirabbit IgG antibody for 1 h (Cell Signaling Technology, Danvers, MA, USA). The immunoreactivity was assessed by using Clarity Western ECL Substrate (Bio-Rad, Hercules, CA, USA). A MicroChemi Imager (DNR Bio-Imaging Systems LTD, Neve Yamin, Israel) was used for developing immunoblotting images, and GelQuant software (DNR Bio-Imaging Systems LTD, Neve Yamin, Israel) was used for the evaluation of the level of protein expression. The results represent the ratio between the expression level of the protein of interest (p38 MAPK, NF-kB/p65, Nrf2) and β-actin.

5.11. Statistical Analyses

The differences for all the investigated parameters were analyzed using one-way ANOVA tests, followed by Fisher's PSLD test.

Author Contributions: Conceptualization, D.E.M. and I.T.; assessment of oxidative stress parameters, M.L.P. and M.I.D., Western blot analyses, C.A.A., C.V.B. and G.C.P.; qPCR analyses C.V.B. and G.C.P., data analysis and statistics, D.E.M.; writing—original draft preparation, D.E.M.; writing—review and editing, I.T.; funding acquisition, D.E.M. and I.T. All authors have read and agreed to the published version of the manuscript.

Funding: This research was funded by National Research Projects PN III—8PCCDI, granted by the Romanian Ministry of Education and Research.

Conflicts of Interest: The authors declare no conflict of interest.

References

1. Grenier, B.; Applegate, T.J. Modulation of intestinal functions following mycotoxin ingestion: Meta-analysis of published experiments in animals. *Toxins* **2013**, *5*, 396–430. [CrossRef]
2. Sarma, U.P.; Bhetaria, P.J.; Devi, P.; Varma, A. Aflatoxins: Implications on health. *Indian J. Clin. Biochem.* **2017**, *32*, 124–133. [CrossRef] [PubMed]
3. Marchese, S.; Polo, A.; Ariano, A.; Velotto, S.; Costantini, S.; Severino, L. Aflatoxin b1 and m1: Biological properties and their involvement in cancer development. *Toxins* **2018**, *10*, 214. [CrossRef] [PubMed]
4. Taniwaki, M.H.; Pitt, J.I.; Magan, N. Aspergillus species and mycotoxins: Occurrence and importance in major food commodities. *Curr. Opin. Food Sci.* **2018**, *23*, 38–43. [CrossRef]
5. Liew, W.-P.-P.; Mohd-Redzwan, S. Mycotoxin: Its impact on gut health and microbiota. *Front. Cell Infect. Microbiol.* **2018**, *8*, 60. [CrossRef]
6. Yin, H.; Jiang, M.; Peng, X.; Cui, H.; Zhou, Y.; He, M.; Zuo, Z.; Ouyang, P.; Fan, J.; Fang, J. The molecular mechanism of g2m cell cycle arrest induced by afb1 in the jejunum. *Oncotarget* **2016**, *7*, 35592–35606. [CrossRef]
7. Peng, X.; Chen, K.; Chen, J.; Fang, J.; Cui, H.; Zuo, Z.; Deng, J.; Chen, Z.; Geng, Y.; Lai, W. Aflatoxin b1 affects apoptosis and expression of bax, bcl-2, and caspase-3 in thymus and bursa of fabricius in broiler chickens. *Environ. Toxicol.* **2016**, *31*, 1113–1120. [CrossRef]
8. Yang, X.; Liu, L.; Chen, J.; Xiao, A. Response of intestinal bacterial flora to the long-term feeding of aflatoxin b1 (afb1) in mice. *Toxins* **2017**, *9*, 317. [CrossRef]
9. Akbari, P.; Braber, S.; Varasteh, S.; Alizadeh, A.; Garssen, J.; Fink-Gremmels, J. The intestinal barrier as an emerging target in the toxicological assessment of mycotoxins. *Arch. Toxicol.* **2017**, *91*, 1007–1029. [CrossRef]
10. Romero, A.; Ares, I.; Ramos, E.; Castellano, V.; Martínez, M.; Martínez-Larrañaga, M.R.; Anadón, A.; Martínez, M.A. Mycotoxins modify the barrier function of caco-2 cells through differential gene expression of specific claudin isoforms: Protective effect of illite mineral clay. *Toxicology* **2016**, *353–354*, 21–33. [CrossRef]
11. Kohan, A.B.; Yoder, S.M.; Tso, P. Using the lymphatics to study nutrient absorption and the secretion of gastrointestinal hormones. *Physiol. Behav.* **2011**, *105*, 82–88. [CrossRef] [PubMed]
12. Alexander, J.S.; Ganta, V.C.; Jordan, P.A.; Witte, M.H. Gastrointestinal lymphatics in health and disease. *Pathophysiology* **2010**, *17*, 315–335. [CrossRef]
13. Worbs, T.; Bode, U.; Yan, S.; Hoffmann, M.W.; Hintzen, G.; Bernhardt, G.; Förster, R.; Pabst, O. Oral tolerance originates in the intestinal immune system and relies on antigen carriage by dendritic cells. *J. Exp. Med.* **2006**, *203*, 519–527. [CrossRef] [PubMed]
14. Pierron, A.; Alassane-Kpembi, I.; Oswald, I.P. Impact of mycotoxin on immune response and consequences for pig health. *Anim. Nutr.* **2016**, *2*, 63–68. [CrossRef] [PubMed]
15. Meissonnier, G.; Pinton, P.; Laffitte, J.; Cossalter, A.-M.; Gong, Y.Y.; Wild, C.; Bertin, G.; Galtier, P.; Oswald, I. Immunotoxicity of aflatoxin b1: Impairment of the cell-mediated response to vaccine antigen and modulation of cytokine expression. *Toxicol. Appl. Pharmacol.* **2008**, *231*, 142–149. [CrossRef] [PubMed]
16. Turcu, R.; Margareta, O.; Criste, R.D.; Mariana, R.; Tatiana, P.; Șoica, C.; Drăgotoiu, D. The effect of using grape seeds meal as natural antioxidant in broiler diets enriched in fatty acids, on meat quality. *J. Hyg. Eng. Des.* **2019**, *35*, 14–20.

17. Chedea, V.S.; Palade, L.M.; Marin, D.E.; Pelmus, R.S.; Habeanu, M.; Rotar, M.C.; Gras, M.A.; Pistol, G.C.; Taranu, I. Intestinal absorption and antioxidant activity of grape pomace polyphenols. *Nutrients* **2018**, *10*, 588. [CrossRef]
18. Veskoukis, A.S.; Kyparos, A.; Nikolaidis, M.G.; Stagos, D.; Aligiannis, N.; Halabalaki, M.; Chronis, K.; Goutzourelas, N.; Skaltsounis, L.; Kouretas, D. The antioxidant effects of a polyphenol-rich grape pomace extract in vitro do not correspond in vivo using exercise as an oxidant stimulus. *Oxid. Med. Cell Longev.* **2012**, *2012*, 185867. [CrossRef]
19. Taranu, I.; Habeanu, M.; Gras, M.A.; Pistol, G.C.; Lefter, N.; Palade, M.; Ropota, M.; Sanda Chedea, V.; Marin, D.E. Assessment of the effect of grape seed cake inclusion in the diet of healthy fattening-finishing pigs. *J. Anim. Physiol. Anim. Nutr.* **2018**, *102*, e30–e42. [CrossRef]
20. Abdel-Wahhab, M.A.; El-Nekeety, A.A.; Hathout, A.S.; Salman, A.S.; Abdel-Aziem, S.H.; Sabry, B.A.; Hassan, N.S.; Abdel-Aziz, M.S.; Aly, S.E.; Jaswir, I. Bioactive compounds from aspergillus niger extract enhance the antioxidant activity and prevent the genotoxicity in aflatoxin b1-treated rats. *Toxicon* **2020**, *181*, 57–68. [CrossRef]
21. Oskoueian, E.; Abdullah, N.; Zulkifli, I.; Ebrahimi, M.; Karimi, E.; Goh, Y.M.; Oskoueian, A.; Shakeri, M. Cytoprotective effect of palm kernel cake phenolics against aflatoxin b1-induced cell damage and its underlying mechanism of action. *BMC Complement. Altern. Med.* **2015**, *15*, 392. [CrossRef] [PubMed]
22. Lu, H.; Liu, F.; Zhu, Q.; Zhang, M.; Li, T.; Chen, J.; Huang, Y.; Wang, X.; Sheng, J. Aflatoxin b1 can be complexed with oxidised tea polyphenols and the absorption of the complexed aflatoxin b1 is inhibited in rats. *J. Sci. Food Agric.* **2017**, *97*, 1910–1915. [CrossRef] [PubMed]
23. Ali Rajput, S.; Sun, L.; Zhang, N.; Mohamed Khalil, M.; Gao, X.; Ling, Z.; Zhu, L.; Khan, F.A.; Zhang, J.; Qi, D. Ameliorative effects of grape seed proanthocyanidin extract on growth performance, immune function, antioxidant capacity, biochemical constituents, liver histopathology and aflatoxin residues in broilers exposed to aflatoxin b_1. *Toxins* **2017**, *9*, 371. [CrossRef] [PubMed]
24. Taranu, I.; Hermenean, A.; Bulgaru, C.; Pistol, G.C.; Ciceu, A.; Grosu, I.A.; Marin, D.E. Diet containing grape seed meal by-product counteracts afb1 toxicity in liver of pig after weaning. *Ecotoxicol. Environ. Saf.* **2020**, *203*, 110899. [CrossRef]
25. Grosu, I.A.; Pistol, G.C.; Taranu, I.; Marin, D.E. The impact of dietary grape seed meal on healthy and aflatoxin b1 afflicted microbiota of pigs after weaning. *Toxins* **2019**, *11*, 25. [CrossRef]
26. Whitlow, L. Evaluation of mycotoxin binders. In Proceedings of the 4th Mid-Atlantic Nutrition Conference, Timonium, MD, USA, 29–30 March 2006.
27. Avantaggiato, G.; Solfrizzo, M.; Visconti, A. Recent advances on the use of adsorbent materials for detoxification of fusarium mycotoxins. *Food Addit. Contam.* **2005**, *22*, 379–388. [CrossRef]
28. Sabater-Vilar, M.; Malekinejad, H.; Selman, M.H.; van der Doelen, M.A.; Fink-Gremmels, J. In vitro assessment of adsorbents aiming to prevent deoxynivalenol and zearalenone mycotoxicoses. *Mycopathologia* **2007**, *163*, 81–90. [CrossRef]
29. Bočarov-Stančić, A.; Adamović, M.; Salma, N.; Bodroža-Solarov, M.; Vučković-Đisalov, J.; Pantić, V. In vitro efficacy of mycotoxins adsorption by natural mineral adsorbents. *Biotechnol. Anim. Husb.* **2011**, *27*, 1241–1251. [CrossRef]
30. Huwig, A.; Freimund, S.; Käppeli, O.; Dutler, H. Mycotoxin detoxication of animal feed by different adsorbents. *Toxicol. Lett.* **2001**, *122*, 179–188. [CrossRef]
31. Di Gregorio, M.C.; Neeff, D.V.D.; Jager, A.V.; Corassin, C.H.; Carão, Á.C.D.P.; Albuquerque, R.D.; Azevedo, A.C.D.; Oliveira, C.A.F. Mineral adsorbents for prevention of mycotoxins in animal feeds. *Toxin Rev.* **2014**, *33*, 125–135. [CrossRef]
32. Teixeira, A.; Baenas, N.; Dominguez-Perles, R.; Barros, A.; Rosa, E.; Moreno, D.A.; Garcia-Viguera, C. Natural bioactive compounds from winery by-products as health promoters: A review. *Int. J. Mol. Sci.* **2014**, *15*, 15638–15678. [CrossRef] [PubMed]
33. Tang, G.-Y.; Zhao, C.-N.; Liu, Q.; Feng, X.-L.; Xu, X.-Y.; Cao, S.-Y.; Meng, X.; Li, S.; Gan, R.-Y.; Li, H.-B. Potential of grape wastes as a natural source of bioactive compounds. *Molecules* **2018**, *23*, 2598. [CrossRef] [PubMed]
34. Chedea, V.S.; Pelmus, R.S.; Lazar, C.; Pistol, G.C.; Calin, L.G.; Toma, S.M.; Dragomir, C.; Taranu, I. Effects of a diet containing dried grape pomace on blood metabolites and milk composition of dairy cows. *J. Sci. Food Agric.* **2017**, *97*, 2516–2523. [CrossRef] [PubMed]

35. Avantaggiato, G.; Greco, D.; Damascelli, A.; Solfrizzo, M.; Visconti, A. Assessment of multi-mycotoxin adsorption efficacy of grape pomace. *J. Agric. Food Chem.* **2014**, *62*, 497–507. [CrossRef] [PubMed]
36. Gambacorta, L.; Pinton, P.; Avantaggiato, G.; Oswald, I.P.; Solfrizzo, M. Grape pomace, an agricultural byproduct reducing mycotoxin absorption: In vivo assessment in pig using urinary biomarkers. *J. Agric. Food Chem.* **2016**, *64*, 6762–6771. [CrossRef] [PubMed]
37. Marin, D.E.; Taranu, I. Overview on aflatoxins and oxidative stress. *Toxin Rev.* **2012**, *31*, 32–43. [CrossRef]
38. Hussain, T.; Tan, B.; Yin, Y.; Blachier, F.; Tossou, M.C.B.; Rahu, N. Oxidative stress and inflammation: What polyphenols can do for us? *Oxid. Med. Cell Longev.* **2016**, *2016*, 7432797. [CrossRef]
39. Marin, D.E.; Pistol, G.C.; Gras, M.; Palade, M.; Taranu, I. A comparison between the effects of ochratoxin a and aristolochic acid on the inflammation and oxidative stress in the liver and kidney of weanling piglets. *Naunyn-Schmiedeberg's Arch. Pharmacol.* **2018**, *391*, 1147–1156. [CrossRef]
40. Marin, D.E.; Pistol, G.C.; Gras, M.A.; Palade, M.L.; Taranu, I. Comparative effect of ochratoxin a on inflammation and oxidative stress parameters in gut and kidney of piglets. *Regul. Toxicol. Pharmacol. RTP* **2017**, *89*, 224–231. [CrossRef]
41. Yunus, A.W.; Razzazi-Fazeli, E.; Bohm, J. Aflatoxin b(1) in affecting broiler's performance, immunity, and gastrointestinal tract: A review of history and contemporary issues. *Toxins* **2011**, *3*, 566–590. [CrossRef]
42. Benkerroum, N. Chronic and acute toxicities of aflatoxins: Mechanisms of action. *Int. J. Environ. Res. Public Health* **2020**, *17*, 423. [CrossRef]
43. Mehrzad, J.; Malvandi, A.M.; Alipour, M.; Hosseinkhani, S. Environmentally relevant level of aflatoxin b(1) elicits toxic pro-inflammatory response in murine cns-derived cells. *Toxicol. Lett.* **2017**, *279*, 96–106. [CrossRef]
44. Sangiovanni, E.; Dell'Agli, M. Special issue: Anti-inflammatory activity of plant polyphenols. *Biomedicines* **2020**, *8*, 64. [CrossRef]
45. Calder, P.C. Immunoregulatory and anti-inflammatory effects of n-3 polyunsaturated fatty acids. *Braz. J. Med. Biol. Res.* **1998**, *31*, 467–490. [CrossRef] [PubMed]
46. Holanda, D.M.; Kim, S.W. Efficacy of mycotoxin detoxifiers on health and growth of newly-weaned pigs under chronic dietary challenge of deoxynivalenol. *Toxins* **2020**, *12*, 311. [CrossRef] [PubMed]
47. Van Le Thanh, B.; Lessard, M.; Chorfi, Y.; Guay, F. The efficacy of anti-mycotoxin feed additives in preventing the adverse effects of wheat naturally contaminated with fusarium mycotoxins on performance, intestinal barrier function and nutrient digestibility and retention in weanling pigs. *Can. J. Anim. Sci.* **2015**, *95*, 197–209. [CrossRef]
48. Solis-Cruz, B.; Hernandez-Patlan, D.; Petrone, V.M.; Pontin, K.P.; Latorre, J.D.; Beyssac, E.; Hernandez-Velasco, X.; Merino-Guzman, R.; Owens, C.; Hargis, B.M.; et al. Evaluation of cellulosic polymers and curcumin to reduce aflatoxin b1 toxic effects on performance, biochemical, and immunological parameters of broiler chickens. *Toxins* **2019**, *11*, 121. [CrossRef]
49. Xu, F.; Wang, P.; Yao, Q.; Shao, B.; Yu, H.; Yu, K.; Li, Y. Lycopene alleviates afb(1)-induced immunosuppression by inhibiting oxidative stress and apoptosis in the spleen of mice. *Food Funct.* **2019**, *10*, 3868–3879. [CrossRef]
50. Taranu, I.; Marin, D.E.; Palade, M.; Pistol, G.C.; Chedea, V.S.; Gras, M.A.; Rotar, C. Assessment of the efficacy of a grape seed waste in counteracting the changes induced by aflatoxin b1 contaminated diet on performance, plasma, liver and intestinal tissues of pigs after weaning. *Toxicon Off. J. Int. Soc. Toxinol.* **2019**, *162*, 24–31. [CrossRef]
51. Taranu, I.; Gras, M.; Pistol, G.C.; Motiu, M.; Marin, D.E.; Lefter, N.; Ropota, M.; Habeanu, M. Omega-3 pufa rich camelina oil by-products improve the systemic metabolism and spleen cell functions in fattening pigs. *PLoS ONE* **2014**, *9*, e110186. [CrossRef]
52. Palade, L.M.; Habeanu, M.; Marin, D.E.; Chedea, V.S.; Pistol, G.C.; Grosu, I.A.; Gheorghe, A.; Ropota, M.; Taranu, I. Effect of dietary hemp seed on oxidative status in sows during late gestation and lactation and their offspring. *Anim. Open Access J.* **2019**, *9*, 194. [CrossRef]
53. Pistol, G.C.; Braicu, C.; Motiu, M.; Gras, M.A.; Marin, D.E.; Stancu, M.; Calin, L.; Israel-Roming, F.; Berindan-Neagoe, I.; Taranu, I. Zearalenone mycotoxin affects immune mediators, mapk signalling molecules, nuclear receptors and genome-wide gene expression in pig spleen. *PLoS ONE* **2015**, *10*, e0127503. [CrossRef] [PubMed]
54. Marin, D.E.; Pistol, G.C.; Neagoe, I.V.; Calin, L.; Taranu, I. Effects of zearalenone on oxidative stress and inflammation in weanling piglets. *Food Chem. Toxicol.* **2013**, *58*, 408–415. [CrossRef] [PubMed]

55. Pistol, G.C.; Gras, M.A.; Marin, D.E.; Israel-Roming, F.; Stancu, M.; Taranu, I. Natural feed contaminant zearalenone decreases the expressions of important pro- and anti-inflammatory mediators and mitogen-activated protein kinase/nf-kappab signalling molecules in pigs. *Br. J. Nutr.* **2014**, *111*, 452–464. [CrossRef] [PubMed]
56. Marin, D.E.; Motiu, M.; Pistol, G.C.; Gras, M.A.; Israel-Roming, F.; Calin, L.; Stancu, M.; Taranu, I. Diet contaminated with ochratoxin a at the highest level allowed by eu recommendation disturbs liver metabolism in weaned piglets. *World Mycotoxin J.* **2016**, *9*, 587–596. [CrossRef]
57. Livak, K.J.; Schmittgen, T.D. Analysis of relative gene expression data using real-time quantitative pcr and the 2(-delta delta c(t)) method. *Methods* **2001**, *25*, 402–408. [CrossRef]

Publisher's Note: MDPI stays neutral with regard to jurisdictional claims in published maps and institutional affiliations.

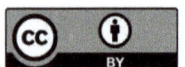

© 2020 by the authors. Licensee MDPI, Basel, Switzerland. This article is an open access article distributed under the terms and conditions of the Creative Commons Attribution (CC BY) license (http://creativecommons.org/licenses/by/4.0/).

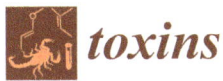

Article

The Effectiveness of Dietary Byproduct Antioxidants on Induced CYP Genes Expression and Histological Alteration in Piglets Liver and Kidney Fed with Aflatoxin B1 and Ochratoxin A

Roua Gabriela Popescu [1], Cristina Bulgaru [2], Arabela Untea [2], Mihaela Vlassa [3], Miuta Filip [3], Anca Hermenean [4], Daniela Marin [2], Ionelia Țăranu [2,*], Sergiu Emil Georgescu [1,*] and Anca Dinischiotu [1]

[1] Department of Biochemistry and Molecular Biology, Faculty of Biology, University of Bucharest, Splaiul Independentei No. 91–95, 050095 Bucharest, Romania; roua.popescu@drd.unibuc.ro (R.G.P.); anca.dinischiotu@bio.unibuc.ro (A.D.)

[2] Laboratory of Animal Biology, National Institute for Research and Development for Biology and Animal Nutrition, Calea Bucuresti No. 1, Balotesti, 077015 Ilfov, Romania; cristina.bulgaru@ibna.ro (C.B.); arabela.untea@ibna.ro (A.U.); daniela.marin@ibna.ro (D.M.)

[3] Raluca Ripan Institute for Research in Chemistry, Babeş Bolyai University, 30 Fântânele Street, 400294 Cluj-Napoca, Romania; mihaela.vlassa@ubbcluj.ro (M.V.); miuta.filip@ubbcluj.ro (M.F.)

[4] "Aurel Ardelean" Institute of Life Sciences, Vasile Godis Western University of Arad, Rebreanu 86, 310414 Arad, Romania; anca.hermenean@gmail.com

* Correspondence: ionelia.taranu@ibna.ro (I.Ț.); sergiu.georgescu@bio.unibuc.ro (S.E.G.); Tel.: +40-213181575 (ext.112) (S.E.G.)

Citation: Popescu, R.G.; Bulgaru, C.; Untea, A.; Vlassa, M.; Filip, M.; Hermenean, A.; Marin, D.; Țăranu, I.; Georgescu, S.E.; Dinischiotu, A. The Effectiveness of Dietary Byproduct Antioxidants on Induced CYP Genes Expression and Histological Alteration in Piglets Liver and Kidney Fed with Aflatoxin B1 and Ochratoxin A. *Toxins* **2021**, *13*, 148. https://doi.org/10.3390/toxins13020148

Received: 11 January 2021
Accepted: 13 February 2021
Published: 15 February 2021

Publisher's Note: MDPI stays neutral with regard to jurisdictional claims in published maps and institutional affiliations.

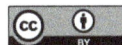

Copyright: © 2021 by the authors. Licensee MDPI, Basel, Switzerland. This article is an open access article distributed under the terms and conditions of the Creative Commons Attribution (CC BY) license (https://creativecommons.org/licenses/by/4.0/).

Abstract: The purpose of this study was to investigate the potential of a byproduct mixture derived from grapeseed and sea buckthorn oil industry to mitigate the harmful damage produced by ochratoxin A and aflatoxin B1 at hepatic and renal level in piglets after weaning. Forty cross-bred TOPIGS-40 hybrid piglets after weaning were assigned to three experimental groups (E1, E2, E3) and one control group (C), and fed with experimental diets for 30 days. The basal diet was served as a control and contained normal compound feed for starter piglets without mycotoxins. The experimental groups were fed as follows: E1—basal diet plus a mixture (1:1) of two byproducts (grapeseed and sea buckthorn meal); E2—the basal diet experimentally contaminated with mycotoxins (479 ppb OTA and 62ppb AFB1); and E3—basal diet containing 5% of the mixture (1:1) of grapeseed and sea buckthorn meal and contaminated with the mix of OTA and AFB1. After 4 weeks, the animals were slaughtered, and tissue samples were taken from liver and kidney in order to perform gene expression and histological analysis. The gene expression analysis showed that when weaned piglets were fed with contaminated diet, the expression of most analyzed genes was downregulated. Among the CYP450 family, *CYP1A2* was the gene with the highest downregulation. According to these results, in liver, we found that mycotoxins induced histomorphological alterations in liver and kidney and had an effect on the expression level of *CYP1A2*, *CYP2A19*, *CYP2E1*, and *CYP3A29*, but we did not detect important changes in the expression level of *CY4A24*, *MRP2* and *GSTA1* genes.

Keywords: piglets; antioxidant effect; feed additives; mycotoxins; CYPs gene expression

Key Contribution: The addition of some plant-derived antioxidants in feed could be a better solution to diminish the deleterious effects of mycotoxins on animal health.

1. Introduction

Mycotoxins are secondary toxic metabolites produced by certain strains of filamentous fungi. These low molecular weight compounds (up to 500 Da) can contaminate a variety of raw materials and cause an increased risk to human and animal health [1]. The number of mycotoxins characterized and with well-known effects is relatively small due to the multitude of metabolites with toxic potential generated by fungi [2–4]. They are classified into five groups, with specific chemical structures that occur frequently in feed and food: trichothecenes, zearalenone, ochratoxins, fumonisins, and aflatoxins. The mycotoxins producing fungi found in food and feed are divided into two groups: those that invade before grain harvesting, called field fungi, and those that grow only after harvesting, called storage fungi [5]. At the European level, there are regulations and recommendations regarding the maximum accepted level for six types of mycotoxins commonly found in pigs' feed: aflatoxins, fumonisins, ochratoxins, deoxynivalenol, T2 toxin, and zearalenone [6–8].

Among the farm animal species, pigs are very sensitive to mycotoxins due to their exposure to cereal-based fodders [9]. Swine metabolism is not effective in detoxifying and excreting mycotoxins, which increases the risk of mycotoxicosis. This susceptibility also varies with age, concentration of mycotoxins in feed, and duration of exposure. Liver is organ most affected by the ingestion of these toxins [10]. Furthermore, these toxins increase the permeability of the intestinal epithelial barrier in swine and poultry, which could generate predisposition for necrotic enteritis [11] and the decrease of innate immunity.

Aflatoxins represent the most abundant mycotoxins found in foodstuffs, oilseeds, cereals, milk, soils, animals, and humans. All types of aflatoxins are derived from fungal species belonging to the genus *Aspergillus* and are considered among the most harmful mycotoxins for animals and humans [4,10–17]. As mentioned above, in suckling piglets and growing, finished, and breeding pigs, the main biological effects of aflatoxins are carcinogenicity, immunosuppression, mutagenicity, teratogenicity, decreased feed efficiency and poor weight gain, impaired liver, and altered serum biochemical parameters [18,19]. Severe effects in swine can lead to acute hepatitis, systemic hemorrhages, nephrosis, and death [20], as well as decreased resistance to stress [21]. Some authors have also shown that swine fed with low levels of aflatoxins presented signs of pulmonary edema, reduced feed consumption and body weight gain, and a decrease in the enzymatic activities implicated in oxidative decarboxylation, as well as total serum protein, blood pressure, and total leukocyte count [18,22–24]. In this context, according to the European Commission Directive 2003/100/EC, the maximum aflatoxin B1 (AFB1) accepted level for pigs is set at 0.02 mg/kg.

Ochratoxins are secondary metabolites produced by fungal species belonging to the genus *Aspergillus* and *Penicillium*. Divergent opinions regarding the genotoxic or nongenotoxic mechanisms of ochratoxins toxicity have been published [25,26]. In vitro and in vivo studies revealed that guanine-OTA-specific DNA adducts persisted for more than 16 days at renal level, whereas in liver and spleen, they were removed after 5 days [27]. Due to this, their main toxic and carcinogenic effects were exerted in kidney [28].

Most metabolites of ochratoxins from Phase I and Phase II detoxification have low toxicity. In the stomach, a part of ochratoxins is hydrolyzed to ochratoxin α by proteolytic enzymes. Another possibility for their hydrolysis is the opening of the lactone ring under alkaline conditions of intestine, thus resulting in a compound with high toxicity. Due to the strong binding to albumin, the elimination of ochratoxins by glomerular filtration is negligible, with the excretion being mainly through tubular secretion. The tubular resorption is considered partially responsible for the intracellular accumulation of ochratoxins [29,30].

Generally, in farm animals, ochratoxins are rapidly absorbed after ingestion through the gastrointestinal tract (stomach and proximal portion of the jejunum) in a passive manner, which is favored by the high affinity of binding of ochratoxins to plasma proteins, and in a nonionized form, which explains their persistence in the body. In porcine serum, ochratoxins bind more specifically to proteins with a molecular mass less than 20 kDa, allowing them to pass through the glomerular basement membrane and exert nephrotoxic effects. Ochratoxins also accumulate in liver and muscles. However, kidneys are the main site of ochratoxins storage, with their reabsorption at the proximal and distal tubules contributing to the body persistence and increased nephrotoxicity [27,31].

On the other hand, once AFB1 is absorbed at the intestinal level, it reaches liver where it is transformed by Phase I metabolizing enzymes by hydroxylation, hydration, demethylation, and epoxidation. The first three reactions generate nontoxic metabolites, whereas the fourth produces AFB1-8,9 epoxide that forms adducts with DNA at the N7 site of guanine [32]. Also, AFB1 can be conjugated with reduced glutathione in a reaction catalyzed by glutathione-S-transferases [33] and glucuronic acid [34]. Excretion of AFB1 occurs primarily through the biliary pathways, followed by the urinary pathway [35].

One of the main difficulties encountered in controlling mycotoxins is that more than one type of mycotoxin is present in a batch of fodder or cereal at the same time. Thus, feeding of piglets and pigs with contaminated feed with several types of mycotoxins, even if they are in minimum concentrations, can cause numerous negative consequences due to their synergistic effect [36–40]. In this context, diminishing and eliminating the negative effects of mycotoxins found in swine feed could decrease production cost and loss in the pig industry.

To date, numerous strategies have been developed to prevent, reduce, or even eliminate mycotoxin contamination from animal feed by biological, chemical, and physical detoxification methods. These methods allow the degradation of mycotoxins and their corresponding metabolites and maintain the nutritional value of the food without introducing other substances with toxic potential into the biological systems [6,14,41].

Biological decontamination of mycotoxins using competitive inhibition by other fungi strains or addition of antioxidant compounds in animal feed in order to reduce the toxic effects of mycotoxins and/or to inhibit the growth of mycotoxin-producing fungus species represents a good solution. The most used method to counteract the negative impact of mycotoxins on farm animals is adding "mycotoxin binders" or "mycotoxin modifiers," which are aluminosilicates with a porous structure that are able to adsorb and trap mycotoxins [42–44]. They are very effective for aflatoxins and have limited activity against other types of mycotoxin. However, being nonspecific, they also bind vitamins and trace elements, generating deficiencies [45–47]. Adding some plant-derived antioxidants in feed could be a better solution [48] to diminish the deleterious effects of mycotoxins on animal health.

P450 cytochromes enzymes, mainly present in liver, intestinal tract, and kidney, play an important role in phase I biotransformation of xenobiotics, especially those belonging to the families 1 and 3 [49]. Mycotoxins can be substrates, inhibitors, or inducers of these metabolizing enzymes. Changes in the specific activity and inducibility of cytochromes P450 will ultimately determine the relative change in the metabolism of a xenobiotic. Mycotoxins may alter the gene expression of these proteins, leading to an altered absorption and biotransformation of nutrients and other substrate drugs from feed. Due to this, the aim of the present study was to investigate the potential of a byproduct mixture derived from *Vitis vinifera* (grapeseed) and *Hippophae rhamnoides* (sea buckthorn) oil industry to mitigate the harmful damage produced by the concomitant presence ochratoxin A (OTA) and aflatoxin B1 (AFB1) in feed at the hepatic and renal level in piglets after weaning.

2. Results
2.1. Diet Composition

The chemical composition of byproducts meal showed that sea buckthorn meal is richer in protein (+38.4%), fat (+66.6%), and carbohydrates and lower in ash than grapeseed meal (Table 1).

Table 1. Chemical composition of grapeseed and sea buckthorn.

Byproducts	DM (103 °C) %	CP (%)	EE (%)	Ash (%)	Carbohydrates (mg/g)			
					Fructose	Glucose	Sucrose	Maltose
Sea buckthorn meal	84.48	15.67	10.28	2.75	9.78	7.68	8.03	0.43
Grapeseed meal	90.85	11.32	6.17	3.34	8.34	5.60	3.49	0.54

DM = Dry matter; CP = Crude protein; EE = Fat (ethyl esters).

The chemical analysis also showed a different profile of the two byproducts in fatty acids, flavonoids, phenolic acids, and minerals. Thus, the sea buckthorn meal has a higher content of saturated fatty acids (palmitic and palmitoleic), omega-9 acids (cis oleic acid), and omega-3 acids (α-linolenic acid) than the grapeseed meal. In contrast, the grapeseed meal has a very high omega-6 acids (linoleic acid) content (67.35% compared to 18.59% in sea buckthorn meal) (Table 2).

Table 2. Fatty acid composition of grapeseed and sea buckthorn (g FAME/100 gTotal FAME).

Saturated Fatty Acids	Sea Buckthorn Meal	Grapeseed Meal	Unsaturated Fatty Acids	Sea Buckthorn Meal	Grapeseed Meal
Butiric (4:0)	0.07	0.12	Miristoleic (14:1)	0.09	0.05
Caproic (6:0)	0.07	0.16	Pentadecenoic (C15:1)	0.00	0.08
Caprilic (10:0)	0.20	0.18	Palmitoleic (C16:1n-7)	14.28	0.33
Capric (10:0)	0.24	0.17	Heptadecenoic (17:1)	0.05	0.00
Lauric (12:0)	0.03	0.03	Oleic cis (C18:1n-9)	31.07	14.66
Miristic (C14:0)	0.93	0.59	Linoleic cis (C18:2n-6)	18.59	67.35
Pentadecanoic (15:0)	0.17	0.07	Linolenic (C18:3n-6)	0.00	0.04
Palmitic (C16:0)	24.32	9.69	α-Linolenic (C18:3n-3)	6.09	0.94
Heptadecanoic (17:0)	0.12	0.09	Octadecatetraenoic (C18:4n-3)	0.28	0.23
Stearic (C18:0)	2.00	3.56	Eicosadienoic (C20:2n-6)	0.44	0.21
			Arachidonic (C20:4n-6)	0.00	0.20
			Eicosapentaenoic (C20:5n-3)	0.19	0.26
			Lignoceric (C24:0)	0.25	0.31
			Nervonic (C24:1n-9)	0.00	0.13
Other fatty acids	0.51	0.55			
Σ SFA	28.40	14.98			
Σ UFA	71.09	84.47			
Σ MUFA	45.49	15.25			
Σ PUFA	25.60	69.23			
SFA/UFA	0.399	0.177			
PUFA/MUFA	0.563	4.541			
Linoleic/α-Linolenic	3.05	71.64			

FAME = Fatty Acid Methyl Esters; SFA = Saturated fatty acids; UFA = Unsaturated fatty acids; MUFA = Monounsaturated fatty acids; PUFA = Polyunsaturated fatty acids.

Both byproducts contain flavonoids and phenolic acids, bioactive compounds known for their antioxidant, anti-inflammatory and immunomodulatory properties [50,51]. Thus, the total concentration of polyphenols was 74.8% higher in grapeseed meal (133.84 mg GAE/L) than in sea buckthorn (76.57 mg GAE/L). Concerning the different classes of polyphenols, grapeseed meal contains higher concentration of catechin and vanillic acid than sea buckthorn, while sea buckthorn is richer in rutin, quercitrin, luteolin, p-coumaric acid, and ferulic acid (Table 3).

Regarding the mineral composition, sea buckthorn meal shoeds a higher content of K, Mg, Fe, Mn, and Zn than grapeseed meal. In contrast, grapeseed meal contained twice as much copper as sea buckthorn meal. Of note is the high concentration of iron from sea buckthorn meal (Table 4).

Table 3. Flavonoids and phenolic acids composition of byproducts.

Flavonoids (mg/g)	Sea Buckthorn Meal	Grapeseed Meal	Phenolic Acids (mg/g)	Sea Buckthorn Meal	Grapeseed Meal
Catechin	0.119	0.378	Vanillic acid	0.008	0.062
Epicatechin	0.397	0.271	Caffeic acid	0.003	0.001
Rutin	0.021	0.009	P-Coumaric acid	0.041	0.005
Quercetin	0.019	0.005	Ferulic acid	0.500	0.063
Luteolin	0.077	0.008			

Table 4. Minerals composition of byproducts.

Macroelements (%)	Sea Buckthorn Meal	Grapeseed Meal	Microelements (ppm)	Sea Buckthorn Meal	Grapeseed Meal
Calcium (Ca)	0.04	0.79	Copper (Cu)	7.26	15.46
Phosphor (P)	0.34	0.35	Iron (Fe)	625.77	89.65
Natrium (Na)	0.117	0127	Manganese (Mn)	22.34	18.27
Kalium (K)	1.69	0.89	Zinc (Zn)	21.90	18.66
Magnesium (Mg)	0.127	0.005			

2.2. Animal Performance

Exposure of piglets from E2 group to ochratoxin plus aflatoxin B1 mixture had no adverse effects on body weight, weight gain, and feed intake, as the differences were not significant compared to the control. In contrast, the administration of the diet containing the byproducts mixture alone (E1) increased significantly the body weight of piglets fed this diet when compared to control (32.14 ± 1.63 vs. 27.09 ± 1.31) and to group E2, which was fed the contaminated diet (32.14 ± 1.63 vs. 28.72 ± 1.07). It should be noted that the group of piglets receiving contaminated feed and the mixture of byproducts had a tendency to gain weight compared to the group of mycotoxin-intoxicated piglets, although the difference was not significant. Biochemical parameters analysis, which characterizes the general state of animal health and the functionality of liver and kidneys, registered normal values for the age and weight category of weaned piglets. No significant differences were identified between groups for most of them (Table 5). However, the mycotoxin mixture increased ALP and gamma GT activity compared to control and decreased activity in the control level in group E3 receiving the byproduct mixture.

Table 5. Biomarkers of liver and kidney function in plasma.

	Control		E1		E2		E3	
	Mean	SEM	Mean	SEM	Mean	SEM	Mean	SEM
Total protein (g/dL)	5.34	0.10	5.08	0.82	5.05	0.18	5.41	0.85
Bilirubin (mg/dL)	0.35	0.04	0.43	0.09	0.31	0.02	0.30	0.06
ALAT (U/L)	49.44	2.36	48.33	1.49	47.22	1.95	50.24	3.56
ASAT (U/L)	38.50	2.92	41.24	3.98	39.96	3.05	41.04	3.28
ALP (U/L)	247.58 [a]	11.1	279.88 [ac]	28.3	311.44 [bc]	25.4	273.22 [ac]	15.9
GGT (U/L)	26.3 [a]	2.55	26.67 [ac]	2.27	34.02 [bc]	3.34	29.92 [ac]	1.88
Albumin (g/L)	3.00	0.00	3.00	0.00	3.02	0.01	3.18	0.02
Creatinine (mg/dL)	0.92	0.33	0.96	0.03	0.94	0.03	0.87	0.05

ALAT = alanine transaminase; ASAT = aspartate transaminase; ALK = alkaline phosphatase; GGT = gamma glutamyl transferase; SEM = standard error of mean; [a,b,c] Mean values within a row with unlike superscript letters were significantly different ($p < 0.05$).

2.3. Histology of Liver and Kidney

Light microscopic analysis of the livers from E2 group, fed with a basal diet contaminated with a mixture of OTA and AFB1, showed focal areas of necrosis, dilatation of sinusoid, and inflammatory parenchymal infiltration. The portal areas revealed mononuclear cellular infiltration and periportal fibrosis. The fibrotic perilobular fibrotic septa were also noticed (Figure 1).

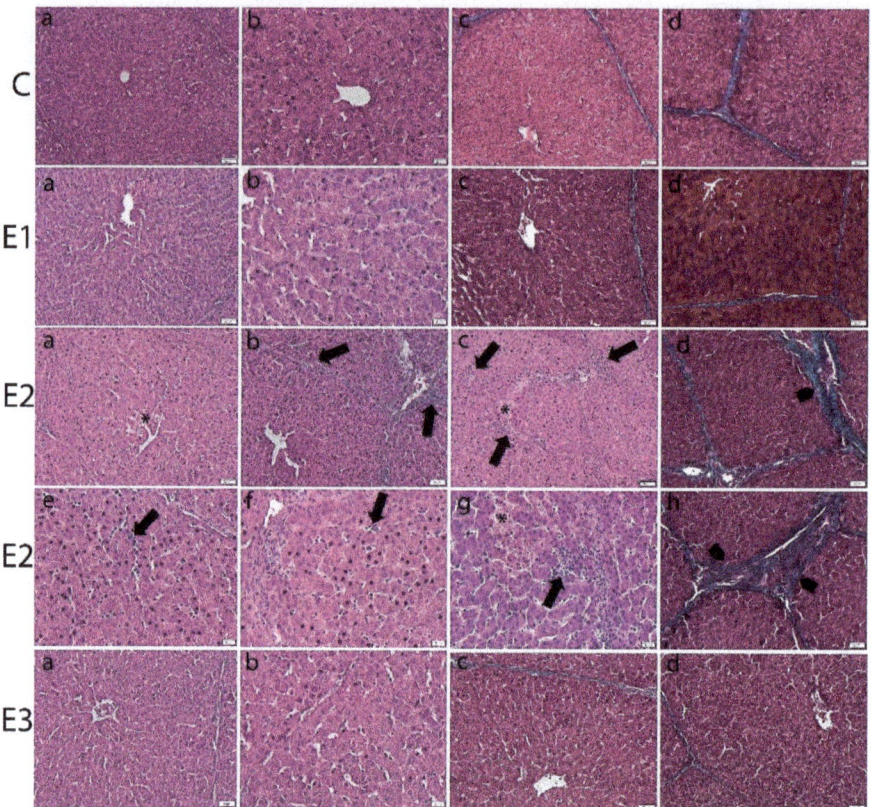

Figure 1. Histopathological changes in liver of weaned piglets subjected to experimental diets. The Control group (C) showed the normal aspect of hepatocytes and sinusoids (**a**,**b**) in the H&E stain and the normal aspect of thin perilobular (**c**) and priportal (**d**) fibrous spikes in Gomori's trichrome stain. The E1 group showed the normal aspect of the liver in the H&E stain (**a**,**b**) and Gomori's trichrome stain (**c**,**d**). The E2 group showed dilated sinusoids and inflammatory infiltrates (arrows) and necrotic hepatocytes (*) in the H&E stain (**a**–**c**,**e**–**g**), and perilobular (**d**) and priportal (**h**) fibrosis (arrowhead) in Gomori's trichrome stain. The E3 group displayed marked improvement of the histological aspect of the liver, which is comparable to that of the control group, in the H&E (**a**,**b**) and Gomori's trichrome stains (**c**,**d**). Scale bar = 50 μm.

Mycotoxin administration caused structural changes in kidneys that affected both the cortex and medulla. Atrophy of the glomerular tufts and alteration of the Bowmann's capsule were noticed (Figure 2). The tubules showed necrosis of lining epithelial cells with inflammatory cells infiltration in between. Focal aggregates of inflammatory cells were observed in between the glomeruli and tubules in association with the focal areas of congestion in blood vessels, especially in the medullary region. Apparently, the collagen proliferation was mainly observed in areas of tubular injury. Furthermore, kidney sections from the E3 groups, the group fed with a basal diet containing a mixture of grapeseed and sea buckthorn meal and contaminated with the mix of OTA and AFB1, revealed minor pathomorphological changes, almost similar to control.

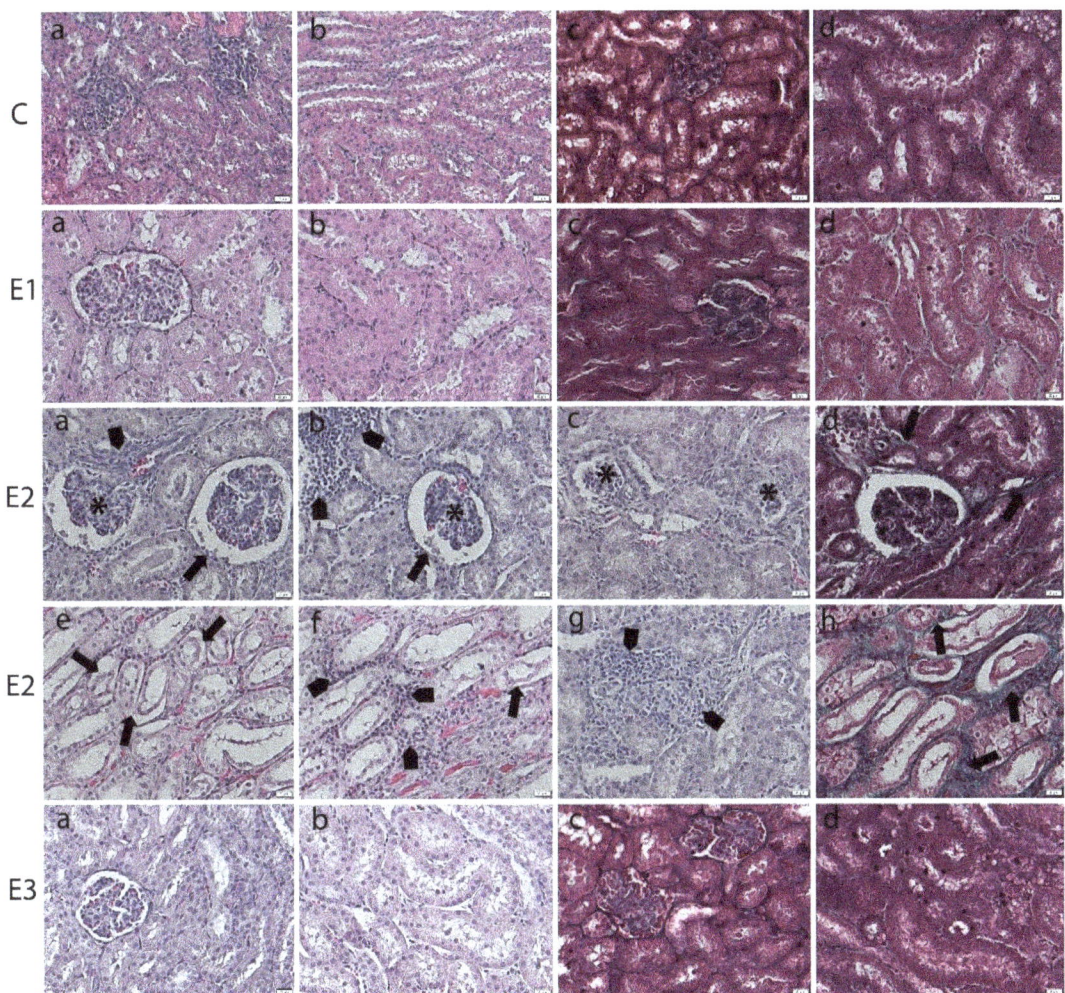

Figure 2. Histopathological changes in kidney of weaned piglets subjected to experimental diets. The Control group (C) showed the normal aspect of kidney cortex (**a**) and medulla (**b**) in the H&E stain and few collagen fibers surrounding glomeruli and tubules in cortex (**c**) and medulla (**d**) in Gomori's trichrome stain. The E1 group showed the normal aspect of kidney cortex (**a**) and medulla (**b**) in the H&E stain and few collagen fibers surrounding glomeruli and tubules in the cortex (**c**) and medulla (**d**) in Gomori's trichrome stain. The E2 group (**a–d**) kidney cortex showed glomerular atrophy (*), Bowmann's capsule injury (arrow), inflammatory cell infiltrates (arrowhead) (**a,b**), or glomerular degeneration (*) in the H&E stain (**a–c**) and slight proliferation of peritubular collagen in Gomori's trichrome stain (arrow) (**d**). (**e–h**) The kidney medulla showed altered tubuli (arrow), inflammatory infiltrates (arrowhead), and congestion in blood vessels in the H&E stain (**e–g**) and the proliferation of peritubular collagen in Gomori's trichrome stain (arrow) (**h**). The E3 group displayed marked improvement of the renal histological aspect, which is comparable to that of the control group, in the kidney cortex (**a**) and medulla (**b**) in the H&E stain and in the cortex (**c**) and medulla (**d**) in Gomori's trichrome stain. Scale bar = 50 μm.

Moreover, the morphometric analysis of the structural injuries in liver and kidney of experimental groups was evaluated (Table 6).

Table 6. The morphometric analysis of the structural injuries in liver and kidney of experimental groups.

MAV	Control Group	E1 Group	E2 Group	E3 Group
Liver	1	1	3.5 ± 0.55 ***	2.5 ± 0.55 ***/^
Kidney	1	1	3.7 ± 0.52 ***	2.3 ± 0.52 ***/^^

One-Way ANOVA test. * (All groups vs. Control group; *** $p < 0.001$). ^ (E3 group vs. E2 group; ^ $p < 0.05$; ^^ $p < 0.01$). MAV = Mean assessment value.

2.4. The Level of Gene Expression

We found that modifying the piglets' diet caused significant liver changes to the *CYP2E1* and *GSTA1* genes in the E1 group fed with a basal diet supplemented with a mixture of grapeseed and sea buckthorn meal, and to the *CYP4A24*, *MRP2*, and *GSTA1* genes in the E2 group fed with a basal diet contaminated with a mixture of AFB1 and OTA. The modifications caused insignificant changes to all the other target genes (Figure 3).

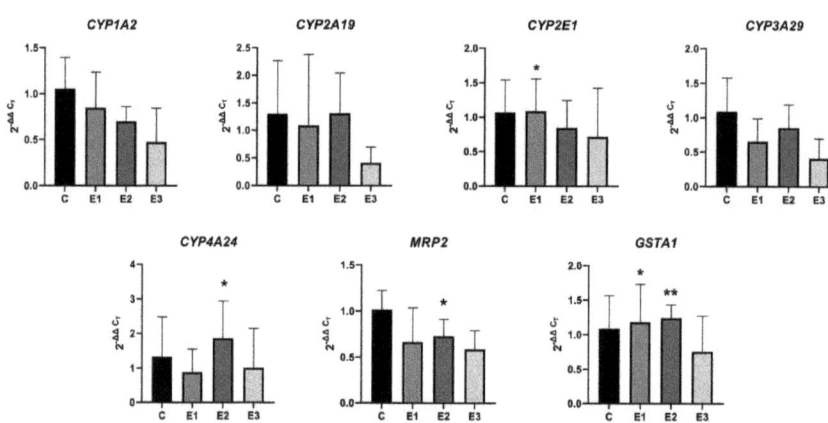

Figure 3. Gene expression level in the liver for *CYP1A2*, *CYP2A19*, *CYP2E1*, *CYP3A29*, *CYP4A24*, *MRP2*, and *GSTA1* of weaned piglets subjected to experimental diets. The data are illustrated as average values of the groups (n = 4) ± standard deviation of the mean (STDEV). Statistical significance: * $p < 0.05$; ** $p < 0.01$. The statistical significance of the changes is related to the control group level.

In liver, the gene expression for *CYP1A2* decreased by 18% for E2 and 44% for E3, respectively, compared to the E1 group. The *CYP2A19* gene expression was unmodified in groups E1 and E2, whereas in group E3, it decreased by almost 62%. A significant increase by 29% was observed in *CYP2E1* gene expression in the E1 group fed with a basal diet supplemented with a mixture of grapeseed and sea buckthorn meal compared to the E2 group. In contrast, the administration of basal diet enriched with a mixture of grapeseed and sea buckthorn meal (E1 group) downregulated the *CYP3A29* gene expression by 24% compared to the E2 group level. Another contrast was observed in the *CYP4A24* gene expression, with a 33% decrease for the E1 group and 24% decrease for the E3 group, and a significant 41% increase in the E2 group fed with a basal diet supplemented with a mixture of AFB1 and OTA, compared to the control level. In the case of *MRP2*, the gene expression pattern was similar to that of the *CYP4A24* gene, with an insignificant 35% decrease for the E1 group and 24% decrease for the E3 group, and a significant 28% increase in the E2 group, compared to the control level. Similarly, to the *CYP4A24* gene expression, the *GSTA1* gene expression showed a significant 14% increase in the E2 group, a 9% increase in the E1 group, and a 30% decrease for the E3 group. Obviously, the concomitant administration of the mixture of grapeseed and sea buckthorn meal and OTA and AFB1 generated a decrease of all analyzed genes expressions in liver compared to control.

Regarding the expression level of these genes in kidneys, compared to liver samples, no statistically significant changes were observed (Figure 4). However, changes in the regulation of gene expression level could be observed.

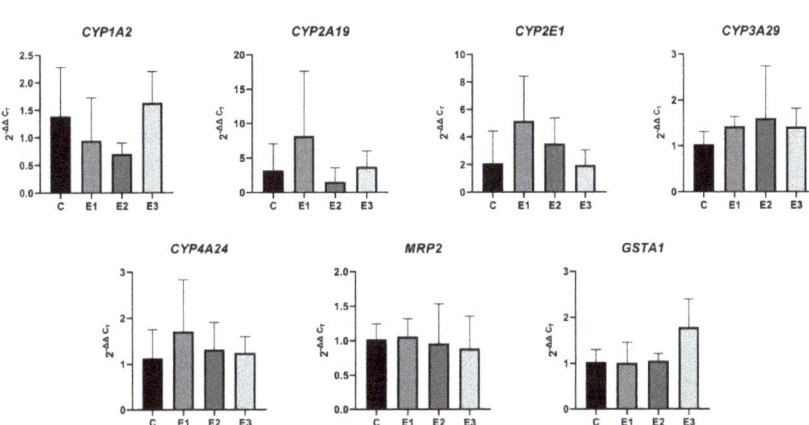

Figure 4. Gene expression level in the kidney for *CYP1A2*, *CYP2A19*, *CYP2E1*, *CYP3A29*, *CYP4A24*, *MRP2*, and *GSTA1* of weaned piglets subjected to experimental diets. The data are illustrated as average values of the groups (n = 4) ± standard deviation of the mean (STDEV).

Analyzing Figure 4, it could be noticed that the mixture of grapeseed and sea buckthorn meal downregulated the *CYP1A2* gene expression and upregulated the *CYP2A19*, *CYP2E1*, *CYP3A29*, and *CYP4A24* gene expression in an insignificant way, whereas *MRP2* and *GSTA1* gene expression remained unmodified. Also, the presence of OTA and AFB1 in piglets feed downregulated *CYP1A2* and *CYP2A19* gene expression in an insignificant way, whereas *MRP2* and *GSTA1* were unmodified. The concomitant administration of the mixture of grapeseed and sea buckthorn meal and OTA and AFB1 determined the return of all genes expression levels to control levels with the exception of *GSTA1*, which presented an important increase compared to E1 group.

3. Discussion

Mycotoxins such as AFB1 and OTA are natural toxins contaminating a large variety of plant products. As a consequence, AFB1, OTA, and their metabolites are present in food and feed, as well as in the products of animal origin [52]. Most of the toxicological studies regarding the effects of mycotoxins have considered the exposure to a single type of mycotoxin without considering the combination and the interaction between them, respectively, the synergistic or antagonistic effects which often occur in nature. Data regarding the toxic effects of mycotoxin combinations are limited, so the risks of exposure to several types of toxins are still unknown.

The occurrence of mycotoxins such as AFB1, DON, ZEA, OTA, FB1, and FB2 in cereal, cereal products, and complementary and complete feeding stuffs for pigs [16] is related to the geographical location and climate change, which increases the risk associated with mycotoxin contamination during the storage and processing of feed products for pigs [53]. The co-contamination of cereals and other raw materials occurs more frequently in real life than single mycotoxin contamination [7]. For example, the co-occurrence of aflatoxin B1 and ochratoxin A has been found in different food or feed ingredients, such as wheat [54], barley [55], cereal flours [56], spice [57], etc. The proportion between AFB1 and OTA in feed was found to be about 1 to 6 [37]. Also, the global feed content in AFB1 and OTA ranged between not determined and 100 ppb and not determined and 211 ppb, respectively [58]. In this context, in order to mimic the field conditions, we studied the effects of these mycotoxins together and to assess the effectiveness of the by-product mix in counteracting the effects of mycotoxins. The natural additives (grapeseed and sea buckthorn byproducts) were selected based on their ability to ameliorate mycotoxicosis upon dietary supplementation [59,60].

In the present study, the exposure of piglets (E2 group) to mycotoxins mixture did not influence the performance of animals (27.83 ± 1.1 vs. 27.09 ± 1.3 for body weight and 1.48 ± 0.9 vs. 1.40 ± 0.8 for feed intake) and biochemical parameters when compared to control. Similarly, Balogh et al. [61] reported that piglets fed with approximately 0.4 mg/kg of OTA during the starter (0–28 days) and grower (29–49 days) period did not register significantly changes in the production traits and clinical signs of toxicity in the grower phase. In contrast, a significant decrease of body weight gain was observed during the starter period when the animals were more sensitive. In this study, the dietary inclusion of the byproduct mixture alone had a significant influence on animal performance (group E1) and tended to increase piglets' weight when the mixture was associated with contaminated food (group E3).

From a toxicological point of view, OTA is classified by IARC (International Agency for Research on Cancer) in the same group (2B) of carcinogenic substances for humans, having a similar toxicity with AFB1 [62]. Toxicokinetic patterns of absorption, distribution, and elimination for these mycotoxins are, for the most part, entirely elucidated. In contrast, despite recent progress, our knowledge of the toxicokinetic biotransformation steps is not elucidated in detail. A number of studies have shown that AFB1 and OTA are metabolized by liver microsomes from humans, pigs, and rats into several epimers [63]. Changes in the specific activity and inducibility of cytochromes P450 ultimately determine the relative change in the metabolism of any xenobiotic.

It has been found that exposure to AFB1 and OTA decreased the gene expression of *CYP1A2, CYP2E1, CYP3A29,* and *MRP2* genes in pig's liver and resulted in several changes in liver histology and ultrastructure, including focal areas of necrosis, dilatation of sinusoid, inflammatory parenchymal infiltration, and periportal fibrosis. Regarding the gene expression level of CYP450 isoforms in pig's kidney, no data were available in the scientific literature.

The *CYP1A2, CYP2A19, CYP2E1, CYP3A29, CYP4A24, MRP2,* and *GSTA1* genes were chosen for this study because they encode proteins with enzymatic activity or transporter function that are involved in Phase I and Phase II of biotransformation and detoxification of xenobiotics to form electrophilic reactive metabolites [64].

According to these results, it appears that the by-product administration determined a decrease in *CYP1A2* gene expression and an increase in *GSTA1* gene expression. Similar results were noticed in HT-29 human colon cancer cells treated with *Salicornia freitagii* extract, known for its antioxidant and anti-inflammatory activity. In this case, due to its content in bioactive phenols, a downregulation of *CYP1A2* mRNA and an upregulation of *GSTA1* mRNA occurred [65]. In contrast to our results, mRNA and protein expression of *CYP1A2* were increased in liver of chicory fed pigs [66]. These different results were probably caused by the different natural compounds present in chicory compared to the byproducts used in the present study, mainly chlorogenic, caffeic, and p-coumaric acids [67].

On the other hand, OTA and AFB1 probably interacted with and activated the aromatic hydrocarbon receptor, leading to its nuclear translocation. After the heterodimerization, OTA and AFB1 probably interacted with hydrocarbon receptor nuclear translocator, the heterodimer, bound to xenobiotic-responsive elements and transactivated genes such as *CYP1A1, CYP1A2,* and *GST* [68]. This xenobiotic-responsive element is shared between *CYP1A1* and *CYP1A2* genes [69], and the two enzymes codified by them present overlapping substrate specificity [70]. In pig liver, only *CYP1A2* activity is present, and its relative amount of total detected CYP450 is 4% [71]. In the human liver, AFB1 and OTA are inducers for CYP1A1, 1A2, 2B6, 2C9, 3A4, and 3A5 [72]. AFB1, as well as OTA exposure, generate mitochondrial dysfunction characterized by an increase in ROS production [14] that could increase TGF-β1 expression or activate latent TGF-β1 [73]. Taking into consideration, the previous evidence that TGF-β1 decreased *CYP1* expression in humans and rats, it is possible that the same mechanism [74] occurred under our conditions. The effects of the concomitant exposure to both mycotoxins and grapeseed and sea buckthorn by-products were probably synergistical, and the expression of *CYP1A2* was lower in E3 compared to E1, E2, and the control group. *CYP1A2* is expressed in lower levels in extrahepatic tissues [75].

The kidney is an organ that receives about 25% of cardiac output and purifies metabolic residue and xenobiotics from the circulatory system. During this discharging process, toxic substances are concentrated in the kidney [76]. In piglet kidneys, the variation of *CYP1A2* gene expression was similar with the expression levels in liver for E1 and E2. Interestingly, in the E3 group, the expression of this gene was at a higher level than the control group. This could possibly be due to the activation of noncanonical signaling pathway for AhR transcription in the kidney cells [77].

In pig liver, the relative amounts of *CYP2A19* and *CYP2E1* represent 31% respectively 13% of total CYP450 [71]. Porcine *CYP2A19* and *CYP2E1* genes are responsible for the biotransformation for endogenous compounds (skatole, sex hormones) as well as exogenous compounds (food components). Both types of compounds are highly expressed in the liver and less in the kidney and adipose tissue. *CYP2A19* transcription is controlled by the CAR transcription factor [78]. Its human orthologue, *CYP2A6* is controlled by CAR, PXR, glucocorticoid receptor (GR), estrogen receptor α, HNF$_4$ α, and PGC-1α [79]. Also, the constitutive hepatic expression of *CYP2A6* in mice is governed by an interplay between HNF$_4$ α, CCAAT-box/enhancer binding protein (C/EBP α, C/EBP β) and octamer transcription factor-1 (Oct-1) [80]. Previously, a positive correlation between mRNA and protein levels for *CYP2A19* gene was observed [81]. Unlike other CYP 450 genes, *CYP2A19* plays a less important role in the xenobiotics' metabolism but is involved in the reaction of cells to stress, Nrf-2, being also involved in *CYP2A19* transcription [82]. The *CYP2A19* gene is probably highly polymorphic compared to the *CYP2A6* gene [83], and an extensive interindividual variation of its product could occur. Previous studies revealed that duck P450 orthologues of the mammalian *CYP2A6* and CYP3A4 are involved in AFB1 bioactivation into its epoxide form [84]. Unlike these results, in the present study, no significant changes of *CYP2A19* gene expression were noticed in the E1 and E2 groups, probably due to the high level of expression of this gene in piglet liver. For now, it is difficult to explain why the co-exposure of both mycotoxins and the mixture of grapeseed and sea buckthorn meal decreased the expression of *CYP2A19*. However, this decrease of expression diminished the risk of generation of toxic metabolites.

In pig kidney, the expression of *CYP2A19* is lower compared to that found in liver [79]. Probably due to this lower expression, animal exposure to the mixture of grapeseed and sea buckthorn meal generated an upregulation of Nrf-2 induced *CYP2A19* gene expression due to the luteolin [85] and ferulic acid [86] content.

On the other hand, there is evidence that only two transcription factors, i.e., chick ovalbumin upstream promoter transcription factor (COUP-TF1) and hepatocyte nuclear factor (HNF-1), are involved in the regulation of *CYP2E1* transcription in pigs [87]. *CYP2E1*, like other xenobiotic-metabolizing P450s, is mainly located in the membrane of the endoplasmic reticulum (ER) and can be induced under a variety of metabolic or nutritional conditions. ER stress can be induced by metabolic stress, which is caused by overload of protein/lipid biosynthesis, and oxidative stress, which could trigger the evolutionarily conserved complex homeostatic signaling pathway known as the unfolded protein response (UPR) [88].

It is likely that the level of *CYP2E1* mRNA was approximately the same in the E1 and control groups due to the antagonistic actions of palmitic acid [89], linoleic, and α-linolenic acids [90] that increased this gene transcription and the actions vanillic and p-coumaric acids which decreased it [65].

Recently, it was proved that OTA-containing feed altered the intestinal microbiota in ducks, affecting the cecum microbiota diversity and composition as well as the intestinal barrier. As a result, Gram-negative bacterial-derived lipopolysaccharides entered the blood and liver, causing liver inflammation [91]. In the case of immune-mediated liver injury, the expression of *CYP2E1* was decreased [92]. This situation could occur in the E2 group. It is likely that the cumulative effects of the two mycotoxins and dietary by-products decreased the expression of *CYP2E1* in liver of the E3 group.

In the kidney, free fatty acids, such as palmitate, oleate, and linoleate, are stored in the nephron [93], and these acids probably increased the expression of the *CYP2E1* gene in the kidneys of the E1 group compared to the control level. According to Pfohl-Leszkowicz and Manderville [25], OTA forms adduct with DNA, generating renal genotoxicity and carcinogenesis. It is likely that high levels of OTA stimulated *CYP2E1* gene expression in the kidneys of the E2 group compared to the control level. In the E3 group, it appears that the coadministration of the two mycotoxins and dietary byproducts had antagonistic effects, with the expression of *CYP2E1* gene returning to the control level. Moreover, histological evaluation for the E3 group showed that the byproduct mixture derived from grapeseed and sea buckthorn oil mitigated the harmful damage produced by aflatoxin B1 and ochratoxin A at the hepatic and renal level in piglets after weaning. CYP2E1, like other xenobiotic-metabolizing P450s, is mainly located in the membrane of the ER and can be induced under a variety of metabolic or nutritional conditions [89]. The regulation of the *CYP2E1* gene in the E1 group was probably due to the hydroxylation of coumarin-derived compounds that were catalyzed by CYP2A enzymes, which are considered to be specific indicators for the presence of CYP2 enzymes [94], with the p-coumaric acid being present in grapeseed and sea buckthorn byproducts.

In the case of pigs, very little is known about the presence of CYP3As enzymes in the renal tissue, and nothing is known about their inducibility [95]. Several genes have been identified in the CYP3A subfamily of mammals (for example, five in rat and four in human), but the expression of these genes in renal tissues has been poorly investigated [96]. In terms of gene expression, Ayed-Boussema et al. (2012) [63] and Gonzalez-Arias et al. [97] described an increase of expression levels in all cytochromes assayed (CYP3A4, 2B6, 3A5, and 2C9) in a primary human hepatocyte culture. Previous studies have reported various results regarding the effects of AFB1 and OTA in primary cultured human hepatocytes in which increasing concentrations of these mycotoxins clearly induced CYP3A4 and CYP2B6 mRNA levels in a dose-dependent manner [63].

In contrast, it has been found that in the presence of OTA and AFB1 in liver (Figure 3, group E2), the *CYP3A29* expression level is decreased compared to the control level, perhaps due to activation of the AhR [98]. These data differ from those of Zepnik et al. [99], who reported an increase of OTA hydrolysis by microsomal enzymes from rat liver, specifically for P450 3A1/2 and 3A4, suggesting that this gene expression is modulated in a species-dependent manner.

In some cases, the inhibition of P450 enzymes by polyphenols may have a chemo-preventive effect due to the potential activation of carcinogens by P450 enzymes within the course of their natural metabolic activity. The inhibition of xenobiotic-metabolizing Phase I enzymes could be one target of the chemo-preventive effects of naturally occurring polyphenols.

The increase of *CYP4A24* observed in liver could be a physiological response in the unusual context of aberrant lipid accumulation and absence of *CYP2E1* activity, due to the fact that *CYP2E1* and CYP4A are inducible hepatic microsomal cytochromes P-450 involved in hydroxylation of fatty acids, and both can initiate the auto-propagative process of lipid peroxidation. They might be complementary, leading to interactions in the regulation of the individual enzymes [100]. It is therefore clear that CYP4A proteins are key intermediaries in an adaptive response to perturbation of hepatic lipid metabolism [101]. The decreased

CYP4A24 level in the kidney probably leads to the toxic effects generated in liver due to the mycotoxin-contaminated diet, which means that *CYP4A24* regulates hepatic ER stress [102,103].

In the present study, the addition of a mixture of grapeseed and sea buckthorn meal by-products increased expression levels in the kidney, which would be expected to favor the elimination processes and maintenance of the balance of intracellular substances [104]. Moreover, OTA was absorbed in the intestine where the multidrug resistance protein 2 (*MRP2* gene) plays an important role, acting as a xenobiotic outward transporter to reduce the oral bioavailability and the toxin load to organs and, thereby, OTA toxicity. Once OTA reaches the bloodstream, it can reach other organs such as liver, and the MRP2 transporter is again a key primary active transporter involved in anionic conjugate and xenobiotic extrusion into the extracellular space which contributes to bile formation and the subsequent elimination of the toxin [97,105]. Also, the MRP2 transporter is present in the apical membranes of enterocytes, kidney-proximal tubules, and other cells [105]. OTA toxicity has been attributed to its isocoumarin moiety, and it is well known that OTA is inactivated or bioactivated by cytochrome P450 enzymes [29]. Previously, the presence of OTA in feed was linked to the development of nephrotoxicity, which, in rats, has been associated with renal adenomas and kidney tumors [97]. In the present study, a decrease of *MRP2* expression in the liver was found, indicating an impairment of the secretion of mycotoxins in the E2 group.

In rats, OTA was observed to be excreted 15% less in the proximal tubules of the kidney, while the proximal tubular transport of amino acids was not impaired [97,106]. Therefore, the decrease of *MRP2* in liver found in this study could be the mechanism through which mycotoxins reach high percentages of bioavailability in vivo. In this way, the AFB1 and OTA exposure of piglets would be magnified, contributing to the hepatotoxicity.

Considering the nephrotoxic potential of OTA and AFB1, the decrease of the *MRP2* gene product may also have a major impact on the proximal tubule, leading to a decreased capacity to eliminate OTA [97]. However, further studies are needed on the AFB1 and OTA transporter mechanism to support this hypothesis.

In Phase II of metabolic detoxification, the original xenobiotic compound or the intermediate metabolites modified during Phase I are conjugated in order to be suitable for excretion. Glutathione S transferases (GSTs) and UDP glycurosyltranferases (UGTs) contribute to Phase II processing [107].

In the presence of a mixture of grapeseed and sea buckthorn meal byproducts in pigs feed, the *GSTA1* expression level in liver is significantly increased, possibly by an antioxidant-responsive element (ARE) and β-NF-responsive element (β-NF-RE), respectively, which, in the presence of phenolic antioxidants, activate the GST isoforms without the need for aryl hydrocarbon (Ah) receptors [108]. Surprisingly, in the study of Ghadiri et al. (2019) [109], the AFB1-mediated mRNA downregulation of *GSTA1* was observed in the cow's liver in the presence of an antioxidant.

Previous studies [110] showed that OTA and AFB1 compete for the same CYP450 enzymes which represent the bioactivation route of AFB1, with less AFB1-DNA adducts being produced. Due to this competition, AFB1 could probably be conjugated with reduced glutathione in a reaction catalyzed by GST enzymes, with their codding genes being upregulated. AFB1 could be involved in other types of Phase II reactions, i.e., glucuronidation and sulfatation, whereas OTA is mainly conjugated with reduced glutathione [72]. Moreover, in response to concomitant administration in the pigs, the feed of two mycotoxins (AFB1 and OTA) increased the generation of the oxidative stress biomarkers. Therefore, defense mechanisms were activated, promoting adaptation and survival in response to oxidative stress [111]. For example, ROS and oxidants could activate the transcription of GST isoforms through ARE [108], as observed in both the liver and kidneys through an increase in the expression level of the *GSTA1* gene.

4. Conclusions

Our data revealed the existence of differences between piglet's kidney and liver regarding the reaction against both mycotoxins and by-products used in this study. Generally, the by-products with antioxidant action decreased the expression of the analyzed CYPs mRNA in liver and increased them in kidney. Also, in both organs, the co-exposure of piglets to OTA and AFB1 generated an increase or a decrease of gene expression dependent on the gene type. The inclusion of grapeseed and sea buckthorn meal in the diet of OTA and AFB1-intoxicated pigs decreased the CYP P450 gene expression, suggesting the decrease of bioactivation of these mycotoxins, probably resulting in a diminished toxicity in both organs, as the histological studies have revealed.

These findings suggest that grapeseed and sea buckthorn meal waste represent a promising source in counteracting the harmful effect of ochratoxin A and aflatoxin B1. Although additional work is needed to unravel the mechanisms by which grapeseed and sea buckthorn byproducts affects AFB1 and OTA biotransformation, and hence the generation of toxic metabolites, the protective effects seem to be at least partly mediated by the enhancement of the antioxidant defense at the liver and kidney level.

5. Materials and Methods

5.1. Experimental Design and Samples Collection

Forty cross-bred TOPIGS-40 hybrid (♀Large White × Hybrid (Large White × Pietrain) × ♂Talent, mainly Duroc) piglets after weaning with an average body weight of 9.11 ± 0.03 kg were assigned to three experimental groups (E1, E2, E3) and one control group (C), housed in pens (two replicates of five pigs per pen per treatment) and fed with experimental diets for 30 days. Feed and water were offered ad libitum during the experiment. The basal diet was served as a control and contained normal compound feed for starter piglets without mycotoxin (corn 68.46%, soya meal 19%, corn gluten 4%, milk replacer 5%, L-lysine 0.3%, DL-methionine 0.1%, limestone 1.57%, monocalcium phosphate 0.35%, salt 0.1%, choline premixes 0.1%, and 1% vitamin-mineral premixes). The experimental groups were fed as follows: E1—basal diet plus a mixture (1:1) of two byproducts (grapeseed and sea buckthorn meal) in a percentage of 5% by replacing corn and soya bean meal; E2—the basal diet artificially contaminated with mycotoxins (a mixture of 62 ppb aflatoxin B1- AFB1 and 479 ppb ochratoxin A-OTA); and E3—basal diet containing 5% of the mixture (1:1) of grapeseed and sea buckthorn meal and contaminated with the mix of AFB1 and OTA. The mixture of OTA and AFB1 mycotoxins was kindly provided by Dr. Boudra and Dr. Morgavi from I. N. R. A, Centre of Clermont Ferrand, and was produced by the cultivation of *Aspergillus flavus* and *Aspergillus ochraceous* on wheat as already described by Boudra et al. [112]. The contaminated material obtained was incorporated in the diets for the E2 and E3 groups, resulting in a final concentration of 479 ppb OTA and 62 ppb AFB1. Animals from all experimental groups had free access to the treatment feed and water every day of the experimental period (30 days). The grapeseed meal and sea buckthorn meal were provided by two local commercials, S.C. OLEOMET-S.R.L. and BIOCATINA, Bucharest, Romania. After 4 weeks, the animals were slaughtered with the approval of the Ethical Committee of the National Research-Development Institute for Animal Nutrition and Biology, Baloteşti, Romania (Ethical Committee no. 118/02.12.2019) and in accordance with the Romanian Law 206/2004 and the EU Council Directive 98/58/EC for handling and protection of animals used for experimental purposes. At the end of the experimental period of this study, the productive parameters, weight, and feed consumption were measured. Liver and kidney samples were collected from four animals per group and perfused with ice-cold saline solution to remove blood. Fragments of ~50 mg from the right liver lobe and renal cortex (three from each) were collected in RNAlater Stabilization Reagent (Qiagen, Germantown, Maryland) and then stored at −80 °C until RNA isolation step.

Due to ethical reasons, maximizing the use of each animal, minimizing the loss of animals, and statistical analysis, the number of individuals was reduced as much as scientifically possible. Good science and good experimental design help to reduce the number of animals used in any research study, allowing scientists to gather data using the minimum number of animals required [113].

5.2. Feed Characterization

Feed diets were analyzed for basal chemical composition (dry matter, crude protein, crude fat, crude fiber, and ash) according to the International Standard Organization methods (SR ISO 6496/2001, Standardized Bulletin (2010). http://www.asro.ro (accessed on 13 February 2021)). Bioactive compounds from byproducts meals, such as polyphenols, polyunsaturated fatty acids (PUFA), and minerals, were determined by Folin-Ciocalteu reaction, HPLC-UV-Vis, and gas chromatography as described by the authors of [113,114]. Antioxidant activity was determined by the DPPH method as described previously by the authors of [115].

5.3. Plasma Biomarkers Analysis

On day 30, blood samples were aseptically collected from fasted piglets. Markers that reflect the functionality of liver (aspartate transaminase-AST, alanine transaminase-ALT, gamma glutamyl transferase-GGT, total protein, alkaline phosphatase-AKL), and kidneys (albumin, creatinine) were determined after blood centrifugation using a Clinical Chemistry benchtop analyser Horiba Medical—ABX Pentra 400, (Irvine, CA, USA).

5.4. Light Microscopy Examination

Liver and kidney biopsies were fixed in 4% phosphate-buffered formaldehyde solution, dehydrated, clarified, and included in paraffin blocks. The 5 µm sections were processed routinely for hematoxylin-eosin and Gomori trichrome (Leica Biosystems, 38016SS1, Nussloch, Germany) staining, respectively, according to Leica's protocol. Microscopic sections were analyzed with an Olympus BX43 microscope equipped with a digital camera Olympus XC30. The histopathological alterations of liver and kidney were graded by the severity of lesions as belonging to grades 1–4, as previously described [116]. For liver, grade 1: Normal aspect; grade 2: Normal hepatocytes, slight dilated sinusoids and congestion; grade 3: Vacuolated hepatocytes, dilated sinusoids and congestion; moderate collagen proliferation; grade 4: Necrosis, inflammatory infiltrates, collagen proliferation. For kidney, grade 1: Normal aspect; grade 2: Slight tubular/glomerular injuries, inflammation, and collagen proliferation; grade 3: Mild tubular/glomerular injuries, inflammation, and collagen proliferation; grade 4: Marked tubular/glomerular injuries, inflammation, and collagen proliferation. A "mean assessment value" (MAV) was calculated as a mean of all data per experimental group.

5.5. RNA Isolation

The isolation of total RNA was performed from 10 mg of tissue using the RNeasy Plus Universal Mini Kit (Qiagen) following the manufacturer's protocol. Moreover, it included the On-column DNase digestion step. After RNA isolation, aliquots were made in order to prevent degradation induced by freeze-thaw cycles. The concentration and purity of total RNA were determined using NanoDrop 8000 spectrophotometer (Thermo Scientific, Wilmington, DE, USA).

5.6. RNA Integrity Number (RIN)

RIN values of the RNA samples were determined using the Agilent RNA 6000 Nano Kit (Agilent, Santa Clara, CA, USA) and Agilent 2100 Bioanalyzer using the manufacturer's protocol. Samples with RIN values smaller than 8 were not included in further analysis, and the isolation steps were repeated.

5.7. Reverse Transcription

For cDNA synthesis, 1000 ng of total RNA was subjected to reverse transcription using iScript cDNA synthesis kit (Bio-Rad, Hercules, CA, USA). A 4 µL reaction mix and 1 µL reverse transcriptase were mixed with 1 µL RNA samples and completed with RNase free water to a total volume of 20 µL. The final concentration of RNA was 1000 ng per reaction. The reaction was performed using a Veriti 96-Well thermal cycler (Applied Biosystems, Foster City, CA, USA) with the following program: One cycle of 25 °C for 5 min, one cycle of 42 °C for 30 min and one cycle of 85 °C for 5 min. The concentration and purity of the cDNA samples was determined using NanoDrop 8000 spectrophotometer (Thermo Scientific).

5.8. Primer Design

Because of the lack of data regarding genes involved in the hepato-nephrotoxicity in the mycotoxin exposure of weaned pigs, primer sequences (Table 7) were designed in silico using Primer3Plus [59] and verified by BLAST program [117]. Those with the highest specificity for the target sequence were selected in order to amplify the *CYP1A2, CYP2A19, CYP2E1, CYP3A29, CYP4A24, MRP2*, and *GSTA1* genes and three reference genes encoding for TATA-box binding protein, ribosomal protein L4, and beta-2-microglobulin in *Sus scrofa*. The annealing temperatures of the primers were determined by temperature gradient PCR.

Table 7. Primers for Real-Time PCR analysis.

GenBank Accession Number	Gene	PCR Product Length (bp)	Primer Name	Primer Sequence
XM021085497	TATA-box binding protein	124	tbp-F tbp-R	5′-GATGGACGTTCGGTTTAGG-3′ 5′-AGCAGCACAGTACGAGCAA-3′
XM005659862	ribosomal protein L4	122	rpl4-F rpl4-R	5′-CAAGAGTAACTACAACCTTC-3′ 5′-GAACTCTACGATGAATCTTC-3′
NM213978	beta-2-microglobulin	172	b2m-F b2m-R	5′-CCGCCCCAGATTGAAATTGA-3′ 5′-GCTTATCGAGAGTCACGTGC-3′
NM001159614	cytochrome P450, family 1, subfamily A, polypeptide 2	173	cyp1a2-F cyp1a2-R	5′-CTCTTCCGACACACCTCCTT-3′ 5′-AATCTCTCTGGCCGGAACTC-3′
NM214417	cytochrome P450 2A19	174	cyp2a19-F cyp2a19-R	5′-CTCATGAAGATCAGCCAGCG-3′ 5′-GCCATAGCCTTTGAAGAGCC-3′
XM005657509	cytochrome P450, family 2, subfamily E, polypeptide 1	150	cyp2e1-F cyp2e1-R	5′-ACCTCATTCCCTCCAACCTG-3′ 5′-CTGGCTTAAACTTCTCCGGC-3′
NM214423	cytochrome P450 3A29	205	cyp3a29-F cyp3a29-R	5′-ATTGCTGTCTCCGACCTTCA-3′ 5′-TGGGTTGTTGAGGGAATCGA-3′
XM021096706	cytochrome P450 4A24	157	cyp4a24-F cyp4a24-R	5′-CTCTATCCGCCAGTACCAGG-3′ 5′-ATGGGTCAAACTCCTCTGGG-3′
XM021073710	ATP binding cassette subfamily C member 2	172	mrp2-F mrp2-R	5′-AGCAGTACACCGTTGGAGAA-3′ 5′-ATCACCCCAACACCTGCTAA-3′
NM214389	glutathione S-transferase alpha 1	186	gsta1-F gsta1-R	5′-GCCCATGGTTGAGATTGACG-3′ 5′-TTTTCATTGGGTGGGCACAG-3′

5.9. Real-Time PCR

The Real-Time PCR reaction was carried out on the iCycler iQ Real-Time PCR Detection System (Bio-Rad) using iQ SYBR Green SuperMix (Bio-Rad). In a 96-well plate, 1 µL of 100 ng/µL cDNA, 12.5 µL iQ SYBR Green SuperMix (Bio-Rad), 0.5 µL of 20 pmol/µL forward primer, 0.5 µL of 20 pmol/µL reverse primer, and 10.5 µL of MilliQ water were added. The total volume was 25 µL. The amplification program was comprised of 1 cycle of 95 °C for 5 min, 45 cycles of 95 °C for 30 s 55/56 °C for 30 s, 72 °C for 45 s, and 85 cycles of 55 °C, with an increase of set point temperature by 0.5 °C per cycle for 10 s. The samples were run, and the threshold cycles (Ct) values were recorded. Melting curves were also performed.

5.10. Data Analysis

The Ct values were processed as stated in "The MIQE Guidelines: Minimum Information for Publication of Quantitative Real-Time PCR Experiments" [118] using OpenOffice

Calc according to the 2-ΔΔCt method described by Livak and Schmittgen (2001) [119]. The reference genes (TBP, RPL4, and B2M) were chosen in order to be stably expressed across different tissue types and treatments on swine specimens [120,121]. The relative expression value ($2^{-\Delta\Delta Ct}$) was obtained by normalization, subtracting the arithmetic mean of the reference genes from each gene of interest. Technical replicates were averaged before statistical analysis. The data are illustrated as average values of the groups (n = 4) ± standard error deviation of the mean (STDEV). All data were statistically analyzed using a one-way ANOVA method performed with GraphPad Prism 3.03 software (GraphPad Software, La Jolla, CA, USA). Post-hoc comparisons between all groups were run using the Bonferroni test. The statistical significance (p value) was presented for all groups in contrast to the Control group (C).

Author Contributions: Conceptualization, A.D. and S.E.G.; methodology, R.G.P., C.B., A.U., M.V., A.H., D.M. and M.F.; software, R.G.P.; validation, R.G.P. and S.E.G.; formal analysis, R.G.P. and S.E.G.; investigation, R.G.P., C.B., A.U., M.V., A.H. and M.F.; writing—original draft preparation, R.G.P., C.B., A.H. and M.V.; writing—review and editing, A.D., I.T. and S.E.G.; supervision, A.D. and S.E.G.; project administration I.T. and S.E.G.; funding acquisition, R.G.P. and S.E.G. All authors have read and agreed to the published version of the manuscript.

Funding: This research was funded by a grant of the Romanian Ministry of Research and Innovation, CCCDI—UEFISCDI, project number PN-III-P1-1.2-PCCDI-2017-0473/"From classical animal nutrition to precision animal nutrition, scientific foundation for food security", within PNCDI I.

Institutional Review Board Statement: The study was conducted according to the guidelines of the Declaration of Helsinki, and approved by the Ethical Committee of the National Research-Development Institute for Animal Nutrition and Biology, Baloteşti, Romania (Ethical Committee no. 118/02.12.2019) and in accordance with the Romanian Law 206/2004 and the EU Council Directive 98/58/EC for handling and protection of animals used for experimental purposes.

Informed Consent Statement: Not applicable.

Data Availability Statement: The data presented in this study are available on request from the corresponding author. The data are not publicly available due to privacy reason.

Acknowledgments: This work was supported by a grant of the Romanian Ministry of Research and Innovation, CCCDI—UEFISCDI, project number PN-III-P1-1.2-PCCDI-2017-0473/"From classical animal nutrition to precision animal nutrition, scientific foundation for food security", within PNCDI I "Use of agro-food residues by feeding solutions which to control the feed contaminants".

Conflicts of Interest: The authors declare no conflict of interest.

References

1. Liew, W.-P.-P.; Mohd-Redzwan, S. Mycotoxin: Its Impact on Gut Health and Microbiota. *Front. Cell. Infect. Microbiol.* **2018**, *8*, 1–17. [CrossRef] [PubMed]
2. Desjardins, A.E.; Hohn, T.M. Mycotoxins in Plant Pathogenesis. *Mol. Plant.-Microbe Interact.* **2007**, *10*, 147–152. [CrossRef]
3. Riley, R.T.; Pestka, J. Mycotoxins: Metabolism, mechanisms and biochemical markers. In *The Mycotoxin Blue Book*, 2nd ed.; Diaz, D., Ed.; Nottingham University Press: Nottingham, UK, 2005; pp. 279–294.
4. Feddern, V.; Dors, G.C.; Tavernari, F.; Mazzuco, H.; Cunha, J.A.; Krabbe, E.L.; Scheuermann, G.N. Aflatoxins: Importance on animal nutrition. In *Aflatoxins Recent Advances and Future Prospects*; InTech Open Access: London, UK, 2013; pp. 171–195. [CrossRef]
5. Medina, A.; Akbar, A.; Baazeem, A.; Rodriguez, A.; Magan, N. Climate change, food security and mycotoxins: Do we know enough? *Fungal Biol. Rev.* **2017**, *31*, 143–154. [CrossRef]
6. Pierron, A.; Alassane-Kpembi, I.; Oswald, I.P. Impact of mycotoxin on immune response and consequences for pig health. *Anim. Nutr.* **2016**, *2*, 63–68. [CrossRef]
7. Streit, E.; Schatzmayr, G.; Tassis, P.; Tzika, E.; Marin, D.; Taranu, I.; Tabuc, C.; Nicolau, A.; Aprodu, I.; Puel, O.; et al. Current situation of mycotoxin contamination and co-occurrence in animal feed—Focus on Europe. *Toxins* **2012**, *4*, 788–809. [CrossRef] [PubMed]
8. Gruber-Dorninger, C.; Jenkins, T.; Schatzmayr, G. Global Mycotoxin Occurrence in Feed: A Ten-Year Survey. *Toxins* **2020**, *11*, 375. [CrossRef]
9. Marin, D.E.; Motiu, M.; Taranu, I. Food Contaminant Zearalenone and Its Metabolites Affect Cytokine Synthesis and Intestinal Epithelial Integrity of Porcine Cells. *Toxins* **2015**, *7*, 1979–1988. [CrossRef] [PubMed]

10. Alassane-Kpembi, I.; Kolf-clauw, M.; Gauthier, T.; Abrami, R.; Abiola, F.A.; Oswald, I.P.; Puel, O. New insights into mycotoxin mixtures: The toxicity of low doses of Type B trichothecenes on intestinal epithelial cells is synergistic. *Toxicol. Appl. Pharmacol.* **2013**, *272*, 191–198. [CrossRef]
11. Broom, L.J.; Wood, M.; Park, E.; Kingdom, U. Organic acids for improving intestinal health of poultry. *Worlds Poult. Sci. J.* **2015**, *71*, 630–642. [CrossRef]
12. Filazi, A.; Sireli, U.T. Occurrence of aflatoxins in food. In *Aflatoxins: Recent Advances and Future Prospects*; Mehdi, R.-A., Ed.; InTech Open Access: London, UK, 2012; pp. 143–170.
13. Seetha, A.; Munthali, W.; Msere, H.W.; Swai, E.; Muzanila, Y.; Sichone, E.; Tsusaka, T.W.; Rathore, A.; Okori, P. Occurrence of aflatoxins and its management in diverse cropping systems of central Tanzania. *Mycotoxin Res.* **2017**, *33*, 323–331. [CrossRef] [PubMed]
14. Ismail, A.; Gonçalves, B.L.; de Neeff, D.V.; Ponzilacqua, B.; Coppa, C.F.S.C.; Hintzsche, H.; Sajid, M.; Cruz, A.G.; Corassin, C.H.; Oliveira, C.A.F. Aflatoxin in foodstuffs: Occurrence and recent advances in decontamination. *Food Res. Int.* **2018**, *113*, 74–85. [CrossRef]
15. Negash, D. Citation: Negash D (2018) A Review of Aflatoxin: Occurrence, Prevention, and Gaps in Both Food and Feed Safety. *J. Appl. Microbiol. Res.* **2018**, *1*, 1–35. [CrossRef]
16. Arroyo-Manzanares, N.; Rodríguez-Estévez, V.; Arenas-Fernández, P.; García-Campaña, A.M.; Gámiz-Gracia, L. Occurrence of Mycotoxins in Swine Feeding from Spain. *Toxins* **2019**, *11*, 342. [CrossRef]
17. Nazhand, A.; Durazzo, A.; Lucarini, M.; Souto, E.B.; Santini, A. Characteristics, Occurrence, Detection and Detoxification of Aflatoxins in Foods and Feeds. *Foods* **2020**, *9*, 644. [CrossRef] [PubMed]
18. Dhama, K.; Singh, K.P. Aflatoxins- Hazard to Livestock and Poultry Production: A Review. *J. Immunol. Immunopathol.* **2014**, *9*, 1–15. [CrossRef]
19. Devreese, M.; De Backer, P.; Croubels, S. Overview of the most important mycotoxins for the pig and poultry husbandry Overzicht van de meest belangrijke mycotoxines voor de varkens-en pluimveehouderij. *Vlaams Diergeneeskd. Tijdschr.* **2013**, *82*, 171–180. [CrossRef]
20. Jatfa, J.W.; Wachida, N.M.; Ijabo, H.M.; Adamu, S.S. Aflatoxicosis Associated with Swine Stillbirth in the Piggery Farm University of Agriculture Makurdi. *Curr. Trends Biomedical. Eng. Biosci.* **2018**, *13*, 555873.
21. Lee, H.S.; Lindahl, J.; Nguyen-Viet, H.; Khong, N.V.; Nghia, V.B.; Xuan, H.N.; Grace, D. An investigation into aflatoxin M1in slaughtered fattening pigs and awareness of aflatoxins in Vietnam. *BMC Vet. Res.* **2017**, *13*, 1–7. [CrossRef]
22. Wilfred, E.G.; Dungworth, D.L.; Moulton, J.E. Pathologic Effects of Aflatoxin in Pigs. *Vet. Pathol.* **1968**, *5*, 370–384. [CrossRef]
23. Dilkin, P.; Zorzete, P.; Mallmann, C.A.; Gomes, J.D.F.; Utiyama, C.E.; Oetting, L.L.; Corrêa, B. Toxicological effects of chronic low doses of aflatoxin B1 and fumonisin B1-containing Fusarium moniliforme culture material in weaned piglets. *Food Chem. Toxicol.* **2003**, *41*, 1345–1353. [CrossRef]
24. Obuseh, F.A.; Jolly, P.E.; Jiang, Y.; Shuaib, F.M.B.; Waterbor, J.; Ellis, W.O.; Piyathilake, C.J.; Desmond, R.A.; Afriyie-Gyawu, E.; Phillips, T.D. Aflatoxin B1 albumin adducts in plasma and aflatoxin M1 in urine are associated with plasma concentrations of vitamins A and E. *Int. J. Vitam. Nutr. Res.* **2010**, *80*, 355–368. [CrossRef] [PubMed]
25. Pfohl-leszkowicz, A.; Manderville, R.A. An Update on Direct Genotoxicity as a Molecular Mechanism of Ochratoxin A Carcinogenicity. *Chem. Res. Toxicol.* **2012**, *25*, 252–262. [CrossRef]
26. Arbillaga, L.; Azqueta, A.; Van Delft, J.H.M.; López, A.; Cerain, D. In vitro gene expression data supporting a DNA non-reactive genotoxic mechanism for ochratoxin A. *Toxicol. Appl. Pharmacol.* **2007**, *220*, 216–224. [CrossRef]
27. Asrani, R.K.; Patial, V.; Thakur, M. Ochratoxin A: Possible mechanisms of toxicity. In *Ochratoxins-Biosynthesis, Detection and Toxicity*; Porter, D., Ed.; Nova Science Publishers Inc.: New York, NY, USA, 2016; pp. 57–89.
28. Marin, D.E.; Braicu, C.; Gras, M.A.; Pistol, G.C.; Petric, R.C.; Neagoe, I.B.; Palade, M.; Taranu, I.S.C. Low level of ochratoxin A affects genome-wide expression in kidney of pig. *Toxicon* **2017**, *136*, 67–77. [CrossRef]
29. Ringot, D.; Chango, A.; Schneider, Y.J.; Larondelle, Y. Toxicokinetics and toxicodynamics of ochratoxin A, an update. *Chem. Biol. Interact.* **2006**, *159*, 18–46. [CrossRef] [PubMed]
30. Kőszegi, T.; Poór, M. Ochratoxin a: Molecular interactions, mechanisms of toxicity and prevention at the molecular level. *Toxins* **2016**, *8*, 111. [CrossRef]
31. Bayman, P.; Baker, J.L. Ochratoxins: A global perspective. *Mycopathologia* **2006**, *162*, 215–223. [CrossRef] [PubMed]
32. Peeradon, T.; Tichakorn, S.; Anupon, T.; Supatra, P. Modulation of Edible Plants on Hepatocellular Carcinoma Induced by Aflatoxin B. In *Phytochemicals in Human Health*; InTech Open Access: London, UK, 2020; pp. 1–23. [CrossRef]
33. Guyonnet, D.; Belloir, C.; Suschetet, M.; Bon, A. Le Mechanisms of protection against aflatoxin B 1 genotoxicity in rats treated by organosulfur compounds from garlic. *Carcinogenesis* **2002**, *23*, 1335–1341. [CrossRef] [PubMed]
34. Moudgil, V.; Redhu, D.; Dhanda, S.; Singh, J. A review of molecular mechanisms in the development of hepatocellular carcinoma by aflatoxin and hepatitis B and C viruses. *J. Environ. Pathol. Toxicol. Oncol.* **2013**, *32*, 165–175. [CrossRef] [PubMed]
35. Li, H.; Xing, L.; Zhang, M.; Wang, J.; Zheng, N. The Toxic Effects of Aflatoxin B1 and Aflatoxin M1 on Kidney through Regulating L-Proline and Downstream Apoptosis. *BioMed. Res. Intern.* **2018**, *2018*, 1–11. [CrossRef] [PubMed]
36. Kanora, A.; Maes, D. The role of mycotoxins in pig reproduction: A review. *Vet. Med.* **2009**, *54*, 565–576. [CrossRef]
37. Li, X.; Zhao, L.; Fan, Y.; Jia, Y.; Sun, L.; Ma, S.; Ji, C.; Ma, Q.; Zhang, J. Occurrence of mycotoxins in feed ingredients and complete feeds obtained from the Beijing region of China. *J. Anim. Sci. Biotechnol.* **2014**, *5*, 1–8. [CrossRef] [PubMed]

38. Svoboda, M.; Blahová, J.; Honzlová, A.; Kalinová, J.; Macharáčková, P.; Rosmus, J.; Mejzlík, V.; Kúkol, P.; Vlasáková, V.; Mikulková, K. Multiannual occurrence of mycotoxins in feed ingredients and complete feeds for pigs in the Czech Republic. *Acta. Vet. Brno.* **2019**, *88*, 291–301. [CrossRef]
39. Khoshal, A.K.; Novak, B.; Martin, P.G.P.; Jenkins, T.; Neves, M.; Schatzmayr, G.; Oswald, I.P.; Pinton, P. Worldwide Finished Pig Feed and Their Combined Toxicity in Intestinal Cells. *Toxins* **2019**, *11*, 727. [CrossRef]
40. Ma, R.; Zhang, L.; Liu, M.; Su, Y.; Xie, W.; Zhang, N. Individual and Combined Occurrence of Mycotoxins in Feed Ingredients and Complete Feeds in China. *Toxins* **2018**, *10*, 113. [CrossRef] [PubMed]
41. Freitas, B.V.; Mota, M.M.; Del Santo, T.A.; Afonso, E.R.; Silva, C.C.; Utimi, N.B.P.; Barbosa, L.C.G.S.; Vilela, F.G.; Araújo, L.F. Mycotoxicosis in Swine: A Review. *J. Anim. Prod. Adv.* **2012**, *2*, 174–181.
42. Adunphatcharaphon, S.; Petchkongkaew, A.; Greco, D.; D'Ascanio, V.; Visessanguan, W.; Avantaggiato, G. The Effectiveness of Durian Peel as a Multi-Mycotoxin Adsorbent. *Toxins* **2020**, *8*, 108. [CrossRef] [PubMed]
43. Agriopoulou, S.; Stamatelopoulou, E.; Varzakas, T. Advances in Occurrence, Importance, and Mycotoxin Control Strategies: Prevention and Detoxification in Foods. *Foods* **2020**, *28*, 137. [CrossRef] [PubMed]
44. Solís-Cruz, B.; Hernández-Patlán, D.; Beyssac, E.; Latorre, J.D.; Hernandez-Velasco, X.; Merino-Guzman, R.; Tellez, G.; López-Arellano, R. Evaluation of Chitosan and Cellulosic Polymers as Binding Adsorbent Materials to Prevent Aflatoxin B1, Fumonisin B1, Ochratoxin, Trichothecene, Deoxynivalenol, and Zearalenone Mycotoxicoses Through an In Vitro Gastrointestinal Model for Poultry. *Polymers* **2017**, *19*, 529. [CrossRef] [PubMed]
45. Čolović, R.; Puvača, N.; Cheli, F.; Avantaggiato, G.; Greco, D.; Đuragić, O.; Kos, J.; Pinotti, L. Decontamination of Mycotoxin-Contaminated Feedstuffs and Compound Feed. *Toxins* **2019**, *11*, 617. [CrossRef]
46. Vila-Donat, P.; Marín, S.; Sanchis, V.; Ramos, A.J. A review of the mycotoxin adsorbing agents, with an emphasis on their multi-binding capacity, for animal feed decontamination. *Food Chem. Toxicol.* **2018**, *114*, 246–259. [CrossRef] [PubMed]
47. Badr, A.N.; Abdel-Razek, A.G.; Youssef, M.; Shehata, M.; Hassanein, M.M.; Amra, H. Natural Antioxidants: Preservation Roles and Mycotoxicological Safety of Food. *Egypt. J. Chem.* **2021**, *64*, 285–298. [CrossRef]
48. Gugliandolo, E.; Peritore, A.F.; D'Amico, R.; Licata, P.; Crupi, R. Evaluation of Neuroprotective Effects of Quercetin against Aflatoxin B1-Intoxicated Mice. *Animals* **2020**, *21*, 898. [CrossRef] [PubMed]
49. Antonissen, G.; Devreese, M.; De Baere, S.; Martel, A.; Van Immerseel, F.; Croubels, S. Impact of Fusarium mycotoxins on hepatic and intestinal mRNA expression of cytochrome P450 enzymes and drug transporters, and on the pharmacokinetics of oral enrofloxacin in broiler chickens. *Food Chem. Toxicol.* **2017**, *101*, 75–83. [CrossRef] [PubMed]
50. Zaragozá, C.; Villaescusa, L.; Monserrat, J.; Zaragozá, F.; Álvarez-Mon, M. Potential Therapeutic Anti-Inflammatory and Immunomodulatory Effects of Dihydroflavones, Flavones, and Flavonols. *Molecules* **2020**, *25*, 1017. [CrossRef] [PubMed]
51. Yahfoufi, N.; Alsadi, N.; Jambi, M.; Matar, C. The Immunomodulatory and Anti-Inflammatory Role of Polyphenols. *Nutrients* **2018**, *10*, 1618. [CrossRef]
52. World Health Organization. Mycotoxins. Children's Health and the Environment. Available online: https://www.who.int/ceh/capacity/mycotoxins.pdf (accessed on 3 January 2021).
53. Perrone, G.; Ferrara, M.; Medina, A.; Pascale, M.; Magan, N. Toxigenic Fungi and Mycotoxins in a Climate Change Scenario: Ecology, Genomics, Distribution, Prediction and Prevention of the Risk. *Microorganisms* **2020**, *8*, 1496. [CrossRef]
54. Joubrane, K.; Mnayer, D.; El Khoury, A.; El Khoury, A.; Awad, E. Co-Occurrence of Aflatoxin B1 and Ochratoxin A in Lebanese Stored Wheat. *J. Food Prot.* **2020**, *83*, 1547–1552. [CrossRef]
55. Ibañez-Vea, M.; González-Peñas, E.; Lizarraga, E.; López de Cerain, A. Co-occurrence of aflatoxins, ochratoxin A and zearalenone in barley from a northern region of Spain. *Food Chem.* **2012**, *1*, 35–42. [CrossRef]
56. Gamze, N.K.; Fatih, O.; Bulent, K. Co-occurrence of aflatoxins and ochratoxin A in cereal flours commercialised in Turkey. *Food Control.* **2015**, *54*, 275–281. [CrossRef]
57. Ozbey, F.; Kabak, B. Natural co-occurrence of aflatoxins and ochratoxin A in spices. *Food Control.* **2012**, *28*, 354–361. [CrossRef]
58. Santos Pereira, C.; Cunha, S.; Fernandes, J.O. Prevalent Mycotoxins in Animal Feed: Occurrence and Analytical Methods. *Toxins* **2019**, *11*, 290. [CrossRef]
59. Taranu, I.; Marin, D.E.; Palade, M.; Pistol, G.C.; Chedea, V.S.; Gras, M.A.; Rotar, C. Assessment of the efficacy of a grape seed waste in counteracting the changes induced by a flatoxin B1 contaminated diet on performance, plasma, liver and intestinal tissues of pigs after weaning. *Toxicon* **2019**, *162*, 24–31. [CrossRef]
60. Nilova, L.; Malyutenkova, S. The possibility of using powdered sea-buckthorn in the development of bakery products with antioxidant properties. *Agro. Res.* **2018**, *16*, 1444–1456. [CrossRef]
61. Balogh, K.; Hausenblasz, J.; Weber, M.; Erdélyi, M.; Fodor, J.; Mézes, M. Effects of ochratoxin A on some production traits, lipid peroxide and glutathione redox status of weaned piglets. *Acta. Vet. Hung.* **2007**, *55*, 463–470. [CrossRef] [PubMed]
62. Marin, D.E.; Taranu, I. Ochratoxin A and its effects on immunity. *Toxin Rev.* **2015**, *34*, 11–20. [CrossRef]
63. Ayed-Boussema, I.; Pascussi, J.M.; Zaied, C.; Maurel, P.; Bacha, H.; Hassen, W. CYP1A2 gene expression in primary cultured human hepatocytes: A possible activation of nuclear receptors. *Drug Chem. Toxicol.* **2012**, *35*, 71–80. [CrossRef]
64. Jiang, Z.; Gu, L.; Liang, X.; Cao, B.; Zhang, J.; Guo, X. The Effect of Selenium on CYP450 Isoform Activity and Expression in Pigs. *Biol. Trace. Elem. Res.* **2020**, *196*, 454–462. [CrossRef]
65. Altay, A.; Bozoğlu, F. Salvia fruticosa Modulates mRNA Expressions and Activity Levels of Xenobiotic Metabolizing CYP1A2, CYP2E1, NQO1, GPx, and GST Enzymes in Human. *Nutr. Cancer* **2017**, *69*, 892–903. [CrossRef] [PubMed]

66. Rasmussen, M.K.; Zamaratskaia, G.; Ekstrand, B. Gender-related Differences in Cytochrome P450 in Porcine Liver-Implication for Activity, Expression and Inhibition by Testicular Steroids. *Reprod. Domest. Anim.* **2011**, *46*, 616–623. [CrossRef] [PubMed]
67. Nwafor, I.C.; Shale, K.; Achilonu, M.C. Chemical Composition and Nutritive Benefits of Chicory (*Cichorium intybus*) as an Ideal Complementary and/or Alternative Livestock Feed Supplement. *Sci. World J.* **2017**, *2017*, 1–12. [CrossRef] [PubMed]
68. Dietrich, C. Antioxidant Functions of the Aryl Hydrocarbon Receptor. *Stem. Cells. Int.* **2016**, *2016*, 1–11. [CrossRef] [PubMed]
69. Kapelyukh, Y.; Henderson, C.J.; Scheer, N.; Rode, A.; Wolf, C.R. Defining the Contribution of CYP1A1 and CYP1A2 to Drug Metabolism Using Humanized CYP1A1/1A2 and Cyp1a1/Cyp1a2 Knockout Mice. *Drug Metab. Dispos.* **2019**, *47*, 907–918. [CrossRef]
70. Sansen, S.; Yano, J.K.; Rosamund, L.; Schoch, G.A.; Keith, J.; Stout, C.D.; Johnson, E.F.; Sansen, S.; Yano, J.K.; Reynald, R.L.; et al. Adaptations for the Oxidation of Polycyclic Aromatic. *J. Biol. Chem.* **2007**, *282*, 14348–14355. [CrossRef] [PubMed]
71. Schelstraete, W.; De Clerck, L.; Govaert, E.; Mil, J.; Devreese, M.; Deforce, D.; D. Bocxlaer, J.; Croubels, S. Characterization of Porcine Hepatic and Intestinal Drug Metabolizing CYP450: Comparison with Human Orthologues from A Quantitative, Activity and Selectivity Perspective. *Sci. Rep.* **2019**, *9*, 1–14. [CrossRef] [PubMed]
72. Wen, J.; Mu, P.; Deng, Y. Mycotoxins: Cytotoxicity and biotransformation in animal cells. *Toxicol. Res. (Camb.)* **2016**, *5*, 377–387. [CrossRef]
73. Liu, R.; Desai, L.P. Reciprocal regulation of TGF-β and reactive oxygen species: A perverse cycle for fi brosis. *Redox Biol.* **2015**, *6*, 565–577. [CrossRef]
74. Muller, G.F. Effect of transforming growth factor-b 1 on cytochrome P450 expression: Inhibition of CYP1 mRNA and protein expression in primary rat hepatocytes. *Arch. Toxicol* **2000**, *74*, 145–152. [CrossRef] [PubMed]
75. Penner, N.; Woodward, C.; Prakash, C. Appendix: Drug Metabolizing Enzymes and Biotransformation Reactions. *ADME* **2012**, *2012*, 545–565. [CrossRef]
76. Pyo, M.C.; Shin, H.S.; Jeon, G.Y.; Lee, K.-W. Synergistic Interaction of Ochratoxin A and Acrylamide Toxins in Human Kidney and Liver Cells. *Biol Pharm Bull.* **2020**, *43*, 1346–1355. [CrossRef]
77. Zhao, H.; Chen, L.; Yang, T.; Feng, Y.L.; Vaziri, N.D.; Liu, B.L.; Liu, Q.Q.; Guo, Y. Aryl hydrocarbon receptor activation mediates kidney disease and renal cell carcinoma. *J. Transl. Med.* **2019**, *2*, 1–14. [CrossRef] [PubMed]
78. Rasmussen, M.K.; Zamaratskaia, G. Regulation of Porcine Hepatic Cytochrome P450—Implication for Boar Taint. *CSBJ* **2014**, *11*, 106–112. [CrossRef]
79. Burkina, V.; Rasmussen, M.K.; Olünychenko, Y.; Zamaratskaia, G. Porcine cytochrome 2A19 and 2E1. *Basic Clin. Pharmacol. Toxicol.* **2019**, *124*, 32–39. [CrossRef] [PubMed]
80. Pitarque, M.; Rodriguez-Antona, C.; Oscarson, M.; Ingelman-Sundberg, M. Transcriptional regulation of the human CYP2A6 gene. *J. Pharmacol. Exp. Ther.* **2005**, *313*, 814–822. [CrossRef] [PubMed]
81. Brunius, C.; Andersson, K.; Zamaratskaia, G. Expression and activities of hepatic cytochrome P450 (CYP1A, CYP2A and CYP2E1) in entire and castrated male pigs. *Animal* **2012**, *6*, 271–277. [CrossRef] [PubMed]
82. Yokota, S.; Higashi, E.; Fukami, T.; Yokoi, T.; Nakajima, M. Human CYP2A6 is regulated by nuclear factor-erythroid 2 related factor 2. *Biochem. Pharmacol.* **2011**, *81*, 289–294. [CrossRef]
83. Tanner, J.; Tyndale, R.F. Variation in CYP2A6 Activity and Personalized Medicine. *J. Pers Med.* **2017**, *6*, 18. [CrossRef]
84. Diaz, G.J.; Murcia, H.W.; Cepeda, S.M.; Boermans, H.J. The role of selected cytochrome P450 enzymes on the bioactivation of aflatoxin B1 by duck liver microsomes. *Avian Pathol.* **2010**, *39*, 279–286. [CrossRef]
85. Kalbolandi, S.M.; Gorji, A.V.; Babaahmadi-Rezaei, H.; Mansouri, E. Luteolin confers renoprotection against ischemia–reperfusion injury via involving Nrf2 pathway and regulating miR320. *Mol. Biol. Rep.* **2019**, *46*, 4039–4047. [CrossRef]
86. Mahmoud, A.M.; Hussein, O.E.; Abd El-Twab, S.M.; Hozayen, W.G. Ferulic acid protects against methotrexate nephrotoxicity via activation of Nrf2/ARE/HO-1 signaling and PPARγ and suppression of NF-kB/NLRP3 inflammasome axis. *Food Funct.* **2019**, *10*, 4593–4607. [CrossRef]
87. Tambyrajah, W.S.; Doran, E.; Wood, J.D.; Mcgivan, J.D. The pig CYP2E1 promoter is activated by COUP-TF1 and HNF-1 and is inhibited by androstenone. *Arch. Biochem. Biophys.* **2004**, *431*, 252–260. [CrossRef] [PubMed]
88. Park, E.C.; Kim, S.I.; Hong, Y.; Hwang, J.W.; Cho, G.; Cha, H.; Han, J.; Yun, C.; Park, S.; Jang, I.; et al. Inhibition of CYP4A Reduces Hepatic Endoplasmic Reticulum Stress and Features of Diabetes in Mice. *Gastroenterology* **2014**, *147*, 860–869. [CrossRef]
89. Raucy, J.L.; Lasker, J.; Ozaki, K.; Zoleta, V. Regulation of CYP2E1 by Ethanol and Palmitic Acid and CYP4A11 by Clofibrate in Primary Cultures of Human Hepatocytes. *Toxicol. Sci.* **2004**, *241*, 233–241. [CrossRef] [PubMed]
90. Sung, M.; Kim, I.; Park, M.; Whang, Y.; Lee, M. Differential effects of dietary fatty acids on the regulation of CYP2E1 and protein kinase C in human hepatoma HepG2 cells. *J. Med. Food* **2004**, *7*, 197–203. [CrossRef]
91. Wang, W.; Zhai, S.; Xia, Y.; Wang, H.; Ruan, D.; Zhou, T.; Zhu, Y.; Zhang, H.; Zhang, M.; Ye, H.; et al. Ochratoxin A induces liver inflammation: Involvement of intestinal microbiota. *Microbiome* **2019**, *7*, 1–14. [CrossRef]
92. Lin, Q.; Kang, X.; Li, X.; Wang, T.; Liu, F.; Jia, J.; Jin, Z.; Id, Y.X. NF-κB-mediated regulation of rat CYP2E1 by two independent signaling pathways. *PLoS ONE* **2019**, *14*, e0225531. [CrossRef]
93. Meyer, C.; Nadkarni, V.; Nadkarni, K.; Stumvoll, M.; Gerich, J. Human kidney free fatty acid and glucose uptake: Evidence for a renal glucose-fatty acid cycle. *Am. J. Phisiol.* **1997**, *273*, 1–5. [CrossRef] [PubMed]
94. Deng, X.; Pu, Q.; Wang, E.; Yu, C. Celery extract inhibits mouse CYP2A5 and human CYP2A6 activities via different mechanisms. *Oncol. Lett* **2016**, *12*, 5309–5314. [CrossRef] [PubMed]

95. Ling, D.; Salvaterra, P.M. Robust RT-qPCR Data Normalization: Validation and Selection of Internal Reference Genes during Post-Experimental Data Analysis. *PLoS ONE* **2011**, *6*, e17762. [CrossRef]
96. Messina, A.; Nannelli, A.; Fiorio, R.; Longo, V.; Gervasi, P.G. Expression and inducibility of and CYP2B22, 3A22, 3A29, 3A46 by rifampicin in the respiratory and olfactory mucosa of pig. *Toxicology* **2009**, *260*, 47–52. [CrossRef] [PubMed]
97. Gonzalez-Arias, C.A.; Crespo-Sempre, S.; Sanchis, V.; Ramos, A.J. Modulation of the xenobiotic transformation system and inflammatory response by ochratoxin A exposure using a co-culture system of Caco-2 and HepG2 cells. *Food Chem. Toxicol.* **2015**, *86*, 245–252. [CrossRef] [PubMed]
98. Rasmussen, M.K. Porcine cytochrome P450 3A: Current status on expression and regulation. *Arch. Toxicol.* **2020**, *94*, 1899–1914. [CrossRef]
99. Zepnik, H.; Pa, A.; Schauer, U.; Dekant, W. Ochratoxin A-Induced Tumor Formation: Is There a Role of Reactive Ochratoxin A Metabolites? *Toxicol. Sci.* **2001**, *59*, 59–67. [CrossRef]
100. Robertson, G.; Leclercq, I.; Farrell, G.C.; Steatosis, C.F.N.; Ii, S. Nonalcoholic Steatosis and Steatohepatitis II. Cytochrome. *Am. J. Physiol. Gastrointest Liver Pysiol.* **2020**, *281*, 1135–1139. [CrossRef]
101. Leclercq, I.A.; Gonzalez, F.J.; Graham, R.; Leclercq, I.A.; Farrell, G.C.; Field, J.; Bell, D.R.; Gonzalez, F.J.; Robertson, G.R. CYP2E1 and CYP4A as microsomal catalysts of lipid peroxides in murine nonalcoholic steatohepatitis. *J. Clin. Investig.* **2000**, *105*, 1067–1075. [CrossRef] [PubMed]
102. Liu, Y.; Xu, W.; Zhai, T.; You, J.; Chen, Y. Silibinin ameliorates hepatic lipid accumulation and oxidative stress in mice with non-alcoholic steatohepatitis by regulating CFLAR-JNK pathway. *Acta Pharm. Sin. B* **2019**, *9*, 745–757. [CrossRef]
103. Stading, R.; Couroucli, X.; Lingappan, K.; Moorthy, B. The role of cytochrome P450 (CYP) enzymes in hyperoxic lung injury. *Expert Opin. Drug Metab. Toxicol.* **2020**, *13*, 1–8. [CrossRef]
104. Ruan, D.; Zhu, Y.W.; Fouad, A.M.; Yan, S.J.; Chen, W.; Zhang, Y.N.; Xia, W.G.; Wang, S.; Jiang, S.Q.; Yang, L.; et al. Dietary curcumin enhances intestinal antioxidant capacity in ducklings via altering gene expression of antioxidant and key detoxification enzymes. *Poult. Sci.* **2018**, *98*, 3705–3714. [CrossRef] [PubMed]
105. Jedlitschky, G.; Hoffmann, U.; Kroemer, H.K. Structure and function of the MRP2 (ABCC2) protein and its role. *Expert Opin. Drug Metab. Toxicol.* **2006**, *2*, 351–366. [CrossRef]
106. Gekle, M.; Mildenberger, S.; Freudinger, R.; Silbernagl, S. pH of endosomes labelled by receptor-mediated and fluid-phase endocytosis and its possible role for the regulation of endocy-totic uptake. In *Studies in Honour of Karl Julius Ultrich. An Australian Symposium*; Poronnik, P., Cook, D.I., Young, J.A., Eds.; Wild & Woolley: Glebe, Australia, 1994; pp. 45–49.
107. Zhang, J.; Pan, Z.; Moloney, S.; Sheppard, A. RNA-Seq Analysis Implicates Detoxification Pathways in Ovine Mycotoxin Resistance. *PLoS ONE* **2014**, *9*, e99975. [CrossRef] [PubMed]
108. Raghunath, A.; Sundarraj, K.; Nagarajan, R.; Arfuso, F.; Bian, J. Redox Biology Antioxidant response elements: Discovery, classes, regulation and potential applications. *Redox Biol.* **2018**, *17*, 297–314. [CrossRef]
109. Ghadiri, S.; Spalenza, V.; Dellafiora, L.; Badino, P.; Barbarossa, A.; Dall, C.; Nebbia, C.; Girolami, F. Toxicology in Vitro Modulation of aflatoxin B1 cytotoxicity and aflatoxin M1 synthesis by natural antioxidants in a bovine mammary epithelial cell line. *Toxicol. Vitr.* **2019**, *57*, 174–183. [CrossRef] [PubMed]
110. Corcuera, L.; Vettorazzi, A.; Arbillaga, L.; Pérez, N.; Gloria, A.; Azqueta, A.; González-peñas, E.; García-jalón, J.A.; López, A.; Cerain, D. Genotoxicity of Aflatoxin B1 and Ochratoxin A after simultaneous application of the in vivo micronucleus and comet assay. *Food Chem. Toxicol.* **2015**, *76*, 116–124. [CrossRef]
111. Shin, H.S.; Lee, H.J.; Pyo, M.C.; Ryu, D.; Lee, K.-W. Ochratoxin A-Induced Hepatotoxicity through Phase I and Phase II Reactions Regulated by AhR in Liver Cells. *Toxins (Basel)* **2019**, *11*, 377. [CrossRef]
112. Boudra, H.S.; Saivin, S.; Buffiere, C.; Morgavi, D.P. Short communication: Toxicokinetics of ochratoxin A in dairy ewes and carryover to milk following a single or long-term ingestion of contaminated feed. *J. Dairy Sci.* **2013**, *96*, 6690–6696. [CrossRef]
113. Festing, S.; Wilkinson, R. The ethics of animal research. Talking Point on the use of animals in scientific research. *EMBO Rep.* **2007**, *8*, 526–530. [CrossRef]
114. Taranu, I.; Braicu, C.; Marin, D.E.; Pistol, G.C.; Motiu, M.; Balacescu, L.; Beridan Neagoe, I.; Burlacu, R. Exposure to zearalenone mycotoxin alters in vitro porcine intestinal epithelial cells by differential gene expression. *Toxicol. Lett.* **2015**, *232*, 310–325. [CrossRef]
115. Taranu, I.; Habeanu, M.; Gras, M.A.; Pistol, G.C.; Lefter, N.; Palade, M.; Ropota, M.; Chedea, V.S.; Marin, D.E. Assessment of the effect of grape seed cake inclusion in the diet of healthy fattening-finishing pigs. *J. Anim. Physiol. Anim. Nutr. (Berl)* **2017**, *102*, 1–13. [CrossRef] [PubMed]
116. Hermenean, A.; Damache, G.; Albu, P.; Ardelean, A.; Ardelean, G.; Puiu Ardelean, D.; Horge, M.; Nagy, T.; Braun, M.; Zsuga, M.; et al. Histopathological alterations and oxidative stress in liver and kidney of Leuciscus cephalus following exposure to heavy metals in the Tur River, North Western Romania. *Ecotoxicol. Environ. Saf.* **2015**, *119*, 198–205. [CrossRef] [PubMed]
117. Untergasser, A.; Nijveen, H.; Rao, X.; Bisseling, T. Primer3Plus, an enhanced web interface to Primer3. *Nucleic Acids Res.* **2007**, *35*, 71–74. [CrossRef] [PubMed]
118. Altschup, S.F.; Gish, W.; Pennsylvania, T.; Park, U. Basic Local Alignment Search Tool 2Department of Computer Science. *J. Mol. Biol.* **1990**, 403–410. [CrossRef]

119. Bustin, S.A.; Benes, V.; Garson, J.A.; Hellemans, J.; Huggett, J.; Kubista, M.; Mueller, R.; Nolan, T.; Pfaffl, M.W.; Shipley, G.L. The MIQE Guidelines: Minimum Information for Publication of Quantitative Real-Time PCR Experiments. *Clin. Chem.* **2009**, *55*, 611–622. [CrossRef] [PubMed]
120. Livak, K.J.; Schmittgen, T.D. Analysis of Relative Gene Expression Data Using Real-Time Quantitative PCR and the $2^{-\Delta\Delta CT}$ Method. *Methods* **2001**, *25*, 402–408. [CrossRef] [PubMed]
121. Sandercock, D.A.; Coe, J.E.; Di, P.; Edwards, S.A. Research in Veterinary Science Determination of stable reference genes for RT-qPCR expression data in mechanistic pain studies on pig dorsal root ganglia and spinal cord. *Res. Vet. Sci.* **2017**, *114*, 493–501. [CrossRef] [PubMed]

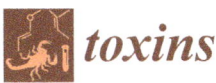

Article

Rat Tumour Histopathology Associated with Experimental Chronic Dietary Exposure to Ochratoxin A in Prediction of the Mycotoxin's Risk for Human Cancers

Diana Herman [1] and Peter Mantle [2,*]

[1] Pathology Department, County Hospital Timisoara, 300736 Timisoara, Romania; diaherman@yahoo.com
[2] Centre for Environmental Policy, Imperial College London, London SW7 2AZ, UK
* Correspondence: p.mantle@imperial.ac.uk

Abstract: Mammalian animal toxicity of ochratoxin A (OTA) has focused largely in the past half-century on pigs because of initial recognition of it as a principal cause of intermittent growth suppression and renal disease caused by mouldy feed. Subsequent classical toxicology has used laboratory rodents because renal pathology in pigs raised questions concerning possible involvement in the human idiopathic bilateral renal atrophy of Balkan endemic nephropathy for which OTA was a focus of attention for human nephropathy through 1980s and into 2000s. Emphasis on human nephropathy has more recently concerned the plant metabolite aristolochic acid. Recognition that agricultural management can often minimise food and feed-stuff spoilage by OTA-producing Aspergilli and Penicillia has moderated some of the risks for animals. Legislation for human food safety combined with sophisticated analysis generally provides safety in the developed world. Chronic experimental exposure of male rats, in the absence of clinical dis-ease, specifically causes renal cancer. The possibility of this as a unique model for the human has generated considerable experimental evidence which may be more directly relevant for carcinogenesis in the complex kidney than that obtained from biochemical toxicities in vitro. Nevertheless, there does not appear to be any case of human renal or urinary tract cancer for which there is verified etiological proof for causation by OTA, contrary to much claim in the literature. To contribute to such debate, histopathology review of OTA/rat renal cancers, augmented where appropriate by immune profiles, has been completed for all remaining tumours in our research archive. Overall consistency of positivity for vimentin, is matched with occasional positives either for CD10 or the cytokeratin MNF 116. The current situation is discussed. Suggestion that OTA could cause human testicular cancer has also been challenged as unsupported by any experimental findings in rats, where the Leydig cell tumour immune profile does not match that of human germ cell neoplasms.

Keywords: vimentin; CD10; MNF 116; renal cell cancer; urothelial cancer; testicular cancer; immunohistochemistry

Key Contribution: Immunohistochemical confirmation of the cytokeratin clone MNF 116 in some ochratoxin/rat kidney cancer contrasts with the protein's apparent absence from human kidney cancer. Experimental animal findings for ochratoxin A toxicity are discussed concerning application to carcinogenesis in humans.

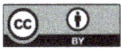

1. Introduction

Ochratoxin A (OTA) was discovered in South Africa in the early 1960s to explain the general toxicity of cultured *Aspergillus ochraceus* as a dietary additive for experimental rats. Concurrently, the term mycotoxins became used to encompass toxic metabolites of other food-spoilage moulds such, as the aflatoxins of *A. flavus*, found to have widespread occurrence. Focus for OTA soon shifted to the spasmodic occurrence of an idiopathic porcine nephropathy in the Danish bacon industry, economically linked to home-grown barley; in some high rainfall years this had been insufficiently dried before storage. Seasonal opportunist moulding by a common *Penicillium*, and chromatographic recognition of OTA partly by its fluorescence under UV_{254} light, revealed another biosynthetic source of the mycotoxin in amounts subsequently demonstrated experimentally as a major cause of the disease in pigs. This had been expressed as reduced growth rate, low carcass weight and mottled and disproportionally enlarged kidneys, readily recognised at meat inspection and the carcass rejected [1].

Several *Aspergillus* and *Penicillium* moulds across both tropical and temperate latitudes were subsequently found to elaborate OTA during spoilage of major staple agricultural products such as cereals, and in crops for high-end commodities such as coffee, cocoa and red wines. Concern that traces of OTA in major cereal products such as pasta might pose a human health risk, and of potential economic threat to commercial images of the high-end commodities, stimulated extensive research into OTA toxicology. Concurrently, worldwide food safety authorities (e.g., for Europe, Joint expert committee on food additives, International agency for research on cancer, European food standards agency) addressed potential health risks and formulated documents to guide regulatory legislations.

Pigs being important in the human food chain in many economies prompted a major US experimental toxicology study in the 1980s with lifetime chronic exposure in rats [2]. The striking finding of renal tumours, expressed late in life mainly in males in the absence of overt toxicity, was the more notable as designating OTA as the most potent chemical for renal carcinoma in rats, although the extensive technical report did not raise any specific concerns for humans. The kidney cancer incidence findings demonstrated across the three gavage dose rates chosen for the NTP study later demonstrated OTA as a model for classic log dose/response for chemical carcinogens [3].

Subsequent developments in sensitive and definitive analytical methodology have shown widespread occurrence of relevant moulds and their mycotoxins, although general occurrence in well-managed agriculture is generally low. For human health, there has been little verified etiological evidence of general toxicities attributable other than to spasmodic episodes. The initial cautious classification of possible carcinogenetic risk [4] seems never subsequently to have had evidence that could stand classical epidemiological scrutiny. Particularly, the relevance of rat and mouse as pathological models for the human has become insecure because of the wide quantitative gulf ($>10^4$-fold) between necessary daily carcinogenic exposure for rodents (>30 µg OTA/kg body weight daily for at least half a rat lifetime, and much more for a mouse) and surveyed average natural daily human intake data (UK, 0.26–3.5 ng/kg b. wt.) [5].

The classical US toxicity study in rats [2] followed strict toxicology protocols involving gavage administration of OTA five days per week for up to 2 years. The more recent London studies, part of a European Commission project on OTA toxicity (2001-4), provided daily dietary ochratoxins as elaborated during moulding of shredded wheat breakfast cereal by *Aspergillus ochraceus* in a shaken solid substrate fermentation. The product, analysed for OTA, was homogenised (c.10^3-fold) into powdered rat diet for consumption during natural diurnal habit for Fischer male rats. Although blood OTA analysis had not been available for the US study, values in London followed a gradual rise to 8–10 µg/mL during the first month. For the highest daily OTA intake employed (300 µg/kg b wt) at least 9 months exposure seemed necessary to initiate kidney cancer, during which the common prevalence of monocytic leukaemia in ageing Fischer males was apparently repressed [6]. The tumour-free outcome for the US study lowest dose (21 µg/kg b wt) was raised to c. 30 µg/kg b wt in a London study in Dark Agouti male rats [7]. The dose/response criteria adopted for OTA's recognition as the model for log dose/response for chemical carcinogens [3] was thus reinforced by all subsequent findings in London [7] describing OTA/rat renal carcinogenicity as thresholded. Notably, this was not considered later in a major analysis of human risk assessment for OTA in Canada [8] in which a curious distorted non-thresholded graphical illustration is presented.

Critical histology review of some OTA/rat renal tumours has been described [9], including exploratory application for the first time of clinical immunohistochemistry where most tumours showed a range of positive responses to the clinical immuno-stains. Although designed for human histopathological diagnosis some immuno-stains helpfully showed cross-reactivity to rats. The primary experimental objective here is to consolidate those findings by completing histology review of all remaining archived cases in our archive.

2. Results

In confirming a renal cell origin for rat/OTA tumours, all four cases were diffusely and intensely positive for vimentin (Figure 1A, Case 1, tumour dimensions 10 × 20 mm)

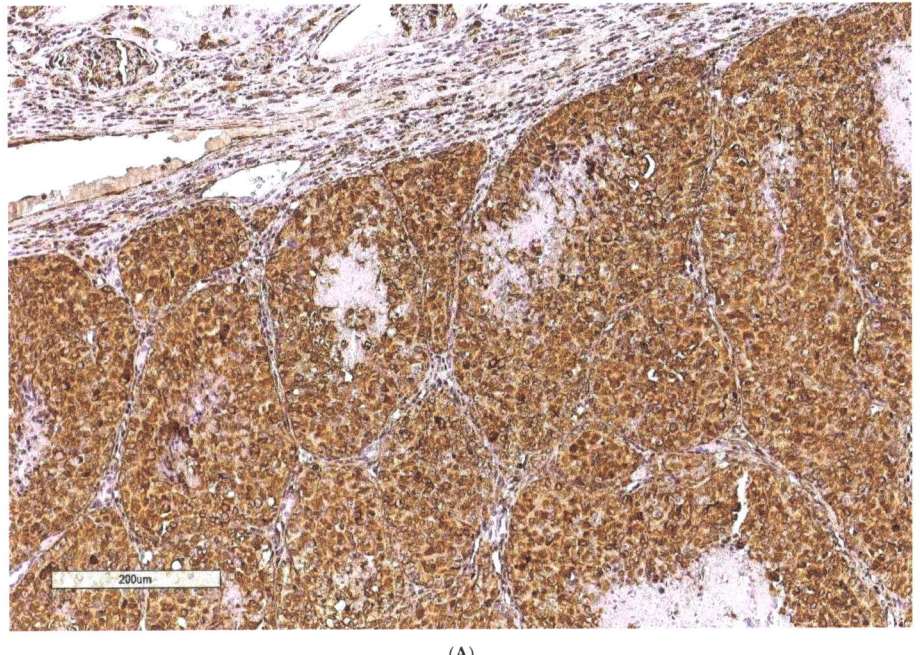

(A)

Figure 1. *Cont.*

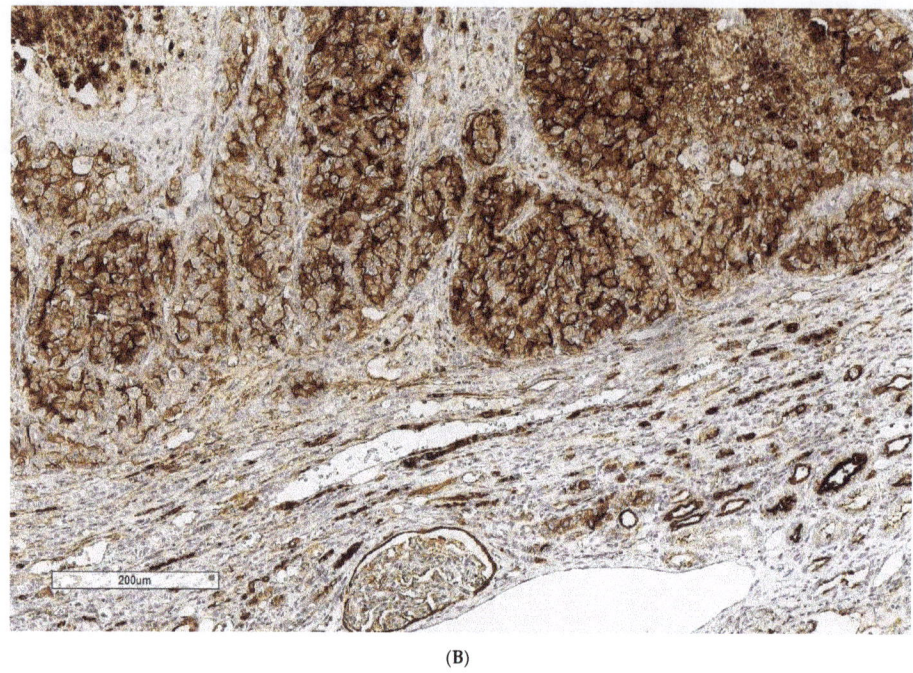

(B)

Figure 1. (**A**) Case 1, Vimentin (100×). (**B**) Case 1, CD10 (100×).

For case 1, CD10 is diffusely and intensely positive, as illustrated on approximately the same area as vimentin, in Figure 1B.

For Case 2, tumour diameter 20 mm, CD10 is negative but cytokeratin clone MNF 116 is diffusely positive, with heterogeneous pattern and variable intensity (Figure 2A, with adjacent Figure 2B as positive control illustrating staining in human tonsil and validating immunostaining cross reactivity in rat).

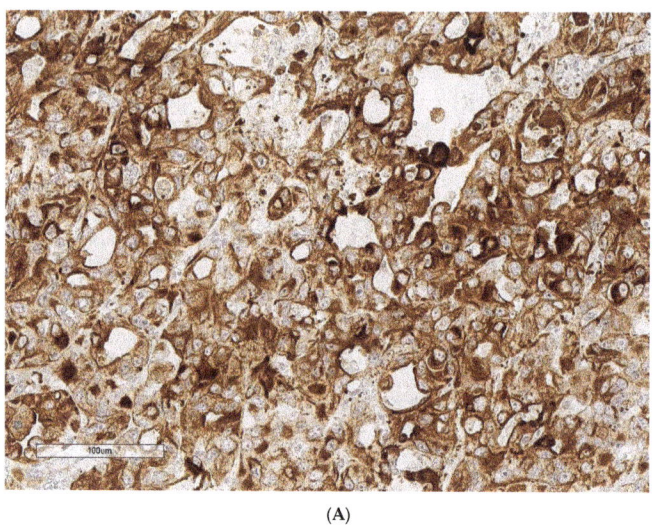

(A)

Figure 2. *Cont.*

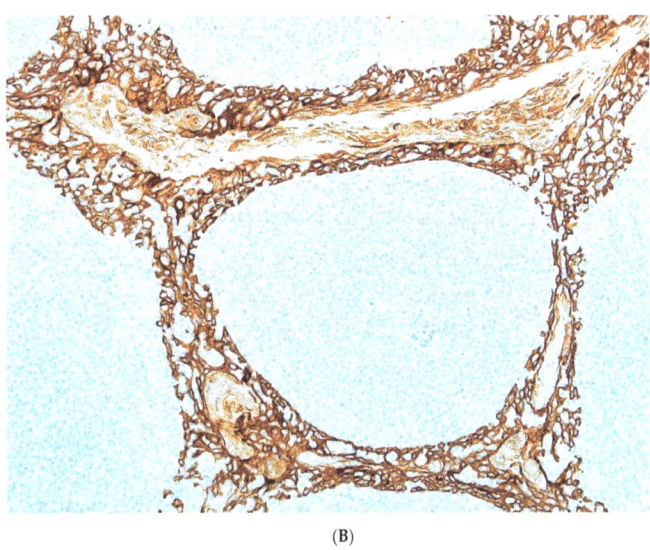

Figure 2. (**A**) Case 2, CK MNF 116 (200×). (**B**) Control (human tonsil), CK MNF 116 (200×).

Case 3 tumour (5 mm) is not immuno-positive other than for vimentin (Figure 3); the diagnosis of renal cell carcinoma is being made on the histological aspect on H&E.

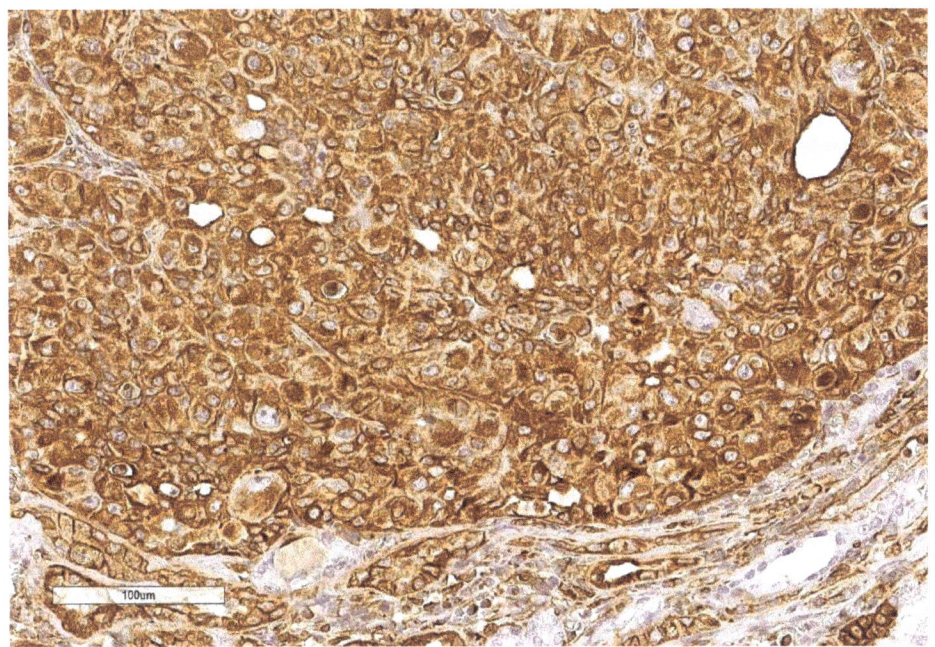

Figure 3. Case 3, Vimentin (200×).

Case 4 tumour (5 mm) is additionally positive for CD10. (not illustrated).

3. Discussion

Histopathology and immune profiles of the present four rat renal tumours caused by chronic exposure to dietary OTA are complementary to our other similar tumours to which immunohistochemical profiles have recently been ascribed [9]. The combined profiles in ten cases dis-associate the rat tumours from implying a model for an etiological role of OTA for the renal pelvic tumours sometimes associated with the Balkan endemic nephropathy. The latter have also recently been shown to have an immune profile indistinguishable from urothelial tumours studied in Slovakia where the Balkan nephropathy has not been reported, thereby dis-associating OTA from urothelial tumours sometimes occurring in Balkan nephropathy cases. A putative model role for human renal cell cancer might still persist if the vital factor of extraordinary dietary exposure to OTA could be established at a plausibly indicative value. Suggestion of OTA involvement in human testicular cancer has also been discounted experimentally in rats.

Immunostaining for vimentin was invariably extensive as is typical for human tissues of mesenchymal origin. The accompanying positivity for CD10 in three of the 10 rat tumours could fit for humans [10]. MNF 116 positivity seems to be a useful characteristic for some rat renal tumours but does not feature for human renal cancer [10]. Immunoprofiles for these renal tumours do not fit easily with the OTA/rat renal expression assisting in predicting OTA as a human carcinogen. Notably, a recent review, co-authored from IARC [11], concludes that defining DNA adducts, oxidative stress and epigenetic factors that operate in humans could lead to reclassification of OTA as a carcinogen. It is not clear whether this indicates official IARC policy. It is unfortunate that authors mis-cite that 'DNA diploidy in OTA-induced rat tumours is associated to genetic change' [12]. It is hoped that any further consideration by IARC would consider that much or most of the in vitro toxicology literature avoids relating the OTA concentration, used to obtain a measured result, to how this relates to kidney parenchyma in vivo during carcinogenesis. It is also important to avoid some literature's assumption of accumulation of OTA in kidney [13].

Gender specificity in rodents is a neglected problem for matching a potential model with the human for whom there seems none for renal cell carcinoma. For the mouse, OTA renal cancer seems specifically male [14] and for the rat is nearly so [2]. A possible explanation for the rat [15] concerns ability of OTA to bind not only to plasma proteins but also to small male-specific urinary peptides in blood. These are subsequently transported through glomerular filtration to pass down nephrons. They follow the usual fate of at least partial salvage absorption in kidney cortex, thereby potentially augmenting delivery of OTA to cortical epithelia. It is hypothesised that the phenylalanine moiety of free OTA predisposes some direct cortical salvage for that essential amino acid in both genders, but that binding to male urinary peptides boosts the overall toxic impact in the potential tissue target for tumorigenesis. Further experimental study could readily detect by analytical gel electrophoresis the extent to which OTA binds to particular urinary proteins, traces of which must escape cortical salvage to appear in urine as pheromones. Such escape is essential in mouse biology, providing the olfactory language of gender and sexuality in the dark. Similarly, in the rat, verification of association of OTA with urinary protein [15] and extension, possibly by use of OTA radiolabelled to high specific activity, could help to clarify some mystery about OTA circulation in blood. OTA binds to serum albumin rather strongly in humans, but the competition in mice and rats between albumin and the smaller proteins that pass though glomeruli is unclear. Some preliminary exploration across puberty in male rats has occurred [16] but there is room for much more in connection with the pharmacokinetics of OTA. Extension of the previous findings [14] was only prevented by the tragic death of the key scientist.

Another way of gaining understanding of the relative dynamics of OTA in blood of male and female rats, to focus on gender differential in renal tumorigenesis, would be by first establishing and quantifying stable circulating OTA in male and female rats during continuous dietary exposure; then to castrate some of the males while continuing the OTA. Predictably, females would have initially attained a higher stable concentration of OTA in blood than males, which were actively excreting more bound to small urinary proteins. Post-castration OTA concentration in male blood could be expected to rise as testosterone-regulated urinary protein synthesis in liver declines. This could be a step towards evaluating the role of urinary proteins in the male rat tendency to develop renal tumours in response to chronic exposure to dietary OTA.

An experimental challenge to explore could be the use of an established technique of rat renal transplantation [17] to study male kidney neoplasia in a female body exposed to dietary OTA for 9–10 months, and vice versa. The graft would have to remain functional for well over a year. However, it is a curious thought that the global concern for OTA as a risk to human health, and the vast expense of analysis and legislation, could be an illusion created experimentally before discovery that small urinary proteins are sex pheromones in mice and rats, where they may transport OTA into kidney.

The above histopathology review [9] also notes that the very small group of female renal tumours in the 1989 NTP study had rather more variable histopathology than males, but the largest example was found to conform to the same immune profile as for males. Qualitative rat renal tumour pathology in response to OTA has thus been found to have a consistent characteristic pattern across genders.

There had been no agreed conclusion in an EU project (European Commission 2001–2004) concerning putative genotoxic, epigenetic or oxidative stress mechanisms in male rat renal carcinogenesis caused experimentally by OTA. However, definitive structural evidence of DNA adduction was subsequently obtained [18] after MS analysis of a synthetic adduct following preparative isolation from photoreaction of OTA and DNA. A previous plan, for MS data of the principal adduct isolated from kidneys of rats given OTA, had failed only due to misunderstanding that all of the extremely small amount of sample would need to go on the MS probe. Unfortunately, this was not practically a repeatable enterprise.

A third lifetime rat study, in Hannover Germany in the 1990s using Dark Agouti rats with gavage exposure to OTA [19] similar to that of the NTP study, also revealed some renal tumours. However, these were noted mainly as indicators of carcinogenicity in six of 15 individuals whose kidneys were subsequently found to contain OTA/DNA adducts. OTA dose was similar in cumulative amount to that in the high dose of the NTP study [2]. Giving OTA in aqueous vehicle, instead of corn oil, would have caused daily surges in circulating toxin concentration with greater toxic impact. Nevertheless, finding consistent occurrence of adducts in elderly rats correlated with continuing exposure to OTA is several months too late to imply an epidemiological role in tumour initiation. The same applies in principle also to human kidney cancer.

Subsequent use also of male Dark Agouti rats [7] generally corroborated the tumour findings in Hannover. However, this was only by doubling the OTA dose through 9 months of dietary exposure in the first year of life, during which OTA was consumed normally and slowly mainly by rat habit during the 12 h human night period. Other gavage regimens have delivered immediately during human daytime. Predictably, no adducts could have been found a year later due to repair of any formed during OTA exposure. In any case, it would be necessary to perfuse-wash tumorous kidneys in situ to remove vascular blood, within which adducts also occur [20], to demonstrate OTA/DNA adducts within kidney or tumour parenchyma. A similar strategy has also been necessary to explain a misconception of accumulation of OTA in mammalian kidney [13].

Across the three main centres for lifetime experiments, there was a consistently lower incidence of renal neoplasms in females than in males for Fischer, Dark Agouti and Lewis rats. A putative mechanism for this differentiation has been proposed [15]. It requires further experimental verification but can not be applied to humans which do not have analogous urinary proteins. This gender focus for OTA also potentially diminishes rat carcinogenicity relevance to humans and is an open question for other mammals.

In recent years ethical considerations have limited some whole animal experimentation, in addition to the economic cost of experimental mycotoxins, and to the lifetime maintenance cost for rodents and particularly for primates. Thus, the scientific literature has reports mainly on tissue culture experiments. Whereas this may provide model information applicable to some mammalian tissues, there is less confidence in application to kidney with its exceptionally complex internal dynamics for sequential stages in filtration, key metabolite recovery, water and ion regulation, metabolic waste excretion and the huge replication of separate nephrons. Particularly, relative roles of trans-membrane ion transfer of OTA, as a phenylalanine derivative, from capillaries to nephron epithelia versus classical understanding of glomerular filtration, are not clear. Very rare finding of very simple early nuclear proliferation in situ within a nephron is tantalising evidence of early neoplasm. We have not yet seen this for OTA, but are aware of a possible model illustrated in a rat in an experiment on chronic exposure to aristolochic acid [21]. In our experience, continuous dietary exposure of male rats to OTA for 6 months, during which nephron epithelia experience millions of OTA molecules, is insufficient to initiate any renal tumour. Nine or ten months is sufficient, but the subsequent point at which pre-cancerous neoplasms might be visible in serial-sectioned kidney is unknown. Is this largely a matter of statistical probability of causing a critical, highly focal, genetic lesion? More experimental understanding is needed for this topic. OTA exposure starting at one year has failed to cause cancers [22]. What factor(s) between 6 and 9 months of age is influential in OTA tumorigenesis?

Experimental evidence shows that the Fischer and other OTA/rat tumours which have generated concern for humans may simply mimic the mechanism operating spontaneously in the EKER strain [23]. The findings are reminiscent of constitutive changes in the rat tuberous sclerosis gene complex which in the EKER strain are correlated with renal neoplasms. Thus, rat renal carcinogenesis caused by OTA does not obviously mimic human urinary tract tumorigenesis.

Another tumorigenesis topic in the literature in the past decade concerns whether OTA is a cause of human testis cancer. This was reiterated prominently in a review abstract [24] with the assertion 'that OTA is a biologically plausible cause of testicular cancer in man'. This was unfortunately based partly on misreading of the literature [22]. There was also insistence that experimental creation of OTA/DNA adducts in testes of newborn mice, from the mother's intrauterine exposure to a quite large OTA insult (2.5 mg/kg b wt) about 4 days previously, without discounting OTA/DNA adducts in newborn blood. Application of immunohistochemistry to histology review of rat testis tumours has since showed [25] the distinctive difference between the natural rat Leydig cell tumours and the germinal cell preponderance of human testicular tumours.

4. Conclusions

Rat and mouse renal tumour response to long-term dietary OTA has cautioned possible analogous cancer risk for humans, but there is yet no verified case of disease. A recent EFSA report [26] expresses continued uncertainty about human risks for OTA contaminations in food. Tumorigenic mechanisms have been proposed from in vitro studies but are unconvincing for tumours of highly focal origin in rodent or human. Review of rat tumour histopathology, including immune profiles, makes the rat a poor model in humans for cancers in kidney and testis. However, several experimental findings for kidney point to OTA mimicking the natural spontaneous renal tumours of the EKER strain. Natural OTA exposure for humans is very much less than that often applied to experimental cells and whole animal carcinogenicity follows a classical log dose/response relationship. Focus on satisfying Bradford Hill criteria for epidemiology of OTA is encouraged to avoid biases.

5. Materials and Methods

Four renal tumours from Fischer male rats given protracted dietary OTA (300 µg/kg body weight daily) [6] were embedded in paraffin blocks. Animals were from the same lifetime experimental group [6] as those whose immunoprofiles were previously described [9]. Ethical review and approval were waived for this study because no new live animals were involved. Sections (3 µm) were mounted on charged slides (TOMO, Matsunami, Japan) and processed for immunohistochemistry in the Cell Pathology Laboratory of South West London Pathology at St George's Hospital, Tooting, variously applying panels of antibodies in fully automated BenchMark ULTRA immunohistochemistry processing, as required to assist clinical diagnoses. Procedures followed exactly those previously described [9]. The following antibodies were used: CK MNF 116, clone MNF 116 (Dako); Vimentin, clone V9 (Dako, Novocastra); CD10, clone 56C6 (Dako). After applying DAB chromogen, nuclei were counterstained blue with haematoxylin. The brown immune reaction product of DAB chromogen is cytoplasmic and/or membranar for the listed antibodies. Haematoxylin and Eosin staining was also performed for preliminary standard tissue differentiation of nuclear (blue) and cytoplasmic components (red).

Author Contributions: Conceptualization, D.H. and P.M. All authors have read and agreed to the published version of the manuscript.

Funding: This research received no external funding.

Institutional Review Board Statement: Ethical review and approval were waived for this study because no new live animals were involved.

Conflicts of Interest: The authors declare no conflict of interest.

References

1. Krogh, P. Porcine nephropathy associated with ochratoxin A. In *Mycotoxins and Animal Foods*; Smith, J.E., Henderson, R.S., Eds.; CRC Press: Boca Raton, Fl, USA, 1991; pp. 627–645.
2. Boorman, G.A. *Toxicology and Carcinogenesis Studies of Ochratoxin A (CAS No. 303-47-9) in F344/N Rats (Gavage Studies)*; Technical Report 358; National Toxicology Program: Durham, NC, USA, 1989.
3. Waddell, W.J. Critique of dose response in carcinogenesis. *Hum. Exp. Toxicol.* **2006**, *25*, 413–436. [CrossRef]
4. IARC (International Agency for Research on Cancer). *Ochratoxin A (Group B)*; Summaries and Evaluations 56: 489; IARC: Lyon, France, 1993. Available online: https://www.ncbi.nlm.nih.gov/books/NBK513594/ (accessed on 10 March 2021).
5. Gilbert, J.; Brereton, P.; MacDonald, S. Assessment of dietary exposure to ochratoxin A in the UK using a duplicate diet approach and analysis of urine and plasma samples. *Food Add. Contam.* **2001**, *18*, 1088–1093. [CrossRef] [PubMed]
6. Mantle, P. Rat kidney cancers determined by dietary ochratoxin A in the first year of life. *J. Kidney Cancer VHL* **2016**, *3*, 1–10. [CrossRef] [PubMed]
7. Mantle, P.G. Minimum tolerable exposure period and maximum threshold dietary intake of ochratoxin A for causing renal cancer in male Dark Agouti rats. *Food Chem. Toxicol.* **2009**, *47*, 2419–2424. [CrossRef] [PubMed]
8. Kuiper-Goodman, T.; Hilts, C.; Hilliard, S.M.; Kiparissis, I.D.K.; Hayward, R.S. Health risk assessment of ochratoxin A for all age-sex strata in a market economy. *Food Add. Contam.* **2010**, *27*, 212–240. [CrossRef] [PubMed]
9. Herman, D.; Mantle, P. Immunohistochemical analysis of rat renal tumours caused by ochratoxin A. *Toxins* **2017**, *9*, 384. [CrossRef]
10. Kim, M.; Joo, J.W.; Lee, S.J.; Park, C.K.; Cho, N.H. Comprehensive immunoprofiles of renal cell carcinoma subtypes. *Cancers* **2020**, *12*, 602. [CrossRef] [PubMed]
11. Ostry, V.; Malir, F.; Toman, J.; Grosse, Y. Mycotoxins as human carcinogens- the IARC monographs classification. *Mycotoxin Res.* **2017**, *33*, 65–73. [CrossRef] [PubMed]
12. Brown, A.L.; Odell, E.W.; Mantle, P.G. DNA ploidy distribution in renal tumours induced in male rats by ochratoxin A. *Exp. Toxicol. Pathol.* **2007**, *59*, 85–95. [CrossRef]
13. Mantle, P.; Kilic, M.A.; Mor, F.; Ozmen, O. Contribution of organ vasculature in rat renal analysis for ochratoxin A: Relevance to toxicology of nephrotoxins. *Toxins* **2015**, *7*, 1005–1017. [CrossRef]
14. Bendele, A.M.; Carlton, W.W.; Krogh, P.; Lillehoj, E.B. Ochratoxin A carcinogenesis in the (C57BL/CJ X C3H)F_1 mouse. *J. Natl. Cancer Inst.* **1985**, *75*, 733–739.
15. Mantle, P.G.; Nagy, J.M. Binding of ochratoxin A to a urinary globulin: A new concept to account for gender difference in rat nephrocarcinogenic responses. *Int. J. Mol. Sci.* **2008**, *9*, 719–735. [CrossRef] [PubMed]
16. Vettorazzi, A.; Wait, R.; Nagy, J.; Monreal, J.I.; Mantle, P. Changes in male rat urinary protein profile during puberty: A pilot study. *BMC Res. Notes* **2013**, *6*, 232. [CrossRef] [PubMed]
17. Spanjol, J.; Celic, T.; Jakljevic, T.; Ivancic, A.; Markic, D. Surgical technique in the rat model for kidney transplantation. *Coll. Anthropol.* **2011**, *35*, 87–90.
18. Mantle, P.G.; Faucet-Marquis, V.; Manderville, R.A.; Squillaci, B.; Pfohl-Leszkowicz, A. Structures of covalent adducts between DNA and ochratoxin A: A new factor in debate about genotoxicity and human risk assessment. *Chem. Res. Toxicol.* **2010**, *23*, 89–98. [CrossRef]
19. Castegnaro, M.; Mohr, U.; Pfohl-Leszkowicz, A.; Esteve, J.; Steinmann, J.; Tillmann, T.; Michelon, J.; Bartsch, H. Sex- and strain-specific induction of renal tumours by ochratoxin in rats correlates with DNA adduction. *Int. J. Cancer* **1998**, *77*, 70–75. [CrossRef]

20. Pfohl-Leszkowicz, A.; Faucet-Marquis, V.; Tozlovanu, M.; Peraica, M.; Stefanovic, V.; Manderville, R. C8-2′-Deoxyguanosine ochratoxin A-adducts and OTA metabolites in biologic fluids as biomarkers of OTA exposure. In Proceedings of the MycoRed International Conference, Mendoza, Argentina, 15–17 November 2011.
21. Gruia, A.; Gazinska, P.; Herman, D.; Ordodi, V.; Tatu, C.; Mantle, P. Revealing a pre-neoplastic renal tubular lesion by p-S6 protein immunohistochemistry after rat exposure to aristolochic acid. *J. Kidney Cancer VHL* **2015**, *2*, 153–162. [CrossRef] [PubMed]
22. Mantle, P.G.; Nolan, C.C. Pathological outcomes in kidney and brain in male Fischer rats given dietary ochratoxin A, commencing at one year of age. *Toxins* **2010**, *2*, 1100–1110. [CrossRef] [PubMed]
23. Gazinska, P.; Herman, D.; Gillett, C.; Pinder, S.; Mantle, P. Comparative immunohistochemical analysis of ochratoxin A tumourigenesis in rats and urinary tract carcinoma in humans; mechanistic significance of p-S6 ribosomal protein expression. *Toxins* **2012**, *4*, 643–662. [CrossRef]
24. Malir, F.; Ostry, V.; Pfohl-Leszkowicz, A.; Novotna, E. Ochratoxin A: Development and reproductive toxicity-an overview. *Birth Defects Res.* **2013**, *98*, 493–502. [CrossRef]
25. Herman, D.; Mantle, P. Immunohistochemical review of Leydig cell lesions in ochratoxin A-treated Fischer rats and controls. *Toxins* **2019**, *11*, 480. [CrossRef] [PubMed]
26. EFSA panel on contaminants in the food chain. Risk assessment of ochratoxin A in food. *EFSA J.* **2020**, *15*, 5. [CrossRef]

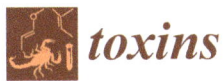

Article

The Impact of the Nephrotoxin Ochratoxin A on Human Renal Cells Studied by a Novel Co-Culture Model Is Influenced by the Presence of Fibroblasts

Gerald Schwerdt *, Michael Kopf and Michael Gekle

Julius-Bernstein-Institut für Physiologie, 06112 Halle, Germany; michael.kopf@uk-halle.de (M.K.); michael.gekle@medizin.uni-halle.de (M.G.)
* Correspondence: gerald.schwerdt@medizin.uni-halle.de

Abstract: The kidney is threatened by a lot of potentially toxic substances. To study the influence of the nephrotoxin ochratoxin A (OTA) we established a cell co-culture model consisting of human renal proximal tubule cells and fibroblasts. We studied the effect of OTA on cell survival, the expression of genes and/or proteins related to cell death, extracellular matrix and energy homeostasis. OTA-induced necrosis was enhanced in both cell types in the presence of the respective other cell type, whereas OTA-induced apoptosis was independent therefrom. In fibroblasts, but not in tubule cells, a co-culture effect was visible concerning the expression of the cell-cycle-related protein p21. The expression of the epithelial-to-mesenchymal transition-indicating protein vimentin was independent from the culture-condition. The expression of the OTA-induced lncRNA WISP1-AS1 was enhanced in co-culture. OTA exposure led to alterations in the expression of genes related to energy metabolism with a glucose-mobilizing effect and a reduced expression of mitochondrial proteins. Together we demonstrate that the reaction of cells can be different in the presence of cells which naturally are close-by, thus enabling a cellular cross-talk. Therefore, to evaluate the toxicity of a substance, it would be an advantage to consider the use of co-cultures instead of mono-cultures.

Keywords: ochratoxin A; cell culture; energy metabolism; apoptosis-necrosis balance; mitochondria

Key Contribution: Co-culture of human renal tubule cells with human fibroblasts demonstrate that the impact of a toxic substance, here ochratoxin A (OTA), can be underestimated when only one cell type is used. Based on gene expression studies, OTA interferes with energy metabolism leading to disturbed mitochondrial function and enhanced glucose mobilization from glycogen stores.

Citation: Schwerdt, G.; Kopf, M.; Gekle, M. The Impact of the Nephrotoxin Ochratoxin A on Human Renal Cells Studied by a Novel Co-Culture Model Is Influenced by the Presence of Fibroblasts. *Toxins* **2021**, *13*, 219. https://doi.org/10.3390/toxins13030219

Received: 25 February 2021
Accepted: 16 March 2021
Published: 18 March 2021

Publisher's Note: MDPI stays neutral with regard to jurisdictional claims in published maps and institutional affiliations.

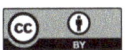

Copyright: © 2021 by the authors. Licensee MDPI, Basel, Switzerland. This article is an open access article distributed under the terms and conditions of the Creative Commons Attribution (CC BY) license (https://creativecommons.org/licenses/by/4.0/).

1. Introduction

Due to its excretory function, the kidney is threatened by a variety of harmful substances such as drugs or food contaminants, like mycotoxins leading to acute or—even worse—chronic kidney diseases with a prevalence of about 10% [1,2]. To understand the mechanisms of the nephrotoxic action it is helpful to find strategies to alleviate these detrimental scenarios and many studies have been performed to solve the question of why and how kidneys are endangered [3–5].

To study the influences of a substance on an organism, it is often difficult to use whole animals because of ethical concerns and organizational, costly and elaborate prerequisites. Furthermore, a transfer of knowledge to the human situation is associated with uncertainties. Therefore, cell culture models have been established and are used widely, and have the advantage that a specific cell type and its response to a substance or to a treatment can be studied under controlled conditions. Although many and important findings have been made using this approach, some disadvantages are inherent: cells of a cell line often have been immortalized by mutagenesis or other—sometimes drastic—methods [6]. This allows easy handling and long usage but with the hazard that results found in a specific model system may not be transferable to the situation in the whole organ or organism. To overcome this disadvantage, instead of immortalized cell lines, primary cells can be used, but the generation of primary cells is often very difficult and requires advanced technical skills. Additionally, primary cells often do not survive for a long period of time and need special individual culture conditions. But primary cells are a step closer to natural conditions and at least sometimes it turned out that they are more sensitive to, e.g., toxic stimuli as cell lines are [7], meaning that cell lines might be more robust. Another disadvantage is the fact that cells are often kept in monoculture, i.e., without the influences of other cell types, which in their home organ usually are close-by. Therefore, it might be a step towards a more realistic situation to study the response of a cell type to a substance or treatment in the presence of those cells, which are in the native organ in close proximity.

In the kidney, proximal tubule cells are surrounded by fibroblasts and a—probably mutual—influence can be assumed. This is also the case in kidney damaging scenarios that in most cases lead to tubulo-interstitial inflammation and fibrosis [8,9], and are decisive for the decline of kidney function. Because of their transport and enzymatic capabilities, renal proximal tubule cells are endangered by a variety of potential toxic substances such as, e.g., drugs or their remnants or mycotoxins. One role of the surrounding fibroblasts is to furnish the extracellular matrix by release of collagens and other matrix components and therefore to participate in the integrity of the tissue [10]. But they are also—together with epithelial cells—involved in inflammatory processes or in fibrotic kidney diseases [11] with the risk of developing renal failure.

An intensively studied mycotoxin with relevance for human health is ochratoxin A (OTA) [12,13]. It can be found in a variety of foodstuffs [12,14] and to avoid its exposure and uptake is almost impossible [9,15]. This leads to the observation that OTA is detected frequently in human blood in low nanomolar concentrations [16]. In exposed animals, OTA leads to kidney failure and fibrotic changes [17,18]. OTA exposure is assumed to be involved in human kidney diseases [19]. In human primary proximal tubule cells, a toxic effect of OTA has been shown, which is also observable in human primary fibroblasts, although it is not as prominent as in proximal tubule cells [7]. The mechanisms behind the toxic action of OTA are still not completely understood and are subject of many ongoing studies. How far neighboring cells with different functions interfere and thereby modulate cell function is almost not known but is expectable. In a previous study using a co-culture model consisting of rat kidney proximal tubule and fibroblast cells, it turned out that a kind of crosstalk between both cell types takes place, leading to the observation that effects of OTA as epithelial-to-mesenchymal transition (EMT) occurred only under co-culture conditions [20]. Another conclusion drawable from that study and others was that rat cells are more robust concerning the tolerance to OTA as compared to human proximal tubule cells [7,20] and therefore a model system based on human cells is required to closer evaluate the human situation and the risk of OTA exposure.

Therefore, in the present study, we establish an advanced cell co-culture model consisting of human proximal tubule cells (HK2 cells) and human fibroblasts (CCD-1092SK cells) to study the effects of OTA on cell survival (apoptosis, necrosis) and expression of some exemplarily chosen genes related to cell cycle, cell death, extracellular matrix, and metabolism. Similar to previous studies using rat cells [20], the human proximal tubule cells were placed on filter devices and the filters were put above a layer of fibroblasts seeded on the bottom of a petri dish so that the basolateral side of the epithelial cells faces towards the fibroblasts, enabling a kind of conversation between both cell types.

2. Results

2.1. Protein, Lactate Dehydrogenase Release and Caspase-3 Activity

To obtain a first impression about possible effects of culture conditions itself as well as about effects on OTA-induced alterations, we compared caspase-3 activity as a measure for apoptosis of cells grown in monoculture with the activity of cells grown in co-culture incubated with or without 100 nM OTA for two points of time, 24 and 48 h. In addition, lactate dehydrogenase (LDH) release as a measure for necrosis was determined as well as protein content to give an overall impression on cell status. Therefore, equal amounts of cells were placed either in the well bottom (fibroblasts) or onto a filter (proximal tubule cells). After reaching confluence, filters were placed into the wells in which the fibroblasts were located (see graphical abstract). As shown in Figure 1A, almost no culture-condition-dependent effects on protein content could be observed in both cell types after 24 or 48 h (see also Supplementary File S1). In fibroblasts, OTA exposure led to a small increase in protein content whereas in tubule cells OTA led to a slight decrease of protein content showing that OTA might have a negative effect on tubule cells. These effects were almost independent from the culture condition in both cell types.

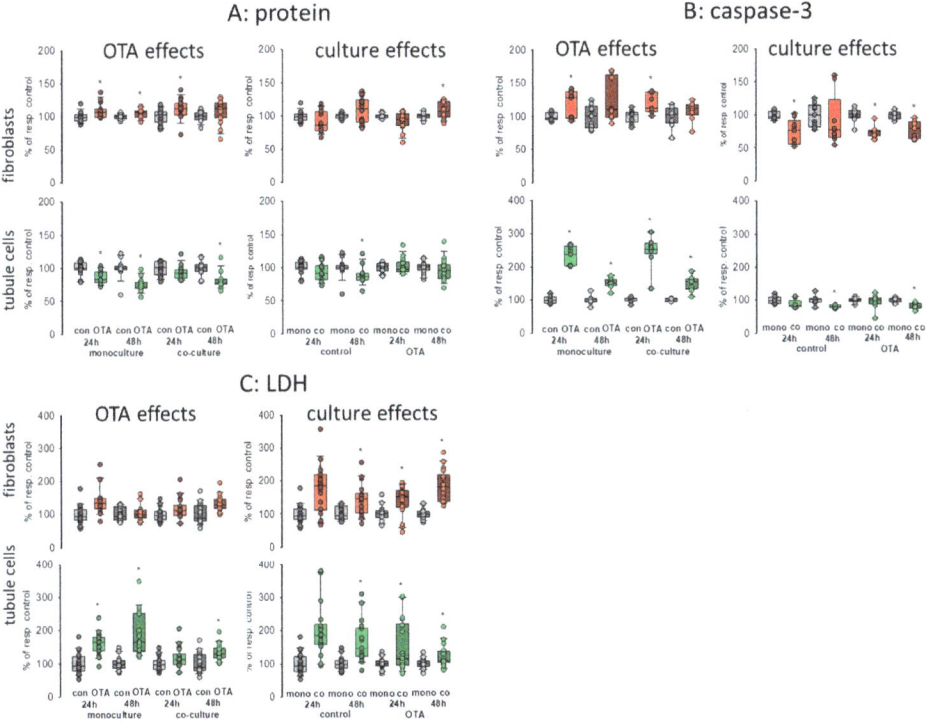

Figure 1. Effects of ochratoxin A (OTA) and/or culture conditions on protein content (**A**), caspase-3 activity (**B**), and lactate dehydrogensase (LDH) release (**C**). Cells were cultivated either in mono- or in co-culture and exposed to 100 nM OTA for 24 or 48 h. $n = 3$–6, $n = 14$–18 (protein, LDH) or 8–9 (caspase-3). * indicates a $p < 0.05$ to non-OTA-exposed cells (comparing the OTA effects, resp. left side) or to cells in mono-culture (comparing culture effects, resp. right side).

To further explain the effect on protein content, we studied apoptosis and necrosis. Compared to fibroblasts, OTA had a clear effect on apoptosis in tubule cells after 24 h exposure with about 2.5-fold increase in activity (Figure 1B). After 48 h exposure the increase was still observable but not as distinctive as after 24 h. However, these increases were almost independent from culture conditions except that after 48 h in the presence of fibroblasts the caspase activity in the tubule cells was slightly reduced, indicating a modest protecting effect of the co-culture. However, a protecting effect of co-culture was observable for the fibroblasts, especially in the presence of OTA.

In Co-culture, LDH release was clearly enhanced in fibroblasts and tubule cells when compared to monoculture conditions independent of the presence of OTA (Figure 1C). In tubule cells, OTA led to an increase of LDH released into the media especially after 48 h exposure, which was not as pronounced in fibroblasts.

Taken together, the presence of the respective other cell type led to enhanced necrosis but to less apoptosis so that the overall protein content was not remarkably changed. The effects of OTA on apoptosis and necrosis were also mostly independent from the presence or absence of the other cell type.

2.2. Western Blot and mRNA Expression

2.2.1. CDKN1A/p21

Cell cycle was shown to be influenced by OTA and it could be shown that the p21 protein which is involved in cell cycle was upregulated by OTA in tubule cells [21]. To investigate how far the protein, as well as the expression of mRNA coding for p21, is influenced by the presence of fibroblasts, we performed Western blots and RT-PCR. As shown in Figures 2A,B and 3, 48 h exposure to 100 nM OTA led to an increase of p21 protein amount in mono but also in co-culture conditions in tubule cells. In fibroblasts under co-culture conditions, OTA had no effect on p21-protein expression although the mRNA expression was increased by OTA independent from the presence of the other cell type. Interestingly, under co-culture conditions, OTA exposure did not further increase p21 protein expression. In tubule cells, the mRNA expression was not altered by the presence of fibroblasts but in fibroblasts in co-culture the p21 mRNA expression was enhanced not only in OTA-exposed but also already in cells not exposed to OTA (see also Supplementary File S1). This shows that the presence of the other cell type has an influence on p21 protein expression, especially in fibroblasts.

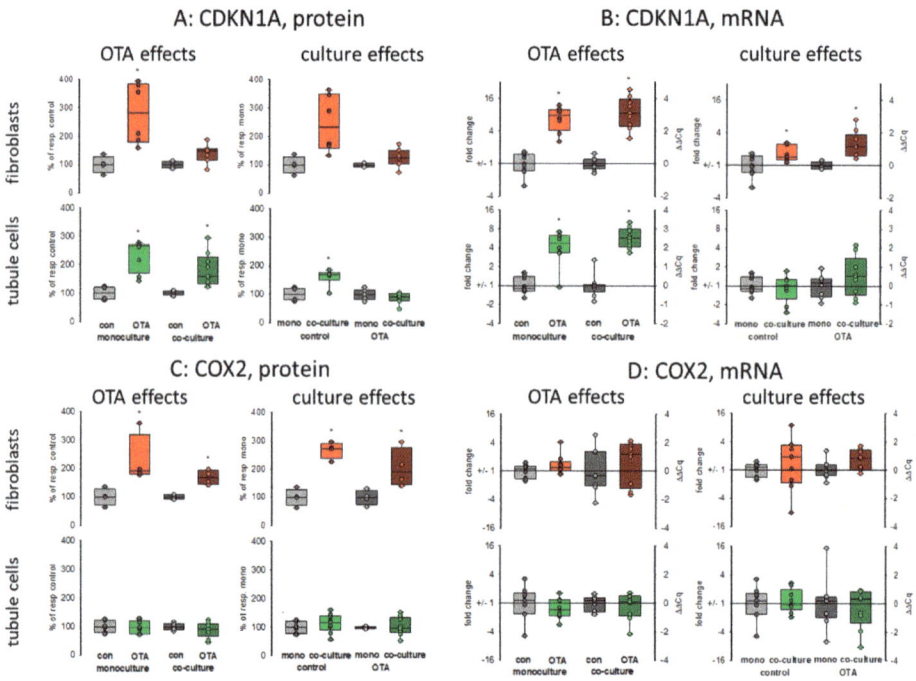

Figure 2. Effects of OTA and/or culture conditions on protein and mRNA expression of CDKN1A/p21 (**A**,**B**) and cyclooxygenase 2 (COX2) (**C**,**D**). Cells were cultivated either in mono- or in co-culture and exposed to 100 nM OTA for or 48 h. $n = 3$, $n = 4–9$ (protein and 8–9 for mRNAs). * indicates a $p < 0.05$ to non-OTA-exposed cells (comparing the OTA effects, resp. left side) or to cells in mono-culture (comparing culture effects, resp. right side).

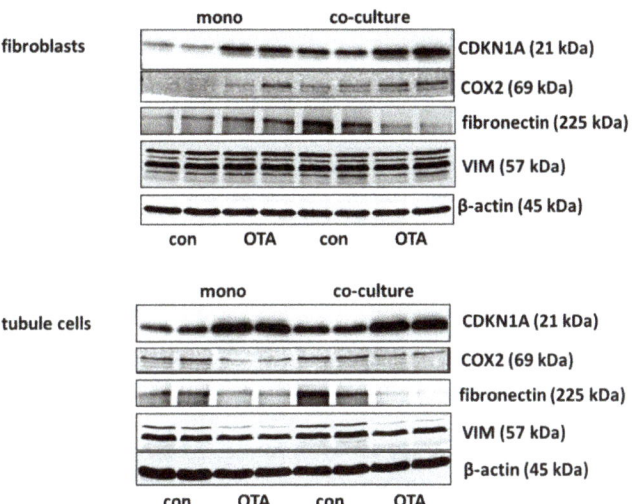

Figure 3. Supplementary representative Western blots to Figures 2A,C and 4A,C.

2.2.2. Cyclooxygenase 2 (COX2)

It has been shown that cyclooxygenase 2 (*COX2*) protein as well as mRNA levels are increased during kidney failure [22]. As shown in Figures 2C,D and 3, only in fibroblasts the protein expression was increased by OTA exposure. In addition, in the presence of tubule cells, COX2 protein expression was enhanced in untreated as well as in OTA-exposed cells, demonstrating a clear influence of tubule cells. The mRNA expression, however, was not influenced by OTA and a very slight effect of co-culture occurred by OTA exposure. In contrast, in tubule cells, the mRNA and protein expression of COX2 was completely independent from OTA or the presence of fibroblasts. That shows that concerning COX2 tubule cells can influence fibroblasts but fibroblasts have no influence on tubule cells.

2.2.3. Fibronectin

Kidney failure is often accompanied by fibrosis. During fibrosis, an accumulation of extracellular matrix takes place and one observation besides other is an increase of fibronectin protein amount [23]. Therefore, the OTA-dependent alteration of fibronectin-coding mRNA and protein expression was determined in mono- or co-culture conditions. As shown in Figures 3 and 4A,B, 48 h exposure of tubule cells to 100 nM OTA led to a decrease of intracellular fibronectin both in mono-and co-culture. The OTA-effect was lower in co-culture. Moreover, the amount of mRNA coding for fibronectin was reduced by OTA exposure independently from the culture conditions and the presence of fibroblasts led to lower mRNA expression in control and OTA-exposed cells. In contrast, in fibroblasts the fibronectin expression was almost not altered neither by OTA nor by culture conditions because of a great variability, especially in the Western blots. A tendency towards OTA-induced expression might be visible in mono-culture.

2.2.4. Vimentin

Vimentin is a protein whose abundance increases when epithelial-to-mesenchymal transition (EMT) takes place and EMT development can lead to kidney failure [23]. Therefore, the OTA-dependent alteration of vimentin mRNA and protein expression was determined in mono- and co-culture conditions. As shown in Figures 3 and 4C,D, 48 h exposure of tubule cells to 100 nM OTA led to a lower abundance of vimentin protein both under mono- and co-culture conditions. However, in the presence of fibroblasts the vimentin protein expression was independent from culture conditions. The expression of mRNA coding for vimentin was almost not altered neither by OTA nor by culture conditions with the exception that OTA exposure in co-culture showed a slight increase. In fibroblasts, the vimentin protein expression was completely independent from OTA exposure as well as from the presence of the tubule cells. In addition, vimentin-coding mRNA expression was almost not altered.

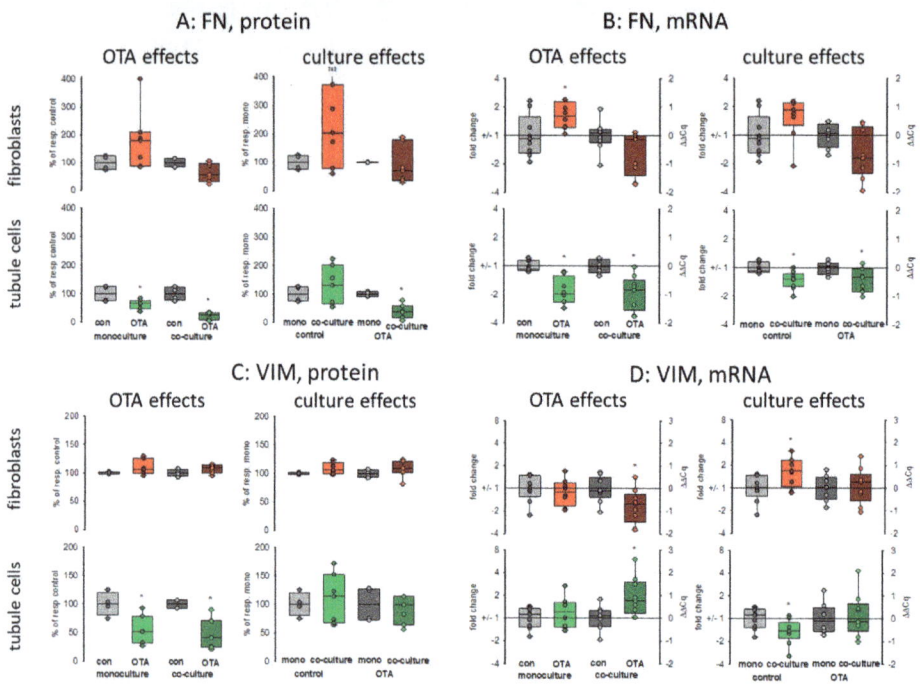

Figure 4. Effects of OTA and/or culture conditions on protein and mRNA expression of fibronectin (*FN*) (**A**,**B**) and vimentin (*VIM*) (**C**,**D**). Cells were cultivated either in mono- or in co-culture and exposed to 100 nM OTA for 48 h. $n = 3$; $n = 4$–8 (FN protein), 4–7 (VIM protein) and 8–9 for mRNAs. * indicates a $p < 0.05$ to non-OTA-exposed cells (comparing the OTA effects, resp. left side) or to cells in mono-culture (comparing culture effects, resp. right side).

2.3. Expression of Some Selected Genes

To further test exemplarily in how far the culture conditions may affect also the expression of other RNAs, we selected some genes, which play a role in apoptosis-necrosis, cancer development, or energy metabolism (see also Supplementary File S1).

2.3.1. WISP1-AS1

WISP1-AS1 is a long non-coding RNA (lncRNA) induced by OTA affecting transcriptional regulation and playing a role in the apoptosis-necrosis balance and probably in cancer development [24]. As seen in Figure 5A, 48 h exposure to 100 nM OTA led in both cell types to a marked increase in the expression of that lncRNA. Without OTA, the presence of the respective other cell type had almost no influence on the expression. However, in the presence of OTA, its expression was higher in co-culture as compared to mono-culture.

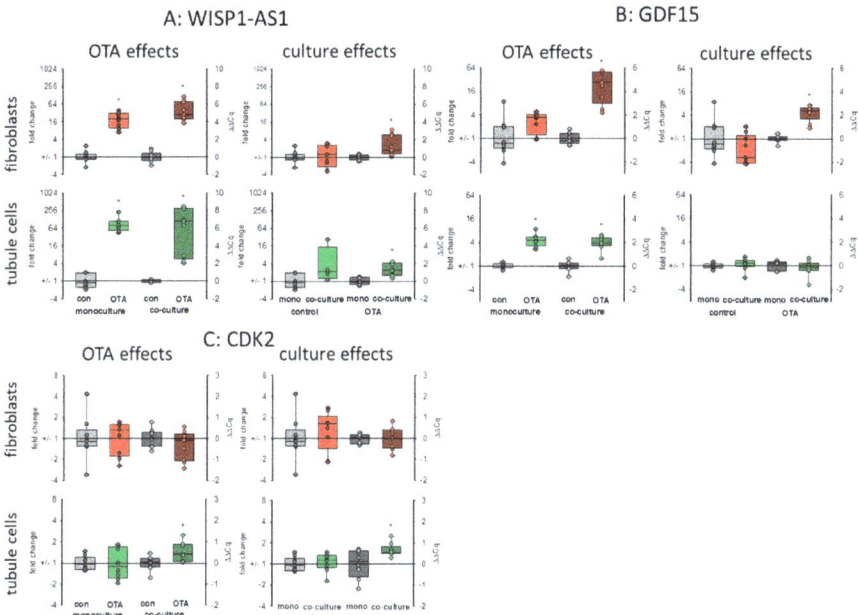

Figure 5. Effects of OTA and/or culture conditions on expression of RNA coding for *WISP1-AS1* (**A**), *GDF15* (**B**), and *CDK2* (**C**). Cells were cultivated either in mono- or in co-culture and exposed to 100 nM OTA for 48 h. $n = 3$, $n = 4$–9. * indicates a $p < 0.05$ to non-OTA-exposed cells (comparing the OTA effects, resp. left side) or to cells in mono-culture (comparing culture effects, resp. right side).

2.3.2. GDF15

Growth differentiation factor 15 (*GDF15*) is a member of the transforming growth factor superfamily responding to stress. It is discussed as a biomarker also for kidney diseases or as a predictor for survival of kidney transplant patients [25,26]. The expression of mRNA coding for *GDF15* was enhanced in both cell types after OTA exposure as shown in Figure 5B. This OTA-induced effect was favored in fibroblasts when tubule cells were in the vicinity. In tubule cells, however, the expression was independent of the presence of fibroblasts (Figure 5B).

2.3.3. CDK2

Cyclin-dependent kinase 2 (*CDK2*) was identified by weighted correlation network analysis as a major regulator of OTA-induced cell cycle dysregulation [21]. In fibroblasts in monoculture the expression of the mRNA coding for *CDK2* was not altered by OTA. Furthermore, the presence of tubule cells did not affect the mRNA expression. However, in tubule cells, OTA led to a slightly enhanced expression only in the presence of fibroblasts (Figure 5C).

2.3.4. Glycogen and Glucose-Related Proteins: *PYGM, GYS1* and *GLUT1 (SLC2A1)*

The kidney is also involved in glucose homeostasis and can provide the body with glucose either by gluconeogenesis or by mobilizing glycogen stores [27]. Glycogen phosphorylase (*PYGM*) plays a role in the decomposition of glycogen stores, thereby mobilizing glucose [28]. As seen in Figure 6A, 48 h exposure to 100 nM OTA led to a marked increase in the expression of the mRNA coding for glycogen phosphorylase, especially in the tubule cells. However, in tubule cells this increase was not dependent on culture condition whereas in fibroblasts the OTA-induced expression was higher in the presence of tubule cells as compared to the condition without tubule cells. Glycogen synthase 1 (*GYS1*) catalyzes the opposite reaction and whereas the expression of the phosphorylase was upregulated, the expression of the synthase was down regulated by OTA in tubule cells and in fibroblasts in co-culture (Figure 6B). This indicates a glucose-mobilizing effect of OTA. Interestingly, the mRNA expression of the glucose transporter GLUT1 (*SLC2A1*) was upregulated by OTA, too (Figure 6C), underlining the idea of an enhanced glucose demand due to OTA exposure maybe due to impaired mitochondria.

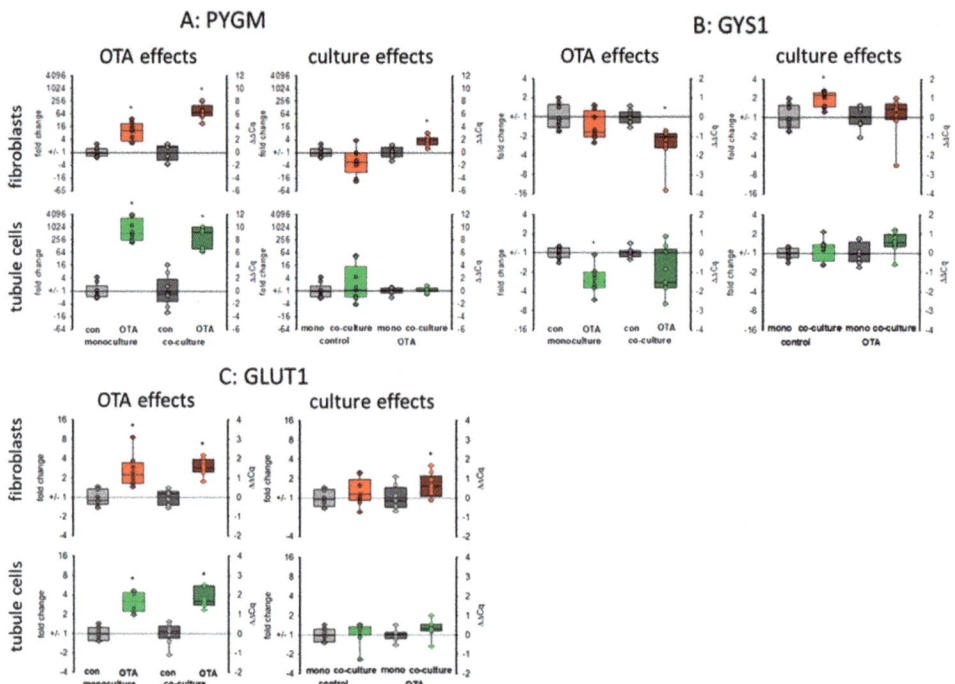

Figure 6. Effects of OTA and/or culture conditions on expression of RNA coding for *PYGM* (**A**), *GYS1* (**B**), and *GLUT1* (**C**). Cells were cultivated either in mono- or in co-culture and exposed to 100 nM OTA for 48 h. $n = 3$, $n = 8$–9. * indicates a $p < 0.05$ to non-OTA-exposed cells (comparing the OTA effects, resp. left side) or to cells in mono-culture (comparing culture effects, resp. right side).

2.3.5. Mitochondria-Related Proteins: *NDUFB10* and *MRPS16*

There are indications that OTA exposure can lead to a decrease of the mitochondrial potential in kidney cells [24] showing that mitochondrial function may be influenced by OTA exposure, which might be additionally influenced by the presence of fibroblasts. Therefore, representative of other RNA coding for mitochondrial proteins, we show here the expression of the mRNAs coding for *NDUFB10* and *MRPS16*. *NDUFB10* codes for the mitochondrial NADH:ubiquinone oxidoreductase subunit B10, which is a part of the mitochondrial respiratory complex I and highly expressed in heart and kidney (NCBI gene. Available online: https://www.ncbi.nlm.nih.gov/gene/4716 (accessed on 17 March 2021)). The *MRPS16* gene codes for the mitochondrial ribosomal protein S16, which plays a role in mitochondrial protein synthesis. As shown in Figure 7, 24 h OTA exposure led in both cell types to a decreased expression of both mRNAs. In tubule cells, the decreased expression of *NDUFB10* gene was not influenced by the presence of fibroblasts, whereas in fibroblasts the OTA-induced reduction of *NDUFB10* expression was slightly rescued in the presence of tubule cells (Figure 7A). In tubule cells, the already lowered expression of the gene coding for the mitochondrial ribosomal subunit by OTA was additionally lower in the presence of fibroblasts, whereas in fibroblasts the presence of tubule cells led to a slightly higher expression of *MRPS16* mRNA (Figure 7B). This shows that mitochondrial function can be affected by OTA but that the OTA effect can additionally be modified when the two cell types are close together.

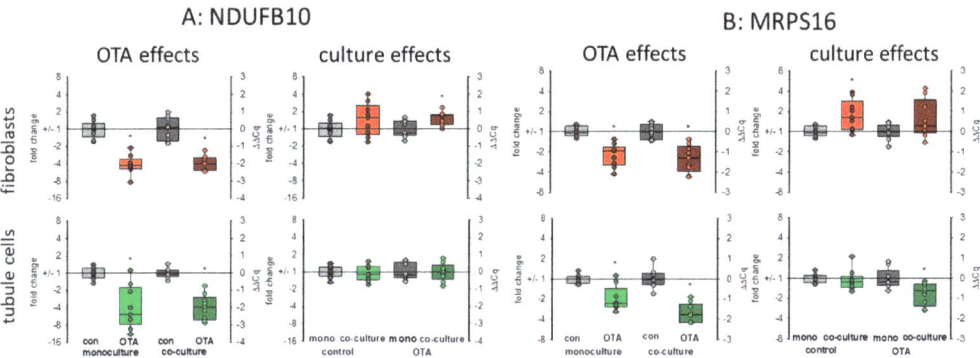

Figure 7. Effects of OTA and/or culture conditions on expression of RNA coding for *NDUFB10* (**A**) and *MRPS16* (**B**). Cells were cultivated either in mono- or in co-culture and exposed to 100 nM OTA for 24 h. $n = 3$, $n = 8$–9. * indicates a $p < 0.05$ to non-OTA-exposed cells (comparing the OTA effects, resp. left side) or to cells in mono-culture (comparing culture effects, resp. right side).

3. Discussion

The kidney is endangered by a variety of nephrotoxic substances with the risk of acute or chronic kidney failure [1]. For the study of the impact of nephrotoxic substances on different cell types and to reduce animal handling, cell cultures have been widely applied. These cell cultures have the additional advantage that experimental conditions can be controlled and specific effects of a substance investigated using a defined cell type. Besides these undisputed advantages, some considerations remain: for example, in the "home organ" one cell type (e.g., proximal tubule cells in the kidney) is surrounded by other cell types (e.g., fibroblasts) with manifold interdependencies. Therefore, the reaction to a substance observed when using only one cell type may not be the same as in the presence of the cells close-by in the original tissue. In a model consisting of two different rat renal cell types, it has been shown that a cross-talk exists between tubule and fibroblast cells, leading to reactions appearing solely when the two cell types were close-together [20]. However, when comparing the results of that study with findings observed using human renal tubule cells it emerges that rat cells obviously are more robust than the human cells concerning their reaction to treatment with a ubiquitous nephrotoxin, ochratoxin A (OTA) [7]. Therefore, a co-culture model consisting of human cells is necessary. We established such a model by using the human proximal tubule cell line HK2 and human fibroblasts. HK2 cells were grown on filter inserts and brought together with fibroblasts, grown on the bottom of a 6-well plate. After recording basic parameters as apoptosis and necrosis, we used this model to obtain initial data on the effect of ochratoxin A on the expression of some proteins and RNAs related to cell cycle, EMT, and cellular metabolism.

3.1. Cell Survival

Based on protein content, it seemed that neither OTA nor the culture-condition had a remarkable effect. However, the relationship between apoptosis and necrosis was shifted towards necrosis in both cell types when cells were cultured together. OTA is known to induce apoptosis in tubule cells [29] and to a lesser extend also in fibroblasts [7]. This is reflected also in the present results. Interestingly, the presence of the respective other cell type led to decreased apoptosis rates in both cell types but to enhanced LDH release. This is a first hint that already the presence of another cell type can influence cellular function and that the reaction of cells to a toxic substance can be different in co-culture compared to mono-culture.

3.2. Protein and RNA Expression

We extended our studies by the determination of protein and RNA expression of some exemplarily chosen proteins and the RNAs coding for them. As OTA was shown to influence cell cycle [21,30], the expression of CDKN1A/p21 was studied. According to the findings by Dubourg et.al [21], OTA led to an enhanced expression not only of *CDKN1A* mRNA but also of CDKN1A/p21 protein in tubule cells. In these cells, the presence of fibroblasts did not influence *CDKN1A* mRNA expression, whereas in fibroblasts a clear co-culture effect was visible with enhanced mRNA abundance only visible in co-culture. However, this increase in mRNA abundance was not completely mirrored by protein expression, suggesting further regulatory mechanisms. Cell cycle studies may be added to get a further insight into the impact on cell cycle. Cyclin-dependent kinase 2 (*CDK2*) was found to play a role in OTA-induced dysregulation of the cell cycle [21]. In tubule cells, its mRNA expression was enhanced by OTA in co-culture whereas fibroblasts were not influenced by tubule cells. Together, the results suggest that the cell cycle in tubule cells is influenced by the presence of fibroblasts.

Another co-culture effect was observed for the expression of *COX2* in fibroblasts. For fibroblasts the presence of tubule cells led to a clearly enhanced protein expression (similar to results observed in rat cells [20]), which was not visible for the tubule cells which did not show any culture-dependency. This indicates that the role of fibroblasts in inflammatory kidney diseases may have been underestimated by studies using fibroblasts in mono-culture.

The intermediate filament protein vimentin is constitutively expressed in fibroblasts and is increasingly expressed during epithelial-to-mesenchymal transition (EMT) in epithelial cells [10]. Although it has been shown that prolonged OTA exposure can lead to enhanced expression of collagen III or fibronectin in tubule cells [7], in the present study the expression of the EMT-indicating protein vimentin in tubule cells was even lower after OTA exposure, independent of culture conditions. In addition, the expression of fibronectin mRNA and protein was rather lower and not enhanced. Furthermore, in fibroblasts, no altered expression was demonstrable so that these findings do not argue in favor of an EMT induced by OTA, as shown by others [31].

To further test whether co culture can influence the cellular answer to stress induced by OTA, we determined the expression of some exemplarily chosen RNAs related to apoptosis-necrosis, cancer development and energy metabolism.

Long non-coding RNAs play a significant role in many cellular regulatory processes and their derailing, and also in renal fibrosis or cancer [32]. *WISP1-AS1* is a long non-coding RNA induced by OTA and expressed in renal tumor cells [24]. We found its upregulation by OTA in both cell types and co-culture enhanced the upregulation. This allows the aggravation of the effect of *WISP1-AS1* on the apoptosis-necrosis balance and probably tumor formation. The enhanced LDH release observed in co-culture can therefore at least partially be explained by the enhanced content of *WISP1-AS1*, which was shown to be necessary for OTA-induced necrosis [24].

WISP1-AS1 was also suspected to play a role in metabolism including mitochondria [24]. In gastric epithelium cells, OTA was shown to cause mitochondrial dysfunction [33]. For kidney cells, there are controversial results as to whether OTA exposure has an influence on mitochondrial potential or not [21,24]. A reduced mitochondrial potential might be the result of impaired mitochondria or might proceed mitochondrial damage. The reduced expression of mitochondrial proteins may lead to impaired function mirrored or followed by altered mitochondrial potential. Impaired mitochondrial function forces the cell to use alternative pathways to assure energy supply. Energy supply under inappropriate mitochondrial contribution can be maintained by an increased use of glycolysis leading to enhanced production of lactate. However, in HEK293 cells, a human embryonic kidney cell line, it was found that OTA led rather to a reduction of glycolysis and the enhanced amount of lactate due to lactate production from glutamine was dependent on the expression of the lncRNA *WISP1-AS1* [24]. In contrast, in gastric epithelia cells, it could be shown that OTA exposure leads to a reprogramming of glucose metabolism towards glycolysis and less tricarboxyic acid cycle activity [34]. We can show here that (1) OTA leads to a reduced mRNA expression of two representatively chosen mitochondrial proteins, which play a role in mitochondrial protein synthesis (*MRPS16*) and energy production (*NDUFB10*) and (2) that glycogen-handling enzymes were regulated in a way that enhanced glucose can be mobilized (*GYS1* down and *PYGM* up). Additionally, a higher GLUT1 transport capacity seems to be induced. However, these OTA-induced alterations were almost independent from culture conditions.

In conclusion, we have shown that under co-culture conditions, the reaction of the cells can be different from the reactions observed in mono-culture, although not all parameters studied here were culture-dependent. However, based on the findings presented here, the use of co-culture should be preferred if possible, thus avoiding the possibility to oversee the effects not taking place when solely one cell type is studied. The question remains of how the cells communicate between each other. Studies in a rat co-culture model revealed a COX2-dependent mechanism [20] and in mice, retinoic acid seems to participate in cellular cross-talk of kidney cells [35]. Additionally, the question remains, if, why and how OTA interferes with cellular energy metabolism and the role of mitochondria therein.

4. Materials and Methods

4.1. Cell Culture

Human proximal tubule cells and fibroblasts were purchased from ATCC (Rockville, MD, USA; HK2: CRL-2190 and CCD-1092SK:CRL-2114). Both were cultured in DMEM-HamF12 media (PAN Biotech, Aidenbach, Germany) containing 10% fetal calf serum. Media were changed every week. 24 h prior to and during OTA exposure, cells were held in serum-free media. For co-culture experiments, HK2 cells were seeded onto a filter (Falcon, Corning GmbH, Wiesbaden, Germany, pore size 0.4 µm) immersed in media in a 6-well-plate whereas fibroblasts were seeded on the well bottom of another 6-well plate. After reaching confluence (usually three days after seeding) the filter with the proximal tubule cells were placed into the well with the fibroblasts in serum-free media. The media volume was 2 mL on the basolateral side of the tubule cells and 900 µL apical. In monoculture, HK2 cells were seeded onto filters, which were further handled as in co-culture except that no fibroblasts were present.

4.2. Determination of LDH and Caspase-3 Activities and of Protein Content

For lysis, cells were washed twice in ice-cold PBS buffer, collected and lysed in MOPS-Triton buffer (20 mM 3-(N-morpholino)propanesulfonic acid, pH 7.4, 0.1% Triton X100). Protein content in cell lysates was determined using bicinchoninic acid [36,37]. LDH activity in media or cell lysates as a measure for necrosis was determined according to Bergmeyer [38] as described in detail in [20]. Caspase-3 activity as a measure for apoptosis was determined using the florigenic caspase-3 substrate (DEVD-AFC) as described in [39]. Briefly, 60 µL cell lysate was incubated with 65 µL reaction buffer (20 mmol/L piperazine-1,4-bis(2ethanesulfonic acid (PIPES), 4 mmol/L EDTA, 0.2% 3-[(3-cholaminopropyl)dimethylammonio]-1-propanesulfate (CHAPS), 10 mmol/L dithiotreitol (DTT), pH 7.4) containing 42 µmol/L DEVD-AFC (Asp-glu-val-asp-7-amino-4-trifluoromethylcoumarin, end-concentration) at 37 °C. Fluorescence of the cleaved product (AFC) was measured at 400 nm excitation and 505 nm emission. Cleaved AFC was quantified by a calibration curve using known AFC concentrations.

4.3. RT-PCR

Isolation of total ribonucleic acid (RNA) was performed using Trizol reagent (Life Technologies, Darmstadt, Germany). Cells were washed and thereafter lysed with Trizol reagent and transferred into a reaction tube. After addition of chloroform and centrifugation ($12,000 \times g$), the upper phase was collected and mixed with ice-cold isopropanol. After centrifugation ($12,000 \times g$) the supernatant was removed and the pellet washed twice with 75% ethanol and finally solved in water. Reverse transcription was performed using a commercial kit from Invitrogen (Thermo Fisher Scientific, Waltham, MA, USA) according to their instructions. Real-time PCR was performed using a SYBR Green reagent (Invitrogen). Primers were synthesized by Microsynth AG, Balgach, Switzerland. Primer sequences are shown in Table 1. Fold change of gene expression was calculated by the $2\Delta\Delta$Ct method using the expression of *EEF2* and *RPS17* as references. The expression of these two genes turned out to be the less altered ones (if at all) in RNA sequencing data when comparing OTA treated with non-treated HK2 cells (non-published results).

Table 1. Primer Sequences (in $5'$–$3'$) used in Real-time-PCR.

Gene Name	Forward	Reverse	Fragment Length
CDKN1A	ACTGTCTTGTACCCTTGTGC	CTCTTGGAGAAGATCAGCCG	144
CDK2	ATTCATGGATGCCTCTGCTC	TTTAAGGTCTCGGTGGAGGA	122
EEF2	GGAGTCGGGAGAGCATATCA	GGGTCAGATTTCTTGATGGG	108
FN	CCATAAAGGGCAACCAAGAG	AAACCAATTCTTGGAGCAGG	142
GDF15	CTCCAGATTCCGAGAGTTGC	CACTTCTGGCGTGAGTATCC	130
GYS1	TTCTACAACAACCTGGAG	CTGAGCAGATAGTTGAGC	404
NDUFB10	ATGATGAAAGCGTTCGACCT	TTGCACTCAGTGATGTCTGG	137
MRPS16	AGAAAAACTCGTTGCCCTCA	AGCAAGACCCAGAAGCTTTT	97
PYGM	TCAATGTCGGTGGCTACATC	CACCACGAAATACTCCTGCT	131
RPS17	TCAGCCTTGGATCAGGAGAT	CATCCCAACTGTAGGCTGAG	114
SLC2A1 (GLUT1)	ACACTGGAGTCATCAATGCC	ACACTGGAGTCATCAATGCC	148
VIM	ATTGCAGGAGGAGATGCTTC	TTCCACTTTGCGTTCAAGGT	112

4.4. Western Blots

After separation of the proteins by sodiumdodecylsulfate-polyacrylamide gel electrophoresis (SDS-PAGE), proteins were transferred onto a nitrocellulose membrane. Thereafter, free binding sites of the membrane were blocked by a 5% solution of non-fat dry milk in TRIS-buffered saline (3 mM TRIS base, 140 mM NaCl, 0.17 mM Tris-HCl, pH 7.4) containing 0.1% Tween20. The first antibodies diluted in TRIS saline + 5% bovine serum albumin (TRIS-BSA, for dilutions see Table 2) were added and membranes incubated overnight. After washing, fluorescence-coupled secondary antibodies in TRIS-BSA were added for 90 min. Fluorescence of the second antibodies was recorded using a LICOR detection system.

Table 2. Antibodies used in Western Blot Experiments.

Antibody Against	Source	Dilution
CDKN1A/p21	Cell Signaling	0.7361111
COX2	Abcam	0.3888889
Fibronectin	Rockland	0.7361111
VIM	Cell Signaling	0.7361111
Beta-Actin	Cell Signaling	0.7361111
Mouse antibody (2nd antibody)	Licor	1:40,000
Rabbit Antibody (2nd antibody)	Licor	1:40,000

4.5. Statistics

The significance of difference was determined by the unpaired Student's *t*-test. $p \leq 0.05$ was considered to be statistically significant and indicated by an * in the figures.

Supplementary Materials: The following are available online at https://www.mdpi.com/2072-6651/13/3/219/s1, File S1: Western Blot, RT-PCR, protein, LDH and caspase-3 raw data excel files.

Author Contributions: Conceptualization: G.S. and M.G.; Methodology: G.S., M.K., M.G.; Formal analysis: G.S., M.K., M.G.; Data Curation: M.K., G.S.; Writing: G.S. M.G.; Original Draft Preparation: G.S.; Supervision: G.S., M.G. All authors have read and agreed to the published version of the manuscript.

Funding: This research received no external funding.

Institutional Review Board Statement: Not applicable.

Informed Consent Statement: Not applicable.

Data Availability Statement: The data presented in this study are available in the Supplementary Materials.

Conflicts of Interest: The authors declare no conflict of interest.

References

1. Ferguson, M.A.; Vaidya, V.S.; Bonventre, J.V. Biomarkers of nephrotoxic acute kidney injury. *Toxicology* **2008**, *245*, 182–193. [CrossRef] [PubMed]
2. Hill, N.R.; Fatoba, S.T.; Oke, J.L.; Hirst, J.A.; O'Callaghan, C.A.; Lasserson, D.S.; Hobbs, F.D.R. Global prevalence of chronic kidney disease—A systematic review and meta-analysis. *PLoS ONE* **2016**, *11*, e0158765. [CrossRef] [PubMed]
3. Damiano, S.; Andretta, E.; Longobardi, C.; Prisco, F.; Paciello, O.; Squillacioti, C.; Mirabella, N.; Florio, S.; Ciarcia, R. Effects of curcumin on the renal toxicity induced by ochratoxin a in rats. *Antioxidants* **2020**, *9*, 332. [CrossRef] [PubMed]
4. Damiano, S.; Navas, L.; Lombari, P.; Montagnaro, S.; Forte, I.M.; Giordano, A.; Florio, S.; Ciarcia, R. Effects of δ-tocotrienol on ochratoxin A-induced nephrotoxicity in rats. *J. Cell Physiol.* **2018**, *233*, 8731–8739. [CrossRef]
5. Yang, X.; Liu, S.; Huang, C.; Wang, H.; Luo, Y.; Xu, W.; Huang, K. Ochratoxin A induced premature senescence in human renal proximal tubular cells. *Toxicology* **2017**, *382*, 75–83. [CrossRef]
6. Haugen, A.; Maehle, L.; Mollerup, S.; Rivedal, E.; Ryberg, D. Nickel-induced alterations in human renal epithelial cells. *Environ. Health Perspect.* **1994**, *102* (Suppl. 3), 117–118. [PubMed]
7. Schwerdt, G.; Holzinger, H.; Sauvant, C.; Königs, M.; Humpf, H.-U.; Gekle, M. Long-term effects of ochratoxin A on fibrosis and cell death in human proximal tubule or fibroblast cells in primary culture. *Toxicology* **2007**, *232*, 57–67. [CrossRef] [PubMed]
8. Tan, R.J.; Zhou, D.; Liu, Y. Signaling crosstalk between tubular epithelial cells and interstitial fibroblasts after Kidney Injury. *Kidney Dis.* **2016**, *2*, 136–144. [CrossRef] [PubMed]
9. Duarte, S.; Pena, A.; Lino, C. A review on ochratoxin A occurrence and effects of processing of cereal and cereal derived food products. *Food Microbiol.* **2010**, *27*, 187–198. [CrossRef]
10. Cruz-Solbes, A.S.; Youker, K. Epithelial to Mesenchymal Transition (EMT) and endothelial to mesenchymal transition (EndMT): Role and implications in kidney fibrosis. *Neurotransm. Interact. Cogn. Funct.* **2017**, *60*, 345–372. [CrossRef]
11. Panizo, S.; Martínez-Arias, L.; Alonso-Montes, C.; Cannata, P.; Martín-Carro, B.; Fernández-Martín, J.L.; Naves-Díaz, M.; Carrillo-López, N.; Cannata-Andía, J.B. Fibrosis in chronic kidney disease: Pathogenesis and consequences. *Int. J. Mol. Sci.* **2021**, *22*, 408. [CrossRef]
12. Malir, F.; Ostry, V.; Pfohl-Leszkowicz, A.; Malir, J.; Toman, J. Ochratoxin A: 50 Years of Research. *Toxins* **2016**, *8*, 191. [CrossRef]
13. Bui-Klimke, T.R.; Wu, F. Ochratoxin A and Human Health Risk: A Review of the Evidence. *Crit. Rev. Food Sci. Nutr.* **2015**, *55*, 1860–1869. [CrossRef]
14. Marin, S.; Ramos, A.; Cano-Sancho, G.; Sanchis, V. Mycotoxins: Occurrence, toxicology, and exposure assessment. *Food Chem. Toxicol.* **2013**, *60*, 218–237. [CrossRef]
15. Duarte, S.C.; Pena, A.; Lino, C.M. Ochratoxin A in Portugal: A Review to assess human exposure. *Toxins* **2010**, *2*, 1225–1249. [CrossRef] [PubMed]
16. Arce-López, B.; Lizarraga, E.; Vettorazzi, A.; González-Peñas, E. Human biomonitoring of mycotoxins in blood, plasma and serum in recent years: A Review. *Toxins* **2020**, *12*, 147. [CrossRef] [PubMed]
17. Pfohl-Leszkowicz, A.; Manderville, R.A. Ochratoxin A: An overview on toxicity and carcinogenicity in animals and humans. *Mol. Nutr. Food Res.* **2007**, *51*, 61–99. [CrossRef] [PubMed]
18. Barnett, L.M.A.; Cummings, B.S. Nephrotoxicity and renal pathophysiology: A contemporary perspective. *Toxicol. Sci.* **2018**, *164*, 379–390. [CrossRef] [PubMed]
19. Fuchs, R.; Peraica, M. Ochratoxin A in human kidney diseases. *Food Addit. Contam.* **2005**, *22*, 53–57. [CrossRef] [PubMed]
20. Schulz, M.-C.; Gekle, M.; Schwerdt, G. Epithelial-fibroblast cross talk aggravates the impact of the nephrotoxin ochratoxin A. *Biochim. Biophys. Acta Bioenergy* **2019**, *1866*, 118528. [CrossRef] [PubMed]
21. Dubourg, V.; Nolze, A.; Kopf, M.; Gekle, M.; Schwerdt, G. Weighted Correlation Network Analysis Reveals CDK2 as a regulator of a ubiquitous environmental toxin-induced cell-cycle arrest. *Cells* **2020**, *9*, 143. [CrossRef] [PubMed]

22. Rios, A.; Vargas-Robles, H.; Gámez-Méndez, A.M.; Escalante, B. Cyclooxygenase-2 and kidney failure. *Prostaglandins Other Lipid Mediat.* **2012**, *98*, 86–90. [CrossRef]
23. Guarino, M.; Tosoni, A.; Nebuloni, M. Direct contribution of epithelium to organ fibrosis: Epithelial-mesenchymal transition. *Hum. Pathol.* **2009**, *40*, 1365–1376. [CrossRef] [PubMed]
24. Polovic, M.; Dittmar, S.; Hennemeier, I.; Humpf, H.-U.; Seliger, B.; Fornara, P.; Theil, G.; Azinovic, P.; Nolze, A.; Köhn, M.; et al. Identification of a novel lncRNA induced by the nephrotoxin ochratoxin A and expressed in human renal tumor tissue. *Cell. Mol. Life Sci.* **2017**, *75*, 2241–2256. [CrossRef] [PubMed]
25. Desmedt, S.; Desmedt, V.; De Vos, L.; Delanghe, J.R.; Speeckaert, R.; Speeckaert, M.M. Growth differentiation factor 15: A novel biomarker with high clinical potential. *Crit. Rev. Clin. Lab. Sci.* **2019**, *56*, 333–350. [CrossRef] [PubMed]
26. De Cos, G.M.; Benito, H.A.; Garcia Unzueta, M.T.; Mazon, R.J.; Lopez Del Moral, C.C.; Perez Canga, J.L.; San Segundo, A.D.; Valero San, C.R.; Ruiz San Millan, J.C.; Rodrigo, C.E. Growth differentiation factor 15: A biomarker with high clinical po-tential in the evaluation of kidney transplant candidates. *J. Clin. Med.* **2020**, *9*, 4112. [CrossRef]
27. Fernandes, R. The controversial role of glucose in the diabetic kidney. *Porto Biomed. J.* **2021**, *6*, e113. [CrossRef] [PubMed]
28. Adeva-Andany, M.M.; Gonzalez-Lucon, M.; Donapetry-Garcia, C.; Fernandez-Fernandez, C.; Ameneiros-Rodriguez, E. Gly-cogen metabolism in humans. *BBA Clin.* **2016**, *5*, 85–100. [CrossRef]
29. Schwerdt, G.; Freudinger, R.; Mildenberger, S.; Silbernagl, S.; Gekle, M. The nephrotoxin ochratoxin A induces apoptosis in cultured human proximal tubule cells. *Cell Biol. Toxicol.* **1999**, *15*, 405–415. [CrossRef] [PubMed]
30. Çelik, D.A.; Gurbuz, N.; Toğay, V.A.; Özçelik, N. Ochratoxin A causes cell cycle arrest in G1 and G1/S phases through p53 in HK-2 cells. *Toxicon* **2020**, *180*, 11–17. [CrossRef]
31. Pyo, M.C.; Chae, S.A.; Yoo, H.J.; Lee, K.W. Ochratoxin A induces epithelial-to-mesenchymal transition and renal fibrosis through TGF-bete/Smad2/3 and Wnt1/beta-catenin signaling pathways in vitro and in vivo. *Arch. Toxicol.* **2020**, *94*, 3329–3342. [CrossRef]
32. Chen, H.; Fan, Y.; Jing, H.; Tang, S.; Zhou, J. Emerging role of lncRNAs in renal fibrosis. *Arch. Biochem. Biophys.* **2020**, *692*, 108530. [CrossRef]
33. Li, Q.; Dong, Z.; Lian, W.; Cui, J.; Wang, J.; Shen, H.; Liu, W.; Yang, J.; Zhang, X.; Cui, H. Ochratoxin A causes mitochondrial dysfunction, apoptotic and autophagic cell death and also induces mitochondrial biogenesis in human gastric epithelial cells. *Arch. Toxicol.* **2019**, *93*, 1141–1155. [CrossRef] [PubMed]
34. Wang, Y.; Zhao, M.; Cui, J.; Wu, X.; Li, Y.; Wu, W.; Zhang, X. Ochratoxin A induces reprogramming of glucose metabolism by switching energy metabolism from oxidative phosphorylation to glycolysis in human gastric epithelium GES-1 cells in vitro. *Toxicol. Lett.* **2020**, *333*, 232–241. [CrossRef]
35. Nakamura, J.; Sato, Y.; Kitai, Y.; Wajima, S.; Yamamoto, S.; Oguchi, A.; Yamada, R.; Kaneko, K.; Kondo, M.; Uchino, E.; et al. Myofibroblasts acquire retinoic acid–producing ability during fibroblast-to-myofibroblast transition following kidney injury. *Kidney Int.* **2019**, *95*, 526–539. [CrossRef] [PubMed]
36. Smith, P.; Krohn, R.; Hermanson, G.; Mallia, A.; Gartner, F.; Provenzano, M.; Fujimoto, E.; Goeke, N.; Olson, B.; Klenk, D. Measurement of protein using bicinchoninic acid. *Anal. Biochem.* **1985**, *150*, 76–85. [CrossRef]
37. Lane, R.D.; Federman, D.; Flora, J.L.; Beck, B.L. Computer-assisted determination of protein concentrations from dye-binding and bicinchoninic acid protein assays performed in microtiter plates. *J. Immunol. Methods* **1986**, *92*, 261–270. [CrossRef]
38. Bergmeyer, H.U.; Bernt, E. Laktat-Dehydrogenase. In *Methoden der Enzymatischen Analyse*, 3rd ed.; Bergmeyer, H.U., Ed.; Verlag Chemie: Weinheim, Germany, 1974; Volume 3, pp. 607–612.
39. Schwerdt, G.; Gordjani, N.; Benesic, A.; Freudinger, R.; Wollny, B.; Kirchhoff, A.; Gekle, M. Chloroacetaldehyde- and acrolein-induced death of human proximal tubule cells. *Pediatr. Nephrol.* **2005**, *21*, 60–67. [CrossRef] [PubMed]

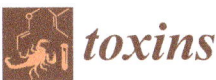

Article

Combining Patulin with Cadmium Induces Enhanced Hepatotoxicity and Nephrotoxicity In Vitro and In Vivo

Jinling Cui [1], Shutao Yin [1], Chong Zhao [1], Lihong Fan [2,*] and Hongbo Hu [1,*]

1. Beijing Advanced Innovation Center for Food Nutrition and Human Health, College of Food Science and Nutritional Engineering, Beijing Key Laboratory for Food Non-Thermal Processing, China Agricultural University, No.17 Qinghua East Road, Haidian District, Beijing 100083, China; cuijinling0420@cau.edu.cn (J.C.); yinshutao@cau.edu.cn (S.Y.); zhaoch0206@cau.edu.cn (C.Z.)
2. College of Veterinary Medicine, China Agricultural University, No.2 Yunamingyuan West Road, Haidian District, Beijing 100193, China
* Correspondence: flh@cau.edu.cn (L.F.); hongbo@cau.edu.cn (H.H.); Tel.: +86-10-6273-8653 (H.H.)

Abstract: Food can be contaminated by various types of contaminants such as mycotoxins and toxic heavy metals. Therefore, it is very likely that simultaneous intake of more than one type of food contaminant by consumers may take place, which provides a strong rationale for investigating the combined toxicities of these food contaminants. Patulin is one of the most common food-borne mycotoxins, whereas cadmium is a representative of toxic heavy metals found in food. The liver and kidneys are the main target organ sites for both patulin and cadmium. We hypothesized that simultaneous exposure to patulin and cadmium could produce synergistic hepatotoxicity and nephrotoxicity. Alpha mouse liver 12 (AML12) and Human embryonic kidney (HEK) 293 (HEK293) cell lines together with a mouse model were used to explore the combination effect and mechanism. The results demonstrated, for the first time, that the co-exposure of liver or renal cells to patulin and cadmium caused synergistic cytotoxicity in vitro and enhanced liver toxicity in vivo. The synergistic toxicity caused by the co-administration of patulin and cadmium was attributed to the boosted reactive oxygen species (ROS) generation. c-Jun N-terminal kinase 1 (JNK1) and p53 as downstream mediators of oxidative stress contributed to the synergistic toxicity by co-exposure of patulin and cadmium, while p53/JNK1 activation promoted the second-round ROS production through a positive feedback loop. The findings of the present study extend the toxicological knowledge about patulin and cadmium, which could be beneficial to more precisely perform risk assessments on these food contaminants.

Keywords: patulin; cadmium; synergistic toxicity; oxidative stress; JNK1; p53

Key Contribution: Co-administration of patulin and cadmium triggered a strong synergistic toxic consequence through increased oxidative stress. JNK1 and p53 as downstream mediators of oxidative stress contributed to the synergistic toxicity by co-exposure of patulin and cadmium.

1. Introduction

Food can be contaminated by various types of contaminants such as mycotoxins, toxic heavy metals, pesticides, veterinary drugs and illegal food additives. Therefore, it is very likely that simultaneous intake of more than one type of food contaminant by consumers may take place, which provides a strong rationale for investigating the combined toxicities of these food contaminants.

Patulin (PAT), which belongs to fungal secondary metabolites (mycotoxins), is a common contaminant of moldy fruits and products based on them [1]. Previous studies have demonstrated that patulin could produce a diverse range of adverse effects on animal and human health, including immunotoxicity, neurotoxicity, hepatotoxicity and nephrotoxicity [2]. Electrophilic patulin forming covalent adducts with glutathione (GSH) results in the generation of ROS, which is crucial to the induction of organ toxicity [3]. In addition, a number of signaling pathways such as mitogen-activated protein kinase (MAPK), p53, v-akt murine thymoma viral oncogene homolog (AKT) and endoplasmic reticulum stress have been identified to be involved in the toxicity of patulin [3–5].

Toxic heavy metals are another major type of food contaminants. Cadmium is one of the most common toxic heavy metals found in food. The toxicities of cadmium mainly include hepatotoxicity, nephrotoxicity, carcinogenicity, teratogenicity and reproductive toxicity [6]. Apoptosis induction in the target organs is considered to be a key event at the cellular level. Oxidative stress induction and MAPK activation have been suggested to contribute to cadmium-induced apoptosis [7,8].

As mentioned above, patulin and cadmium are often found in fruits and rice, respectively; therefore, it is possible that consumers are co-exposed to patulin and cadmium when the meal they eat contains patulin-contaminated fruits and cadmium-contaminated rice. The liver and kidneys are the main target organ sites for both patulin and cadmium. We hypothesized that simultaneous exposure to patulin and cadmium could produce synergistic hepatotoxicity and nephrotoxicity. In our study, this hypothesis was tested using both cell and mouse models.

2. Results

2.1. Combining PAT and $CdCl_2$ Causes a Synergistic Apoptosis Induction In Vitro

For the purpose of assessing the combined toxicity of PAT and cadmium chloride ($CdCl_2$), AML12 mouse liver cells and HEK293 human kidney cells were employed to examine the combined hepatocyte and nephrocyte toxicity, respectively. According to our preliminary dose range finding experiments, we chose dose levels of 2.5 to 4.5 µmol/L PAT and 12.5 to 22.5 µmol/L $CdCl_2$, which, by themselves, caused minimal or modest apoptosis in AML12 cells. As shown in Figure 1A, treatment with PAT or $CdCl_2$ individually induced a slight or modest, but dose-dependent, increase in apoptosis. However, co-treatment caused a significantly higher increase in cell death induction and cleavage of poly(ADP-ribose) polymerase (c-PARP) (Figure 1B). We wondered if the enhanced cell death was a synergistic action. Therefore, the data that the doses of each compound tested covered a range of toxicity from about 30% to 90% were processed to calculate the combination index (CI) using CompuSyn software (see Figure S1 in Supplementary Materials). The values of CI were lower than 1 for all combinations tested, suggesting that a synergistic effect did exist on AML12 cells by co-treatment with PAT/$CdCl_2$ (Figure 1C). For the combined nephrocyte toxicity, the dose levels of 2 to 4 µmol/L PAT and 1 to 2 µmol/L $CdCl_2$ were chosen in HEK293 cells based on the same criteria used for hepatocyte toxicity. As shown in Figure 1D–F and Figure S2 in Supplementary Materials, similar results were found in HEK293 cells. Together, these results indicate that combination of patulin and cadmium induced a synergistic hepatocyte and nephrocyte toxicity in vitro.

2.2. Synergistic Cell Death Caused by PAT and $CdCl_2$ Is Mitochondria-Mediated Caspase-Dependent Apoptosis

It was demonstrated that the mitochondrial pathway was activated in response to either patulin or cadmium [9,10]. To determine the contribution of the mitochondrial pathway to the synergistic cell death mediated by PAT and $CdCl_2$, we measured the levels of cell mitochondrial membrane potential (MMP) by treatment with each agent alone or their combination. The co-treatment caused a significant decrease in MMP, while the level was not significantly altered by either agent alone (Figure 2A). MMP is tightly regulated by b-cell lymphoma-2 (Bcl-2) family proteins. As expected, Bcl-2 interacting mediator of cell death (Bim), a pro-apoptotic Bcl-2 family protein, was upregulated by the combination of PAT and $CdCl_2$, followed by an obvious activation of caspase-9 (Figure 2B,C). These results suggest that the synergistic cell death induced by PAT and $CdCl_2$ is mitochondria-mediated caspase-dependent apoptosis.

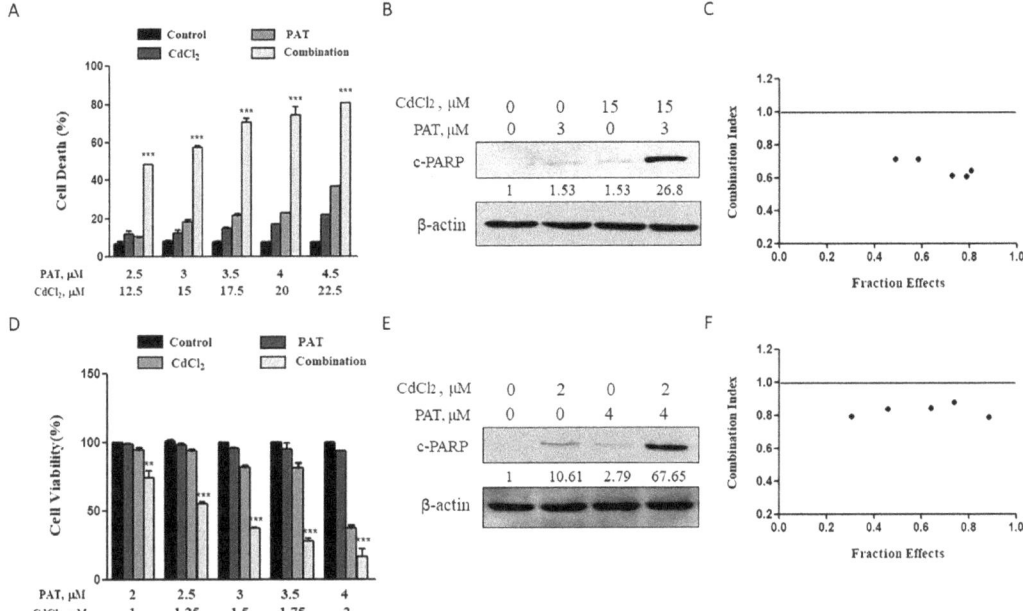

Figure 1. Synergistic effect in cell death can be induced by patulin (PAT) and cadmium chloride (CdCl$_2$) in AML12 and HEK293 cells. (**A**) Cell death caused by PAT with or without CdCl$_2$ in AML12 cells. Cells were incubated with PAT, CdCl$_2$ or both co-administered in a fixed ratio (1:5) for 24 h and cell death was measured. (**B**) Western blot showing the expression of c-PARP in AML12 cells. (**C**) The combination index (CI) was calculated using CompuSyn software. (**D**) Cell death caused by PAT with or without CdCl$_2$ in HEK293 cells. Cells were incubated with PAT, CdCl$_2$ or both co-administered in a fixed ratio (2:1) for 24 h and the cell number was measured. (**E**) Western blot showing the expression of c-PARP in HEK293 cells incubated with PAT and/or CdCl$_2$. (**F**) The combination index (CI) was calculated using CompuSyn software. $n = 3$, ** $P < 0.01$ and *** $P < 0.001$.

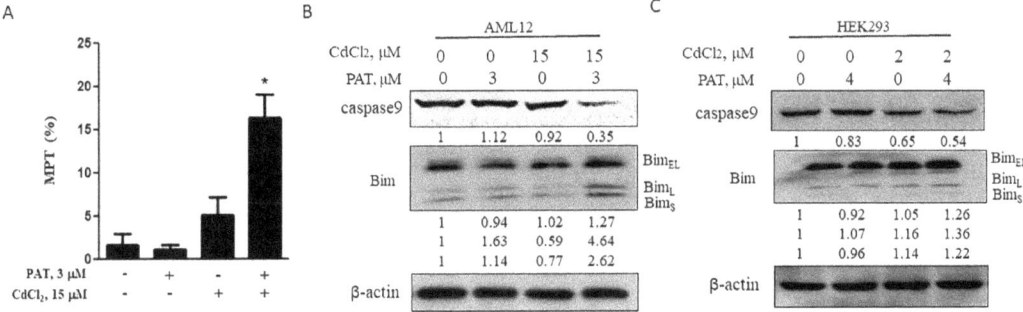

Figure 2. Synergistic cell death induced by PAT and CdCl$_2$ is mitochondria-mediated caspase-dependent apoptosis. (**A**) Effect of PAT/CdCl$_2$ co-administration on mitochondrial permeability transition (MPT) in AML12 cells. The cells were treated with PAT, CdCl$_2$ or their combination for 12 h and the MPT was detected by tetraethyl benzimidazolyl carbocyanine iodide (JC-1) staining. (**B**) Effect of PAT/CdCl$_2$ co-administration on mitochondria-mediated apoptosis. AML12 cells were incubated with PAT with or without CdCl$_2$ for 24 h, and then, Bim and caspase-9 were assessed. (**C**) Effect of PAT/CdCl$_2$ co-administration on mitochondria-mediated apoptosis. HEK293 cells were incubated with PAT with or without CdCl$_2$ for 24 h, and then, Bim and caspase-9 were assessed. $n = 3$, * $P < 0.05$.

2.3. Enhanced ROS Generation Plays a Critical Role in the Cell Death Caused by Co-Treatment with PAT and CdCl₂

It has been shown that ROS generation plays a key role in the cytotoxic effect induced by either patulin or cadmium [5,7]. We thus evaluated whether the co-treatment with PAT and $CdCl_2$ induced a synergistic effect on the level of ROS production. As shown in Figure 3A, combination of PAT and $CdCl_2$ induced a significant elevation of ROS compared with PAT or $CdCl_2$ treatment alone. To investigate the importance of increased ROS levels in the synergistic toxicity, we measured the influence of the ROS inhibitor Nacetyl-1-cysteine (NAC) on the cell death induction. As expected, treatment with NAC dramatically decreased the synergistic cell death caused by the co-administration (Figure 3B). These results demonstrate that the co-administration of patulin and cadmium boosted ROS generation, which, in turn, led to the synergistic cytotoxicity.

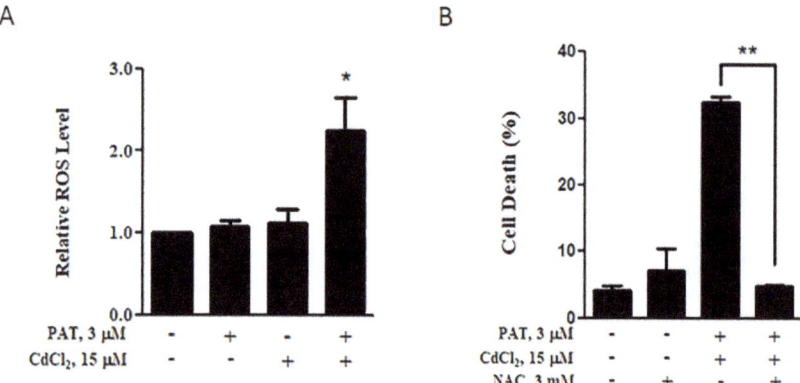

Figure 3. Increased ROS level induced by the co-administration of PAT and $CdCl_2$ in AML12 cells. (**A**) Effect of PAT/$CdCl_2$ co-administration on ROS level. Cells were incubated with PAT with or without $CdCl_2$ for 12 h, and ROS levels were detected using 2′,7′-Dichlorodihydrofluorescein diacetate (DCFH-DA). (**B**) Effect of Nacetyl-1-cysteine (NAC) on PAT/$CdCl_2$-induced cell death. Cells were incubated with a combination of PAT and $CdCl_2$ or the combination plus NAC for 24 h, and then, cell death was measured. $n = 3$, * $P < 0.05$ and ** $P < 0.01$.

2.4. p53 Contributes to the Synergistic Effect Induced by the Combination of PAT and CdCl₂

It was shown that activated p53 was involved in patulin- or cadmium-mediated toxicity [4,11,12]; therefore, we wondered if p53 was involved in the synergistic cytotoxicity induced by PAT and $CdCl_2$. The results showed that co-treatment with PAT and $CdCl_2$ increased the expression of p53 and p-JNK but reduced phosphor-extracellular regulated protein kinase (p-ERK) (Figure 4A). As shown in Figure 4B, pretreatment with NAC dramatically decreased the phosphorylation of p53 and JNK induced by the combination. Our previous study showed that p53 plays a pro-oxidant role by patulin treatment [4]. We next investigated the contribution of p53 to the enhanced oxidative stress by combining patulin with cadmium. Cell death induction was decreased in p53-/- mouse embryonic fibroblast (MEF) cells in comparison with that in p53+/+ MEF cells (Figure 4C). Consistent with the reduction in apoptosis, a decreased ROS level was detected in p53-/-MEF cells than that found in p53+/+ MEF cells (Figure 4D). The results indicate that p53 activation exerts a pro-oxidant function that leads to ROS generation by co-administration of PAT and $CdCl_2$.

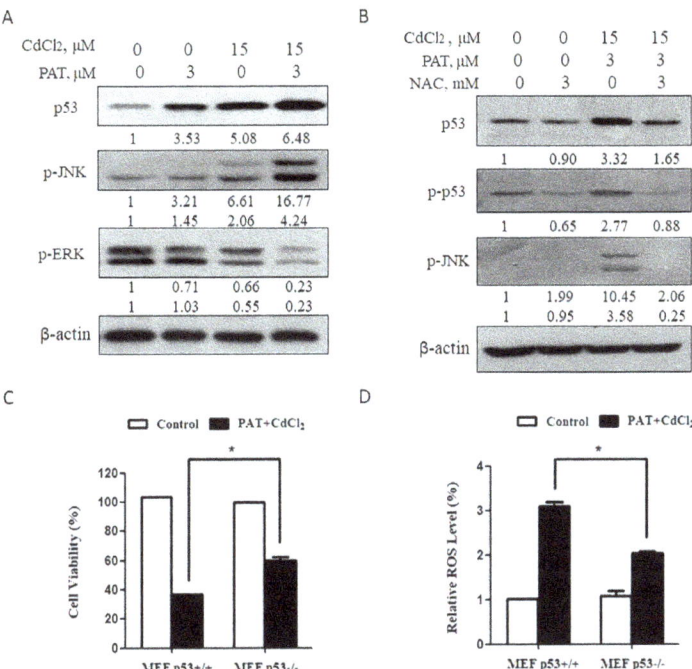

Figure 4. p53 contributes to the synergistic effect induced by the combination of PAT and CdCl$_2$. (**A**) Effect of the combination of PAT and CdCl$_2$ on p53 and MAPK pathway. Western blot showing the expression of p53, p-JNK and p-ERK in AML12 and HEK293 cells treated with PAT and/or CdCl$_2$. (**B**) Effect of NAC on PAT/CdCl$_2$-induced activation of p53 and JNK. AML12 cells were incubated with the combination of PAT and CdCl$_2$ or the combination plus NAC for 24 h, and then, p53, p-p53 and p-JNK were assessed. (**C**) Co-treatment of PAT and CdCl$_2$ induced growth inhibition in p53+/+ or p53-/- MEF cells. The cells were incubated with PAT and CdCl$_2$ for 24 h, and cell viability was measured. (**D**) ROS levels were detected in p53 knockout/wild-type MEF cells by co-treatment of PAT and CdCl$_2$. The cells were incubated with PAT and CdCl$_2$ for 12 h; then, the ROS levels were detected by using DCFH-DA. $n = 3$, * $P < 0.05$.

2.5. JNK1 Activation Contributes to the Synergistic Effect Caused by the Combination of PAT and CdCl$_2$

Having found p-JNK induction obviously by PAT/CdCl$_2$ combination, we used a JNK inhibitor to see if it protected against cell death as JNK exerted its pro-apoptotic function generally. As expected, the JNK1 inhibitor DB07268 reduced the combination-induced cell death significantly (Figure 5A). Consistent with the reduction in apoptosis, a significantly decreased ROS level was detected by pretreatment with DB07268 (Figure 5B). Meanwhile, the activation of p53 and Bim induced by the combination was nearly reduced to control level (Figure 5C). These results suggest a crucial role for JNK1 in the synergetic cell death induced by PAT and CdCl$_2$.

2.6. Combination of PAT and CdCl$_2$ Caused Hepatic and Renal Injury In Vivo

After investigating the toxicological mechanism of co-administration of PAT and CdCl$_2$ in vitro, we further validated these findings in vivo. The combination of PAT and CdCl$_2$ decreased the body weight of mice compared with PAT or CdCl$_2$ treatment alone (Figure 6A). Biochemical parameters of liver damage, serum alanine transaminase (ALT) and aspartate transaminase (AST) were significantly increased by the co-administration (Figure 6B,C). Acidophilic change was only found in PAT/CdCl$_2$ combination (Figure 6E), suggesting a severe liver injury compared with PAT or CdCl$_2$ treatment alone. The key kidney damage marker, serum urea, was increased significantly, suggesting a severe kidney injury induced by co-treatment with PAT and CdCl$_2$ (Figure 6F). Hematoxylin–eosin (H&E) staining showed that treatment with CdCl$_2$ resulted in mild tubule swelling and protein casts. The co-administration group showed serious tubule swelling, protein casts and infiltrate of neutrophil polymorphs (Figure 6G). Consistent with the change in protein expression in vitro, p53 and p-JNK were upregulated following co-administration of PAT and CdCl$_2$ in mice (Figure 6D).

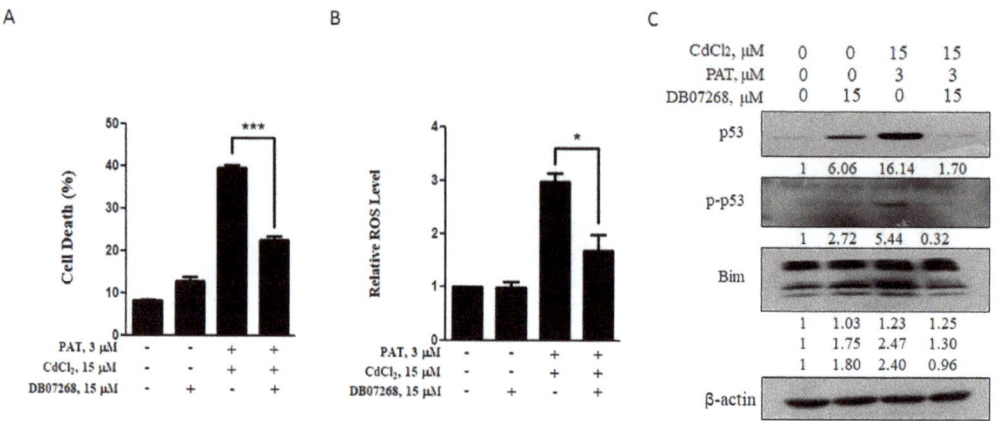

Figure 5. JNK1 inhibitor (DB07268) can rescue the synergistic effect caused by co-treatment with PAT and CdCl$_2$. (**A**) Effect of DB07268 on PAT/CdCl$_2$-induced cell death. The cells were treated with the combination of PAT and CdCl$_2$ or the combination plus DB07268 for 24 h, and then, cell death was measured. (**B**) Effect of DB07268 on PAT/CdCl$_2$-induced ROS generation. The cells were incubated with the combination of PAT and CdCl$_2$ or the combination plus DB07268 for 12 h, and ROS levels were detected by using DCFH-DA. (**C**) Effect of DB07268 on activation of p53 and Bim induced by PAT and CdCl$_2$. AML12 cells were incubated with the combination of PAT and CdCl$_2$ or the combination plus DB07268 for 24 h, and then, p53, p-p53 and Bim were measured by Western blotting. $n = 3$, * $P < 0.05$ and *** $P < 0.001$.

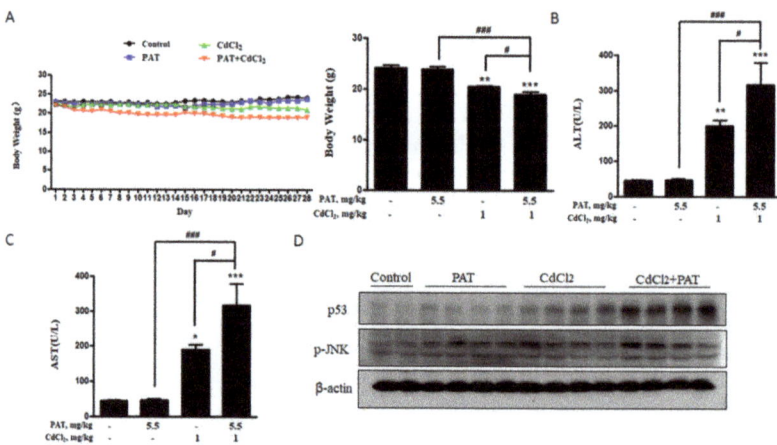

Figure 6. Cont.

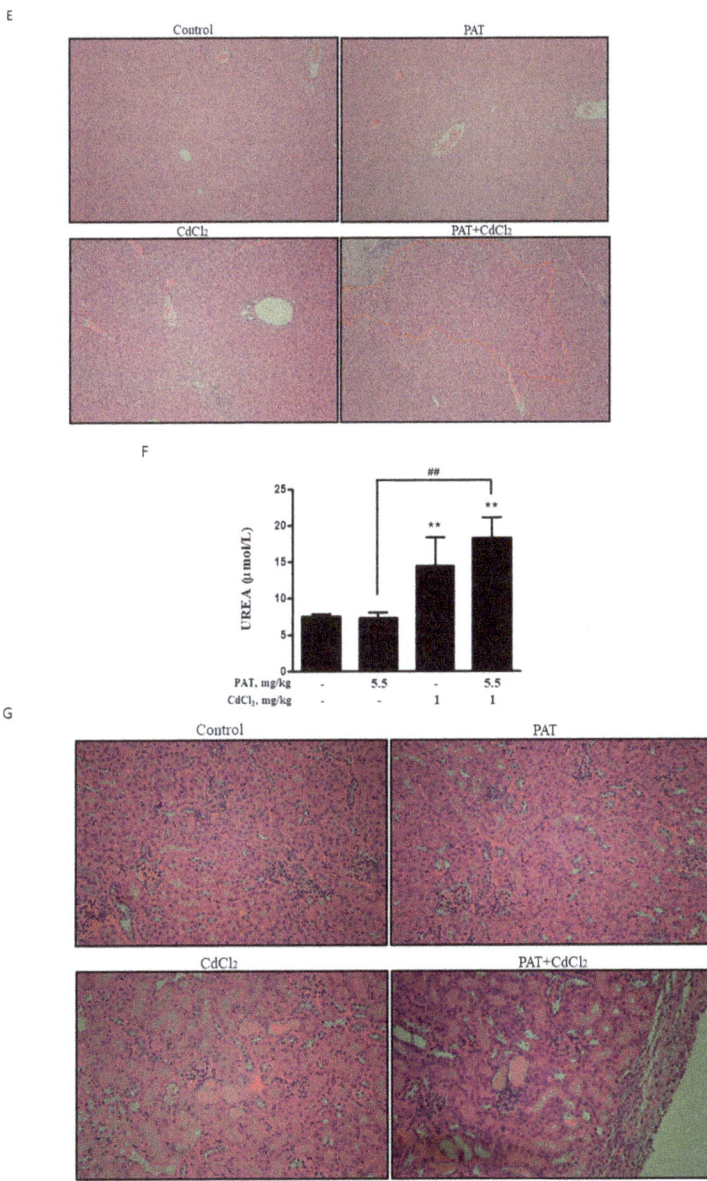

Figure 6. Combination of PAT and CdCl$_2$ causes liver and kidney damage in vivo. (**A**) Body weight of mice. (**B**,**C**) Effects of PAT and/or CdCl$_2$ on serum alanine transaminase (ALT) and aspartate transaminase (AST). (**D**) Western blot showing the effects of PAT and/or CdCl$_2$ on p53 and p-JNK of liver tissues. (**E**) Liver pathological damage caused by PAT and/or CdCl$_2$ combination as measured by hematoxylin–eosin (H&E) staining of sections of liver tissues. (**F**) Effects of PAT and/or CdCl$_2$ on serum urea. (**G**) Kidney pathological injury caused by PAT and/or CdCl$_2$ as assessed by H&E staining of sections of kidney tissues. $n = 5$, "*" represents the significance compared with control group, where * $P < 0.05$, ** $P < 0.01$ and *** $P < 0.001$. "#" represents the significance compared between cotreatment of PAT and CdCl$_2$ with PAT or CdCl$_2$ treatment alone. # $P < 0.05$, ## $P < 0.01$ and ### $P < 0.001$.

3. Discussion

Previously, toxicological evaluation of food contaminants was generally performed under a single exposure setting. Recently, the combined toxic effect of food contaminants has drawn increasing attention due to the fact that consumers are often exposed not to a single contaminant but to a combination of contaminants. However, most of the studies have focused on the interaction among same the class of food contaminants such as the combined toxicity of mycotoxins [13,14] or the combined toxicity of heavy metals [15,16]. Due to the co-occurrence of mycotoxins in food, co-exposure to mycotoxins was considered a severe issue. Studies have elucidated the toxicological interactions between them. Patulin and ochratoxin A induced a synergistic effect at low doses but antagonistic action at higher levels [13]. The toxicity, higher than additive toxicity, was induced by citrinin and patulin when combined with ochratoxin A or ochratoxin B in Lilly Laboratories cell porcine kidney 1 (LLC-PK1) cells [17]. As, Cd and Pb induced synergistic action in glial and neuronal functions [18]. The combination of cadmium and molybdenum caused synergistic toxicity through mitochondria-mediated oxidative stress and apoptosis [19]. However, data on the combined toxicity of different types of food contaminants are rarely available. Given the possibility that consumers are often exposed to multiple types of contaminants, investigations on the toxicological interactions among different types of food contaminants are clearly needed, especially for contaminants that share the same toxic target organs. Patulin is one of the most common food-borne mycotoxins, whereas cadmium is a representative of toxic heavy metals found in food. The toxicities of single exposure have been well documented, and hepatotoxicity and nephrotoxicity are the major adverse effects of either patulin or cadmium [2,6,20]. The present study moved from single exposure to combined exposure, and the results demonstrated, for the first time, that the co-exposure of liver or renal cells to patulin and cadmium caused synergistic cytotoxicity in vitro and enhanced hepatotoxicity in vivo. The findings of our results extend the toxicological knowledge about patulin or cadmium, which could be beneficial to more precisely perform risk assessment on these food contaminants.

It was reported that patulin has a strong affinity for SH groups due to its electrophilic attribute [21,22], which was proven by the research showing that patulin induced a significant decrease in GSH activity by forming an adduct with SH groups [23]. In addition, a disrupted cellular GSH system contributes to ROS formation, which is suggested to play a critical role in cadmium-induced toxicity [24]. We speculated that the synergistic cytotoxicity caused by co-administration of patulin and cadmium was probably attributed to augmented ROS generation. Indeed, the results showed that a significantly elevated ROS level was induced in response to the co-occurrence in comparison with exposure to each agent alone, whereas suppression of ROS by an antioxidant abolished the combination-induced cell death. The data clearly support our hypothesis. To decipher the downstream signaling pathway that contributed to the combination-induced ROS-mediated cytotoxicity, a number of apoptosis-related molecules were analyzed, and the results demonstrated that an enhanced phosphorylation of p53 and JNK was detected in the combination-treated cells compared with that found in the treatment with either agent alone. Inhibition of ROS led to abolishment of the activation of p53 and JNK, while inhibiting JNK1 activation resulted in inactivating p53. The functional role of p53 or JNK was further validated by p53 knockout/wild-type MEF cell system or JNK1 inhibitor. In addition, inhibiting either JNK1 or p53 caused significant attenuation of the combination-induced ROS generation. These results together indicate that increased activation of the ROS-JNK1-p53 axis contributed to the synergistic toxicity caused by co-administration of patulin and cadmium, while p53/JNK1 activation promoted the second-round ROS generation through a positive feedback loop. In our finding, the combination of patulin and cadmium activated Bim, with obvious increased L and S subunits but little change to the EL subunit. As demonstrated in a previous study, L and S subunits of Bim are more potent inducers of cell death than the EL subunit [25]. We also found that ERK phosphorylation was decreased by the combination. ERK has been reported to mediate the phosphorylation and degradation of Bim [26]. The decrease in p-ERK might be one of the reasons for Bim upregulation by co-administration of patulin and cadmium. Collectively, the data provided a mechanistic explanation for the synergistically toxic interaction between patulin and cadmium.

4. Conclusions

In summary, the present study demonstrated that co-administration of patulin and cadmium triggered a strong synergistic toxic consequence through increased oxidative stress. JNK1 and p53 as downstream mediators of oxidative stress contributed to the synergistic toxicity by co-exposure of patulin and cadmium. The findings implied that the combined toxicity should be taken into account when performing risk assessments for the presence of patulin and cadmium in food.

5. Materials and Methods

5.1. Chemicals and Reagents

Patulin (PAT), cadmium chloride ($CdCl_2$), Nacetyl-1-cysteine (NAC) and 2′,7′-Dichlorodihydrofluorescein diacetate (DCFH-DA) were purchased from Sigma-Aldrich (St. Louis, MO, USA.). DB07268 was purchased from Med Chem Express (Danvers, MA, USA.). Antibodies specific for cleaved PARP (9532), p53(2524), p-p53(9284), p-JNK (9251), p-ERK (9101), caspase-9 (9508), Bim (2933) and β-actin were purchased from Cell Signaling Technology (Beverly, MA, USA.). PAT (10 mg) was dissolved in 1.3 mL ultrapure water to make it a 50-mM solution. PAT (2 mM) was obtained by mixing 100 μL PAT (10 mM) with 400 μL ultrapure water. $CdCl_2$ (18 mg) was dissolved in 1.23 mL ultrapure water to make it a 80-mM solution. $CdCl_2$ (10 mM) was obtained by mixing 100 μL $CdCl_2$ (80 mM) with 700 μL ultrapure water. $CdCl_2$ (1 mM) was obtained by mixing 50 μL $CdCl_2$ (10 mM) with 450 μL ultrapure water.

5.2. Cell Culture and Treatments

AML12 cells were obtained from the American Type Culture Collection (ATCC), which were cultured in Dulbecco's Modified Eagle Medium (DMEM)/F12 medium (HyClone, Logan, UT, USA) with 1% insulin transferrin selenium (ITS) and supplemented with 10% fetal bovine serum. HEK293 and MEF cells were obtained from ATCC, which were cultured in Dulbecco's Modified Eagle Medium (DMEM) (HyClone, Logan, UT, USA) supplemented with 10% fetal bovine serum. After plating for 24 h, the cultured cells were grown to 50% confluence. Then, the medium was aspirated, and the treatment with different agents was given.

5.3. Apoptosis Evaluation

Treated cells were analyzed by flow cytometry after staining with Annexin V and PI (MBL International Corporation, Boston, MA, USA) for 30 min. The second method was immunoblot analysis of PARP cleavage.

5.4. Crystal Violet Staining

After treatment, the medium was removed and 1% glutaraldehyde solution was added to fix the cells for 15 min. After washing with phosphate buffer saline (PBS), the cells were stained with a 0.02% crystal violet solution for 30 min. After air-drying, 70% ethanol was added for solubilization. The absorbance at 570 nm was examined using a microplate reader with a 405-nm reference filter.

5.5. Western Blotting

Cells were lysed with radio-immuno-precipitation assay (RIPA) buffer containing protease inhibitor. The denatured proteins were loaded onto the gel and assessed by SDS-PAGE electrophoresis. After transferring onto a nitrocellulose membrane, the membrane was incubated with primary antibodies followed by the corresponding secondary antibody. The blots were recorded on X-ray film using enhanced chemiluminescence. The quantification of Western blot can be found in Figure S3.

5.6. Measurement of ROS

Cells were incubated with PAT (3 μM) and/or $CdCl_2$ (15 μM) for 12 h. Thirty minutes before harvesting the cells, free medium containing DCFH-DA (20 μM) was added. After washing with PBS, the cells were harvested and resuspended. The fluorescent dichlorodihydrofluorescein (DCF) was examined using a flow cytometer.

5.7. Measurement of MMP

Cells were incubated with PAT (3 μM) and/or $CdCl_2$ (15 μM) for 12 h. Mitochondrial membrane potential (MMP) was analyzed by flow cytometry after staining with JC-1 according to the manufacturer's instructions (JC-1 kit, Solarbio Life Science, Beijing, China).

5.8. Combination Index Calculation

The synergistic effects between PAT and $CdCl_2$ were analyzed by calculating the combination index (*CI*) using CompuSyn 2.0 software (CompuSyn, Paramus, NJ, USA). The cells were incubated with various concentrations of PAT, $CdCl_2$ and their combination, and the total inhibitory effect was assessed by cell viability or cell death (see Figures S1 and S2 in Supplementary Materials). $CI < 1$, $CI = 1$ and $CI > 1$ indicate synergism, additive effect and antagonism, respectively.

5.9. Animals and Treatments

Male C57BL/6N mice weighing 20.5 ± 1.0 g were purchased from Vital River (Beijing, China) and were employed in the present study. The mice received a commercial standard mouse cube diet (Beijing Keaoxieli Feed Company, China). After acclimatization, the mice were randomly divided into 4 groups ($n = 5$): Control group, PAT group (5.5 mg/kg/i.g.), $CdCl_2$ group (1 mg/kg/i.p.) and combination group. The mice were administrated with agents every day for 27 d continuously. Male mice and the doses were chosen according to previous toxicological studies of PAT or $CdCl_2$. The mice were sacrificed 24 h after the last administration for the collection of plasma, liver and kidney tissues. Sera received from centrifugal plasma were stored at -80 °C. Except for fixing in neutral buffered formalin for H&E staining, liver and kidney tissues were stored at -80 °C for Western blotting.

5.10. Biochemical Assay

Serum levels of ALT, AST and urea were measured according to the manufacturer's instructions (Nanjing Jiancheng Institute of Biotechnology, Nanjing, China).

5.11. Histopathology

Fixed liver and kidney tissues were processed to 5-μm thick paraffin sections and stained with hematoxylin and eosin (H&E).

5.12. Statistical Analysis

The results were obtained three times and data were presented as mean ± standard deviation (SD). The data were evaluated using a one-way ANOVA followed by Tukey's post-hoc test. $P < 0.05$ was considered statistically significant.

Supplementary Materials: The following are available online at https://www.mdpi.com/2072-6651/13/3/221/s1, Figure S1: CompuSyn report—AML12, Figure S2: CompuSyn report—HEK293, Figure S3: Quantification of Western blot.

Author Contributions: Conceptualization, H.H.; methodology, J.C.; investigation, J.C.; data analysis, J.C., S.Y. and C.Z.; writing—original draft preparation, J.C.; writing—review and editing, H.H., S.Y. and L.F.; supervision, H.H. All authors have read and agreed to the published version of the manuscript.

Funding: This study was funded by the National Key Research and Development Program, 2018YFC1603706.

Institutional Review Board Statement: This study was approved by the Institutional Animal Care and Use Committee of China Agricultural University (approval code: AW62010202-4; approval date: 26 October 2020).

Informed Consent Statement: Not applicable.

Data Availability Statement: Data is contained within the article or supplementary material.

Conflicts of Interest: The authors declare no conflict of interest.

References

1. Puel, O.; Galtier, P.; Oswald, I.P. Biosynthesis and Toxicological Effects of Patulin. *Toxins* **2010**, *2*, 613–631. [CrossRef] [PubMed]
2. Pal, S.; Singh, N.; Ansari, K.M. Toxicological effects of patulin mycotoxin on the mammalian system: An overview. *Toxicol. Res.* **2017**, *6*, 764–771. [CrossRef] [PubMed]
3. Liu, B.H.; Wu, T.S.; Yu, F.Y.; Wang, C.H. Mycotoxin patulin activates the p38 kinase and JNK signaling pathways in human embryonic kidney cells. *Toxicol. Sci.* **2006**, *89*, 423–430. [CrossRef] [PubMed]
4. Jin, H.; Yin, S.; Song, X.; Zhang, E.; Fan, L.; Hu, H. 53 activation contributes to patulin-induced nephrotoxicity via modulation of reactive oxygen species generation. *Sci. Rep.* **2016**, *13*, 24455. [CrossRef] [PubMed]
5. Manel, B.; Intidhar, B.S.; Alexandre, P.; Arnaud, G.; Hassen, B.; Salwa, A.E.; Christophe, L. Patulin induces apoptosis through ROS-mediated endoplasmic reticulum stress pathway. *Toxicol. Sci.* **2015**, *144*, 328–337. [CrossRef]
6. Thévenod, F.; Lee, W.K. Toxicology of Cadmium and Its Damage to Mammalian Organs. *Met. Ions Life Sci.* **2013**, *11*, 415–490. [CrossRef] [PubMed]
7. Zhang, J.; Zheng, S.; Wang, S.; Liu, Q.; Xu, S. Cadmium-induced oxidative stress promotes apoptosis and necrosis through the regulation of the miR-216a-PI3K/AKT axis in common carp lymphocytes and antagonized by selenium. *Chemosphere* **2020**, *258*, 127341. [CrossRef]
8. Chuang, S.M.; Wang, I.C.; Yang, J.L. Roles of JNK, p38 and ERK mitogen-activated protein kinases in the growth inhibition and apoptosis induced by cadmium. *Carcinogenesis* **2000**, *21*, 1423–1432. [CrossRef] [PubMed]
9. Wu, T.S.; Liao, Y.C.; Yu, F.Y.; Chang, C.H.; Liu, B.H. Mechanism of patulin-induced apoptosis in human leukemia cells (HL-60). *Toxicol. Lett.* **2009**, *183*, 105–111. [CrossRef]
10. Cao, X.; Fu, M.; Bi, R.; Zheng, X.; Fu, B.; Tian, S.; Liu, C.; Li, Q.; Liu, J. Cadmium induced BEAS-2B cells apoptosis and mitochondria damage via MAPK signaling pathway. *Chemosphere* **2021**, *263*, 128346. [CrossRef]
11. Lee, J.Y.; Tokumoto, M.; Fujiwara, Y.; Hasegawa, T.; Seko, Y.; Shimada, A.; Satoh, M. Accumulation of p53 via down-regulation of UBE2D family genes is a critical pathway for cadmium-induced renal toxicity. *Sci. Rep.* **2016**, *25*, 21968. [CrossRef] [PubMed]
12. Son, Y.O.; Lee, J.C.; Hitron, J.A.; Pan, J.; Zhang, Z.; Shi, X. Cadmium induces intracellular Ca^{2+}- and H_2O_2-dependent apoptosis through JNK- and p53-mediated pathways in skin epidermal cell line. *Toxicol. Sci.* **2010**, *113*, 127–137. [CrossRef]
13. Assunção, R.; Pinhão, M.; Loureiro, S.; Alvito, P.; Silva, M.J. A multi-endpoint approach to the combined toxic effects of patulin and ochratoxin a in human intestinal cells. *Toxicol. Lett.* **2019**, *313*, 120–129. [CrossRef] [PubMed]
14. Ruiz, M.J.; Macáková, P.; Juan-García, A.; Font, G. Cytotoxic effects of mycotoxin combinations in mammalian kidney cells. *Food Chem. Toxicol.* **2011**, *49*, 2718–2724. [CrossRef] [PubMed]
15. Matović, V.; Buha, A.; Đukić-Ćosić, D.; Bulat, Z. Insight into the oxidative stress induced by lead and/or cadmium in blood, liver and kidneys. *Food Chem. Toxicol.* **2015**, *78*, 130–140. [CrossRef]
16. Dai, X.; Xing, C.; Cao, H.; Luo, J.; Wang, T.; Liu, P.; Guo, X.; Hu, G.; Zhang, C. Alterations of mitochondrial antioxidant indexes and apoptosis in duck livers caused by Molybdenum or/and cadmium. *Chemosphere* **2018**, *193*, 574–580. [CrossRef]
17. Heussner, A.H.; Dietrich, D.R.; O' Brien, E. In vitro investigation of individual and combined cytotoxic effects of ochratoxin A and other selected mycotoxins on renal cells. *Toxicol. In Vitro* **2006**, *20*, 332–333. [CrossRef]
18. Rai, A.; Maurya, S.K.; Khare, P.; Srivastava, A.; Bandyopadhyay, S. Characterization of developmental neurotoxicity of As, Cd, and Pb mixture: Synergistic action of metal mixture in glial and neuronal functions. *Toxicol. Sci.* **2010**, *118*, 586–601. [CrossRef] [PubMed]
19. Wang, C.; Nie, G.; Yang, F.; Chen, J.; Zhuang, Y.; Dai, X.; Liao, Z.; Yang, Z.; Cao, H.; Xing, C.; et al. Molybdenum and cadmium co-induce oxidative stress and apoptosis through mitochondria-mediated pathway in duck renal tubular epithelial cells. *J. Hazard. Mater.* **2020**, *383*, 121157. [CrossRef] [PubMed]
20. Rinaldi, M.; Micali, A.; Marini, H.; Adamo, E.B.; Puzzolo, D.; Pisani, A.; Trichilo, V.; Altavilla, D.; Squadrito, F.; Minutoli, L. Cadmium, Organ Toxicity and Therapeutic Approaches: A Review on Brain, Kidney and Testis Damage. *Curr. Med. Chem.* **2017**, *24*, 3879–3893. [CrossRef] [PubMed]
21. Fliege, R.; Metzler, M. Electrophilic properties of patulin. N-acetylcysteine and glutathione adducts. *Chem. Res. Toxicol.* **2000**, *13*, 373–381. [CrossRef] [PubMed]
22. Fliege, R.; Metzler, M. The mycotoxin patulin induces intra- and intermolecular protein crosslinks in vitro involving cysteine, lysine, and histidine side chains, and alpha-amino groups. *Chem. Biol. Interact.* **1999**, *123*, 85–103. [CrossRef]

23. Mahfoud, R.; Maresca, M.; Garmy, N.; Fantini, J. The mycotoxin patulin alters the barrier function of the intestinal epithelium: Mechanism of action of the toxin and protective effects of glutathione. *Toxicol. Appl. Pharmacol.* **2002**, *181*, 209–218. [CrossRef] [PubMed]
24. Liu, J.; Qian, S.Y.; Guo, Q.; Jiang, J.; Waalkes, M.P.; Mason, R.P.; Kadiiska, M.B. Cadmium generates reactive oxygen- and carbon-centered radical species in rats: Insights from in vivo spin-trapping studies. *Free Radic. Biol. Med.* **2008**, *45*, 475–481. [CrossRef]
25. O' Connor, L.; Strasser, A.; O' Reilly, L.A.; Hausmann, G.; Adams, J.M.; Cory, S.; Huang, D.C. Bim: A novel member of the Bcl-2 family that promotes apoptosis. *EMBO J.* **1998**, *17*, 384–395. [CrossRef]
26. Kennedy, D.; Mnich, K.; Oommen, D.; Chakravarthy, R.; Almeida-Souza, L.; Krols, M.; Saveljeva, S.; Doyle, K.; Gupta, S.; Timmerman, V.; et al. HSPB1 facilitates ERK-mediated phosphorylation and degradation of BIM to attenuate endoplasmic reticulum stress-induced apoptosis. *Cell Death Dis.* **2017**, *8*, e3026. [CrossRef]

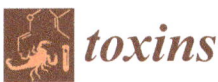

Review

Zearalenone and the Immune Response

Cristina Valeria Bulgaru [1,2], Daniela Eliza Marin [1,*], Gina Cecilia Pistol [1] and Ionelia Taranu [1,*]

[1] Laboratory of Animal Biology, National Institute of Research and Development for Biology and Animal Nutrition, 077015 Balotesti, Romania; cristina.bulgaru@ibna.ro (C.V.B.); gina.pistol@ibna.ro (G.C.P.)
[2] Faculty of Biology, University of Bucharest, Splaiul Independentei 91-95, R-050095 Bucharest, Romania
* Correspondence: daniela.marin@ibna.ro (D.E.M.); ionelia.taranu@ibna.ro (I.T.)

Abstract: Zearalenone (ZEA) is an estrogenic fusariotoxin, being classified as a phytoestrogen, or as a mycoestrogen. ZEA and its metabolites are able to bind to estrogen receptors, 17β-estradiol specific receptors, leading to reproductive disorders which include low fertility, abnormal fetal development, reduced litter size and modification at the level of reproductive hormones especially in female pigs. ZEA has also significant effects on immune response with immunostimulatory or immunosuppressive results. This review presents the effects of ZEA and its derivatives on all levels of the immune response such as innate immunity with its principal component inflammatory response as well as the acquired immunity with two components, humoral and cellular immune response. The mechanisms involved by ZEA in triggering its effects are addressed. The review cited more than 150 publications and discuss the results obtained from in vitro and in vivo experiments exploring the immunotoxicity produced by ZEA on different type of immune cells (phagocytes related to innate immunity and lymphocytes related to acquired immunity) as well as on immune organs. The review indicates that despite the increasing number of studies analyzing the mechanisms used by ZEA to modulate the immune response the available data are unsubstantial and needs further works.

Keywords: zearalenone; metabolites; innate immunity; cell immunity; humoral immunity

Key Contribution: The review presents the results obtained from in vitro and in vivo experiments exploring the ZEA and its metabolites effects on the immune response and propose some mechanisms responsible for the immunotoxicity produced by the toxin in the immune cells.

1. Introduction

Fusariotoxins are secondary metabolites originate from fungi of the *Fusarium* and *Gibberella* species which represent the largest group of mycotoxins (more than 140). Of these the most widespread and also of primary concern are the trichothecenes, fumonisins, and zearalenone [1,2]. Despite the mitigation efforts, exposure of crops to mycotoxins is indeed inevitable and decontamination is very difficult [3,4]. Even though numerous studies concerning the effect of mycotoxins are reported in the specific literature, the contamination of cereals with fusariotoxins, the impact on animal health and the economic losses they imply [5–7], the transmission of fusariotoxins into the target organism and the potential existence of toxic components in meat and dairy products remain unknown and need further investigations [8].

Zearalenone (ZEA) is a fusariotoxin that belongs to the class of xenoestrogens due to its structural similarity to 17β-estradiol (Figure 1), but also due to the binding affinity to estrogen receptors [9]. It is a resorcyclic acid lactone [10], produced by *Fusarium graminearum*, *Fusarium cerealis*, *Fusarium semitectum*, *Fusarium culmorum* and *Fusarium equiseti* [11] which binds to estrogen receptors in mammalians target cells leading to reproductive disorders especially in female pigs [12]. In terms of physicochemical properties, ZEA has been shown to have high stability, being resistant to high temperatures and UV radiation, making it almost impossible to decontaminate crops on a large scale [13].

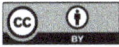

ZEA is metabolized mainly at the intestinal and hepatic level and transformed in several metabolites by hydroxylation, glucuronidation or conjugation reactions [14]. Biotransformation of ZEA lead primarily to the formation of two metabolites, α-zearalenol (α-ZOL) and β-zearalenol (β-ZOL) which can be further reduced to α-zearalanol (α-ZAL) and β-zearalanol (β-ZAL) [15].

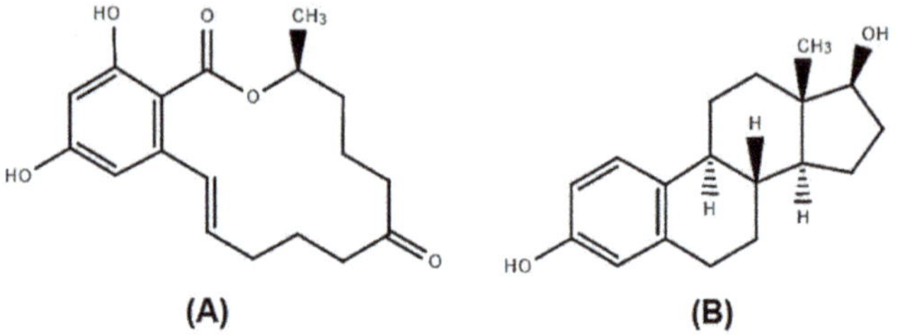

Figure 1. Chemical structures of Zearalenone (ZEA) (**A**) and 17β-estradiol (**B**).

After oral contamination, zearalenone is rapidly absorbed in mammals (rabbits, rats, humans and pigs, 80–85%) [16,17]. As mentioned above, structurally, ZEA has a strong similarity with 17 β-estradiol, and is able to bind to estrogen receptors, being also classified as a phytoestrogen, or as a mycoestrogen [18]. From this reason ZEA intoxication most often leads to disorders of the reproductive system. The changes involve low fertility, abnormal fetal development, reduce litter size and modification in the level of specific reproductive hormones: Estradiol and progesterone [19]. But, ZEA manifests its toxicity on many other systems besides the reproductive one. Studies show that the liver and spleen are also affected when exposed to this mycotoxin. It has been demonstrated in an experiment on female piglets that excessive amounts of ZEA raises the key liver enzymes level such as glutathione peroxidase and decreases spleen weight [20]. ZEA exerts significant effects on immune response, the major defense mechanism against pathogens, toxins and other antigens in all mammals with immunostimulatory or immunosuppressive results [21]. The cellular mechanisms activated by zearalenone in triggering its different effects are not yet well understood.

This review presents the effect of ZEA and its derivatives on all levels of the immune response such as innate immunity with its principal component inflammatory response as well as the acquired immunity with two components, humoral and cellular immune response. The mechanisms involved by ZEA in triggering its effects are also addressed in this review. The gut is the first organ exposed to mycotoxins, after oral contamination [22]. For this reason, the review presents initially the effect of ZEA on the gut.

2. Effect of ZEA on Gut Immunity

The gut represents a physical barrier that ensure the body's protection against environmental agents, mycotoxins included [23]. This barrier involves intestinal epithelial cells (IECs), but also components of both innate and adaptive immunity, as IgA and pro-inflammatory cytokines or molecules involved in the inhibition of bacterial colonization (mucins and antimicrobial peptides) [24].

A recent study of Lahjouji et al. [25] reported that the intestine is a target of ZEA which cause pathological intestinal changes. Depending on different factors as specie, sex, dose or time of exposure, ZEA can affect or not the normal anatomic structure of the intestine. For example, ZEA (40 µg/kg b.w.) did not change the mucosa thickness, the height of villi or the number of goblet cells in swine [26,27], but the ingestion of ZEA (0.3–146 mg/kg feed) in pregnant rats modified the structure of villi and decrease the junction proteins expression [28]. Also, in the first week of a chronic exposure of pigs to ZEA (40 µg/kg b.w.) produced transitory morphological modifications of small intestine and an increase in Paneth cell numbers in the crypt [25].

Exposure to ZEA was associated with the impairment of cell viability, apoptosis and necrosis in different organs including gut [29,30]. For example, recent studies have shown that treatment with ZEA at 10–100 µM for 24h decreased viability of porcine intestinal epithelial cells IPEC-J2 [31] and IPEC-1 [32,33] and increase LDH activity [31]. Apoptosis is one of the main mechanisms involved by ZEA induced toxicity in the gut and it was shown that ZEA can cause apoptosis in various intestinal epithelial cells as IPEC-J2 [34], MODE-K [35] and HCT116 [36]. Sub-chronic exposure of female Polish Large White pigs to low doses of ZEA increased apoptosis and decreased the ileal Peyer's patches lymphocytes proliferation [37].

Some recent studies have shown that ZEA exposure alters or not the T- and B-cell subtype populations in small intestine. The administration of ZEA (5 or 20 mg/kg b.w.) to female BALB/C mice increased the percentages of CD8+ and decreased the percentages of CD4+ cells in the lamina propria and intra-epithelium lymphocytes, while no effect on CD8+ and CD19+ lymphocytes was observed in the Peyer' patches [38]. Also, the exposure of prepubertal gilts to 100mg ZEA/kg feed decreased the percentage of CD21+ lymphocytes in pig ileum [37].

Endoplasmic reticulum stress (ERS) pathway seems to be the main signaling pathway involved in ZEA induced apoptosis. In MODE-K mouse cells exposed to zearalenone, the toxin increased the gene expression and protein synthesis of molecules involved in ERS-induced apoptosis pathway as: c-Jun N-terminal kinase, C/EBP homologous protein, GRP78, caspase-1 and the anti-apoptotic protein Bax, while decreasing the levels of the pro-apoptotic related protein Bcl-2 [35]. Similarly, an increased number of apoptotic cells were observed in the Peyer' patches of the 20 mg/kg ZEA-treated mice associated with a significantly increase of Bax gene expression and of the ratio of Bax:Bcl-2 [38].

Mucosal IgA protects the intestinal epithelium from xenobiotics, viruses and bacteria and maintains also the homeostasis of the intestinal environment [39]. Indeed, previous studies have linked the increase of IgAs to repeated exposure to environmental toxins or to chronic infections [40]. The effect of ZEA on IgAs synthesis is controversial. ZEA administered by oral gavage to female BALB/c mice for two weeks at a dose of 5 or 20 mg/kg b.w. provokes a significantly decrease of the mucosal IgA antibody level in mice duodenum [38]. On the other side, the administration of 20 mg of ZEA/kg b.w. for only one week to male BALB/c mice significantly increased fecal IgA levels in the jejunum (1.5-fold higher that in the control group) [41]. Because the same concentration of ZEA (20 mg/kg b.w.) and the same way of administration (oral gavage) were used in both experiments, the different results could be related to the experiment duration (one week vs. two weeks) or could be influenced by the sex of the animals (male vs. female) and the intestinal segment.

Mucin glycoproteins are produced by epithelial or submucosal mucus-producing cells and represents the principal constituent of mucus [42]. The mucus structure is permanently renewed and could be rapidly adjusted to respond to the changes of the environment, as for example in response to microbial infection or to exposure to contaminants [30]. Recent studies have shown that ZEA (20 mg/kg b.w.) is responsible for intestinal mucosa abnormalities [41] as mice exposure for a short period (one week) to ZEA significantly increased the expression of mucin 1 and mucin 2 genes in the gut. Results on in vitro cell cultures also indicates that ZEA interferes with the mucin synthesis since the toxin increased the concentration of these molecules in Caco-2/HT29-MTX cells [43]. In vitro exposure of swine IPEC-J2 cells to 40 µM ZEA [44], and in vivo exposure of mice to 20 mg ZEA/kg b.w. [41] resulted in the upregulation of β-defensin, an important antimicrobial peptide, with important consequences for the defense against intestinal infection.

The effect of ZEA on the intestinal inflammatory response is not very clear, and this fact is due probably to the different experimental models and various ZEA concentrations used in several studies. Thus, in vitro studies showed that the incubation of porcine intestinal cells with 10 and 40 µM of zearalenone respectively lead to the increased expression of genes encoding for molecules involved in inflammation such as TLRs and the cytokines: *IL-1β, TNF-α, IL-6, IL-8, IL-12p40* in IPEC-1 [22] and of *IL-1β* and *TNF-α* in IPEC-J2 cells [44].

The increase in the expression of pro-inflammatory cytokines (IL-1β and TNF-α) was also registered in the in vivo studies, in jejunum of mice intoxicated with 20 mg ZEA/kg b.w. Also, prepubertal gilts exposed to 100 mg ZEA/kg feed for 42 days had elevated ileum concentrations of IL-12/23 40p and IL-1β [37]. By contrast, other researchers found that ZEA had no effect on proinflammatory IL-8 cytokine synthesis by IPEC-1 cells [32] or decreased the gene expression of *IL-1β*, *TNF-α* and *IL-8* in the jejunum of rats when administered in different doses (0.3–146.0 mg/kg feed) [28]. As well, a microarray study performed on IPEC-1 cells exposed to ZEA (25 μM) found a decrease of the expression of pro-inflammatory cytokines *IL-8*, *TNF-α* and *IL-6* [45]. The inflammatory effect produced by ZEA can be transmitted from mother to offspring. Piglets derived from sows fed 300 ppb zearalenone one week before farrowing and during the lactation period developed gut inflammation [46].

3. Effect of ZEA on Innate Immune Response

Innate or nonspecific immunity is the first form of defense for multicellular organisms. The innate immune response is triggered by receptors that recognize the pathogen and activate a series of signaling pathways that control the immune response [47]. Neutrophils, NK and NKT cells, monocytes/macrophages and dendritic cells that mediate interactions with pathogens are the innate immune system components able to form networks with key role in the initial immune response to infection and tissue damages [48]. They are phagocytic cells that when stimulated can produce reactive oxygen species (ROS), important in cell signaling and homeostasis [49,50]. An imbalance between ROS production and its inefficient elimination drives to a dramatic increase in ROS levels leading to cells damage, known as oxidative stress [49]. Recently, Wang et al., reported that ZEA (5, 10, 20 μM) increased ROS production in bovine neutrophils and decreased antioxidant enzymes (SOD and CAT) activity by involving NADPH, ERK and p38 activation followed by the formation of neutrophil extracellular traps (NETs), a network of DNA extracellular fibbers which help neutrophil cells to kill extracellular pathogens [51]. This could have significant cytotoxic and pro-inflammatory consequences.

According with the study of Marin et al., zearalenone and its metabolites decreased cells viability of porcine polymorphonuclear cells, interleukine-8 synthesis and increased superoxide production, ZEA metabolites being more immunotoxic than ZEA [52]. Moreover, Murata et al., found that the effect of ZEA and its metabolites on bovine neutrophiles depend on their chemical structure [53]. Thus, these authors found that zearalenone and its derivatives α- and β-zearalenol suppressed luminol dependent PMA chemiluminescence in neutrophils due to their C1′-2′ double bonds while, zearalanone, α- and β-zearalanols did not exert this effect because they possess a hydrogenated C1′-2′ bond instead of the double bond. In vivo experimentation conducted on Ross 308 hybrid broilers fed with two concentration of deoxynivalenol and zearalenone after hatching showed that the toxins induced oxidative stress and inhibited significantly the blood cells phagocytic activity [54]. In combination with other mycotoxins (alternariol, deoxynivalenol), ZEA affect innate immune functions by inhibited for example the differentiation of monocyte into macrophages (THP-1 cell line). Moreover, the combination of ZEA with alternariol at low concentration lead to synergistic effect on CD14 expression [55]. The combination of the two toxins altered the macrophages functions by the inhibition of TNF-α secretion. The primary function of RAW 264.7 macrophages such as proliferation was reduced and apoptosis was induced in a dose-dependent manner by zearalenone (from 0 to 100 μM) via the ERS pathway [56]. Three milligrams of ZEA /kg b.w. altered in in vivo treated rats the hydrogen peroxide release by peritoneal macrophages [57]. Also in vivo, the low concentrations of ZEA (40 μg/kg b.w. per day) alone or in combination with deoxynivalenol (DON, 12 μg/kg b.w. per day), another *Fusarium* mycotoxin, produced changes in the morphology of pig Kupffer cells (stellate macrophages) with consequences on their activity [58].

Inflammation represents a rapidly nonspecific immune response through which the phagocytic cells are activated and produce bioactive molecules (inflammatory cytokines, prostaglandins and leukotrienes) as well as oxygen and nitrogen metabolites [59]. Being an agonist of the estrogenic receptors, ZEA can modulate similarly the in vitro and in vivo inflammatory response depending on its concentration, time of exposure and immune indices investigated.

In vitro studies highlight an increase or a decline of inflammatory response induced or not by ZEA depending on the immune cell type. Thus, the in vitro study of Marin et al., in which swine PBMCs were exposed to ZEA and its metabolites for 48h showed that ZEA decreased significantly at 5 and 10 μM the TNF-α response of these cells and had no significantly effect on IL-1β and IL-8, while zearalanone decreased also the production of IL-8 at 10 μM [19]. Interleukin 8 (IL-8) is a common inflammatory cytokine important in the recruitment of the immune cells, a key parameter in localized inflammation which induced after that an increase of oxidative stress mediators [60]. The same authors reported later [32] that ZEA derivatives, alpha-zearalenol (α-ZOL), beta-zearalenol (β-ZOL), and zearalanone (ZAN) decreased in a dose dependent manner the IL-8 synthesis in polymorphonuclear cells (PMN), significantly at 10 μM (−49.2% for α-ZOL; −45.6% for β-ZOL and −45.1% for ZAN respectively) after 3 h of exposure. No effect of ZEA on IL-8 concentration registered. Similarly, ZEA metabolites were more potent than ZEA itself in decreasing the IL-8 synthesis in porcine epithelial cells (IPEC-1) [32]. By contrast, Ding e al. [61] found that the level of IL-1β and IL-18 increased significantly in peritoneal mouse macrophages isolated from mice receiving ZEA by gavage (4.5 mg/kg b.w.) once a day for 9 days and treated in vitro with 8 μg/mL for 24h. In a model monocytic cell line, hER + IL-1β-CAT+, the exposure of the cells to low level 50 ng/mL of zearalenone and α-zearalenol resulted in a pro-inflammatory effect as 17β-estradiol by modulating and promoting IL-1β synthesis. The toxins manifested full agonist activity with 17β-estradiol but at lower potency [62] exposure of human placental choriocarcinoma (BeWo) cells to different concentrations of ZEA (2–16μM) increased the IL-6 production [63].

In vivo studies confirmed the biphasic effect of zearalenone on inflammation. Experiments performed on piglets found that in spleen and blood, ZEA increased the gene expression of pro-inflammatory *TNF-α, IL-6, IL-8* and *IL-1β*, while in liver the toxin decreased dramatically the expression of these cytokine which might have consequences on immune homeostasis taking into account that liver is considered a key organ for immune homeostasis [64]. It seems that the pro- or anti-inflammatory effect of ZEA depend on the organ involved. The earlier results of Salah-Abbes [65,66] showed a significant reduction of TNF-α, IL-1β and IL-12 in plasma of mice treated with 40 mg ZEA /kg b.w. as well as an increase of the cytokines (TNF-α, IL-6, IL-10) in kidney of mice fed the same concentration of toxin [67]. The inflammatory reaction in kidney is produced through the activation of macrophages which, once activated, will further produce inflammatory cytokines and chemokines subsequently responsible for different reactions and effects such as apoptosis and necrosis, the up- or down regulation of pro- and anti- apoptotic genes [67]. In testicular tissue of mice exposed for 48h to ZEA (40mg/kg b.w.) the toxin increased the level of TNF-α, IL-1β, IL-6 and decreased the level of anti-inflammatory IL-10 cytokine [68].

4. Effect of Zearalenone on Adaptive Immune Response
4.1. Effect of Zearalenone on Humoral Immune Response

Animal exposure to different doses of zearalenone has resulted in an alteration of humoral immunity as can be seen in Table 1. Literature studies show that ZEA leads to a decrease in serum IgG levels regardless the animal species (mice, rat or swine), toxin concentration or the duration of the exposure. Similarly, most studies have shown that the level of IgM in serum decreases no matter the species (mice or rats), time of exposure (12–36 days) and mycotoxin concentration (5–30 mg/kg b.w.). However, sub-chronic exposure (3–4 weeks) of rats to lower concentrations of ZEA (2–4 mg/kg b.w.) was associated with an increase in serum IgM concentration [69,70]. It seems that the effect of ZEA on IgM concentration is correlated with the sex of animal, since male piglets exposed to low concentration of toxin (0.8 mg/kg feed) resulted in a decreased in IgM level, while no significant changes were observed in serum IgM concentration of gilts receiving ZEA higher concentrations (1.1–3.2 mg/kg feed). Serum IgA concentration was not affected in mice, rats or swine after the exposure to low and medium concentration of the toxin (0.08–30 mg/kg feed) as resulted from most studies (Table 1) and it is not related to the time of exposure (18–42 days). BALB/c female mice fed higher concentration of ZEA (40 mg/kg feed) for 48h showed a decrease of IgA concentration [71].

Table 1. Effect of ZEA on the humoral immune response.

Effect (s)	Species/Cell Type	Dose/Time of ZEA Administration	References
↑ IgE, ↓ IgM no changes of IgG and IgA	BALB/c mice female	20 mg/kg b.w. 14 days	[38]
↓ IgG, IgA ↑ IgM	Pregnant rats	100,150 mg/kg feed 7 days	[70]
↓ IgG, IgM, IgE no changes of IgA	Wistar rats female	0, 1, 5, 30 mg/kg b.w. 36 days	[72]
↓ Ig A, Ig G	BALB/c mice, female	40 mg/kg b.w. 48h	[71]
↓ IgG ↑ Ig M	Wistar rats male	2 mg/kg b.w./week 3 weeks	[69]
↓ Ig G no changes of IgA, IgM	Prepubertal gilts	200, 800, 1600 µg/kg feed 14 days	[73]
↓ IgG, IgM no changes of IgA	Piglets male	0.8 mg/kg feed 4 weeks	[74]
↓ IgG, IgM in serum ↑ IgA in serum	Kunming mice, female	30 mg/kg b.w. 12 days	[75]
↓ IgG in serum no changes on IgA, IgM	post-weaning female piglets	1.1-3.2 mg/kg feed 18 days	[76]
no effect of serum IgG, IgM, IgA	B6C3F1 mice	10 mg/kg feed 6 weeks	[77]
↓ IgG, IgA, IgM in cell SN	Swine PBMC	10 mM 7 days	[19]
↓ IgG ↓ IgM	BALB/c mice	5, 10, 15 mg/kg b.w./day 2 weeks	[66]

Moreover, ZEA metabolites interfere with immunoglobulin synthesis. As it was shown in an in vitro study using swine peripheral blood mononuclear cells, both ZEA and its metabolites (α-ZOL, β-ZOL and ZAN) significantly decreased the immunoglobulins IgG, IgM and IgA synthesis at concentrations higher that 5 µM [19].

It was observed that the consumption of contaminated feed led to an increase of toxin concentration in the serum of intoxicated animals before farrowing and during lactation suggesting that ZEA or its metabolites can interfere with immunoglobulin secretion in colostrum/milk and in offspring. Also, α-zearalenol metabolite was found in the colostrum and milk of the sows [46], but in our knowledge no data concerning this interference are available until now in the literature. However, feeding sows with a dietary mixture of mycotoxins containing DON, ZEA and fusaric acid resulted in a decrease of the concentration of IgA in the colostrum and of IgA and IgG in serum of their offspring [78].

A common method for the assessment of the T-cell-dependent antibody responses is represented by the sheep red blood cells (SRBCs) assay. Few data (Table 2) concerning this type of immune response related to ZEA exposure are available. For example, exposure to 10 mg ZEA /kg b.w. of female B6C3F1 mice had no effect on the splenic plaque forming cells in response to SRBC [79] while a decrease of the B cells producing immunoglobulin M antibody to SRBC was observed in female Wistar rats exposed for 28 days to 3 mg of ZEA/kg b.w. [57].

In a recent review concerning the impact of *Fusarium* mycotoxins on human and animal host susceptibility to infectious diseases, it was shown that in contrast to other fusariotoxins, the interaction between zearalenone and infectious disease was less studied [80]. Pestka and collaborators showed that mice fed 10 mg ZEA/kg feed for 2 weeks and infected with *Listeria monocytogenes*, registered a decreased resistance to Listeria and an increase of the bacterial count in spleen as compared with control animals [79]. It can be claimed that ZEA exposure interferes with the capacity of organism to realize an adequate immune response to vaccination and that the toxin can alter the specific antibody synthesis. Indeed, several studies have shown a decrease of antibody titer to porcine parvovirus [72] or to swine plague [76] in zearalenone intoxicated animals, but however more studies are needed in order to better understand the relation between zearalenone and the response to infectious disease.

Table 2. Humoral immunity with specific antibody/in vaccination.

Effect (s)	Species/Cell Type	Dose/Time of ZEA Administration	References
↓ B cells producing IgM to SRBC [1]	Wistar rats female	3 mg/kg b.w. 28 days	[57]
No differences in humoral immune response against SRBC [1]	prepubertal gilts	0.75 mg/kg feed 21 days	[81]
↓ Ab titer to porcine parvovirus	Wistar rats	5 mg/kg b.w. 36 days	[72]
↓ Ab titer to swine plague	post-weaning female piglets	1.1–3.2 mg/kg feed 18 days	[76]
No effect on the splenic PFC [2] response to SRBC [1] Delayed hypersensitivity response to keyhole limpet hemocyanin	B6C3F1 female mice	10 mg/kg b.w. 2–8 weeks	[79]

[1] SRBC (sheep red blood cell); [2] PFC (plaque forming cells).

4.2. Effect of Zearalenone on Cellular Immune Response

Beside its effect on humoral immune response, ZEA cause negative effects on cellular immune response (e.g., cell viability and proliferation, apoptosis and necrosis, and cytokine production) due to the fact that most of the cells involved in the immune response have estrogenic receptors on their surface [82]. A disturbance of cell proliferation and apoptosis was reported in a number of studies investigating ZEA toxicity. As proved by many studies zearalenone is an inductor of apoptosis and necrosis in different type of immune cells. B and T lymphocytes are among the immune cells affected by the action of ZEA. It seems in fact that the immunosuppression produced by ZEA is caused by the decrease in B and T lymphocytes viability and proliferation [66,83]. These authors reported that ZEA (0.2–1800 ng/mL) produced a reduction of peripheral lymphocytes and this was a consequence of apoptosis and cell death triggered by ZEA at the spleen level knowing that spleen is one of the most important organs for maturing lymphocytes [66,71]. The death of spleen lymphocytes leads to the decrease of the peripheral lymphocytes. Zearalenone metabolites also reduced the lymphocytes proliferation. EFSA Scientific Opinion (2011) [84] cited the work of Forsell [85] in which the proliferation of human lymphocytes stimulated with different mitogens was reduced with 50% by 3.5 µg/mL zearalenone, 6.3 µg/mL α-zearalenol, 36 µg/mL β-zearalenol, 3.8 µg/mL α-zearalanol and 33 µg/mL β-zearalanol. The inhibition of proliferation was not related to the estrogenic potential of ZEA and its derivatives, but to their structure and the presence of a single or double bond. The presence in C-6′ of a keto parent molecule (ZEA) or alpha-hydroxyl substituents (alpha-ZEL and alpha-ZAL) led to a 10-fold higher toxicity [86]. Comparing the in vitro effect of zearalenone and is derivatives α-zearalenol and β-zearalenol with that of trichothecenes on proliferation of human peripheral mononuclear cells (PBMC) [83] observed that only the high concentration of these toxins had significant immunosuppressive effect. Indeed, in vitro investigation of Vlata et al. [87] on freshly human PBMC using increased concentration of zearalenone (0.1, 1, 5, 10, 30 μg/mL) showed that the highest concentration of ZEA (30 μg/mL) inhibited the proliferation of B and T lymphocytes and induced also a necrotic effect. A clear necrotic effect was also found irrespective of cells stimulation. The study of Zhang et al. [88] demonstrated that ZEA at 10–50 μg/mL had a time and dose dependent inhibitory action on mouse thymic epithelial cells proliferation and arrested thymic cells in G2/M phase of cellular cycle. Studies performed on TM3 cells shows that low doses of ZEA increases cell proliferation [89].

ZEA decrease not only the lymphocytes viability and proliferation but also lymphocytes phenotype number. A decreased expression of T (CD3+, CD4+, CD8+), NK and B lymphocytes was observed by Salah-Abbes et al. [66], when BALB c male mice were treated with ZEA 40 mg/kg. In the same line, Swamy et al. [90] pointed out that a diet naturally contaminated with *Fusarium* mycotoxins, ZEA (0.4 mg/kg and 0.7mg/kg) among them decreased linearly the number of B-cells, CD3+, CD4+, CD8+ lymphocytes and NK cells in broiler chickens via the reduction of interferon-β levels and IL-2 expression. Studies in mice, rats or pigs indicated a decrease in splenic coefficients, including proliferation and cell viability, the most affected cell populations being CD4+ and CD8+.

CDs (Clusters of Differentiation) are glycoproteins expressed on the surface of the immune cells. T cells are characterized by the expression of CD3, CD4 and CD8 markers [91,92] which are involved in in the transduction of signals from T cell surfaces (CD4 and CD8), while CD3 markers activate both the cytotoxic and helper T cells. As can be seen also in Table 3, there are conflicting data concerning the effect of ZEA on T cells subpopulations. While, most studies indicate a decrease in CD4+, CD8+ and CD3+ expression under the influence of ZEA, regardless of the animal species, other studies suggest an increase in CD4+ and CD8+ expression. However, any change in the CD4/CD8 ratio may indicate an immune dysfunction [91,92].

Induction of cellular death and proliferation inhibition was also found on other type of immune cells than lymphocytes. Viability of polymorphonuclear cells was decreased after 24h by 50 μM of ZEA and its metabolites α-ZOL, β-ZOL and ZAN action [52] and the exposure of RAW 264.7 macrophages to 10 to 100 μM ZEA for 24h diminished the cell viability in a dose dependent manner through apoptosis and necrosis [56,93].

By its estrogenic like-effects, ZEA impacts the development of reproductive organs irrespective of animal species, but with a different sensitivity of cells.

In weaned piglets, ZEA (0.5, 1.0 and 1.5 mg/kg) induces ovarian development by accelerating ovarian follicles proliferation through the activation of ERs/GSK-3β-dependent Wnt-1/β-catenin signaling pathway [94]. Also, ZEA (0.5–1.5 mg/kg) determined an abnormal uterine proliferation through TGF signaling pathway [95]. Investigating other regulatory pathways involved by ZEA in uterine hypertrophy, these authors exposed porcine endometrial epithelial cells to ZEA 0, 5, 20 and 80 μmol/L for 24 h and cell cycle was analyzed. A significant lower proportion of cells in S and G2 phases and an increase in the phase of G1 was found at ZEA 80 μmol/L [95]. The related mechanism involved also the activation of Wnt/β-catenin signaling pathway.

In mouse ovarian granulosa cells Chen et al. [96] and Zhang et al. [97] demonstrated by MTT, EdU and flow cytometry that ZEA suppressed in vitro cell viability at 30–150 μM and increased apoptosis at 15–60 μM after 24 or 72h of exposure. Close to the results recorded by Song et al. [95] in pig (a decreased of cell proportion in the S and G2 phase at ZEA 80 μmol/L), Zhang et al. [97], found that mouse granulosa cells were arrested in G1 phase of cell cycle and the cells proportion decreased in phase S and G2 after 30 μM ZEA treatment. However, in another study this author [98] found species specific ZEA effect, pig being more sensitive than mouse. Thus, ZEA 10 μM significantly increased the percentage of TUNEL porcine positive cells while the TUNEL percentage of granulosa mouse cells increased only at 30 µM.

Also, it has been observed that the metabolite of ZEA, α-ZOL at 9.4 µM concentration induces an increase in porcine granulosa cell proliferation and in progesterone levels [99].

In rats, ZEA perturb cell proliferation in both female and males. In Sprague Dawley males receiving by gavage 10 or 20 mg ZEA/kg b.w., the toxin significantly decreased the numbers of Leydig cells (adjacent cells to the testicle seminiferous tubules) which could produce anomalies of the male reproductive tract [100]. Similar results on Leydig cells were found by Wang et al. [101], with ZEA 50 µM. By contrast, Zheng et al. [89], found that low doses of zearalenone (0.01, 0.02, 0.03, 0.04, and 0.05 µmol/L) stimulated cell viability of TM3 cells (Leydig cells) measured by using the xCELLigence real-time cell analysis. Also, under the action of ZEA (20µM), cell viability of Sertoli cells derived from Male Wistar, which are important for male reproductive system, increased over control [102].

In human, study of Marton et al. [103], on ovarian epithelial cells investigating the effect of several compounds, ZEA among them on miRNA expression in correlation with cells estrogenic sensitivity observed that ZEA (1, 10, 100, 1000 nM) increased the rate of cell proliferation in direct proportion to ZEA concentration and depending on the presence of ER-α. By contrast, 30 µM of ZEA in prostate cancer cells induced G2/M cell cycle arrest and decreased cell viability compared to control [104].

Table 3. Effect of ZEA on cellular immune response.

Effect (s)	Species/Cell Type	Dose/Time of ZEA Administration	References
↓ $CD4^+$, $CD8^+$, $CD11c^+$ in spleen ↓ $CD4^+$, $CD8^+$, $F4/80^+$ and ↑ $CD19^+$ and $CD11c^+$ in the mesenteric lymph nodes ↑TNFα and apoptosis, ↓ IL-6	BALB/c mice (female, 7-week-old)	5,20 mg/kg b.w. 2 weeks	[38]
ZEA 100 and 150 mg/kg: ↓ viability of splenocytes ↓ T-cell proliferation Induce histopathological damage in spleen ZEA 150mg/kg: ↑ interleukin IL-6, IL-18 and IL-1β ↓ interferon-γ, TNFα and IL-10 in spleen	Sprague Dawley Pregnant Rats	50, 100, 150 mg/kg b.w. 7 days	[70]
disrupt the proliferation of $CD4^+8+$ in peripheral blood cells	Polish Landrace x Polish Large White crossbreeds	0.5 mg/kg 6 weeks	[105]
↓ IL-1 in thymus and spleen ↓ IFN-γ in serum ↓ IL-2, IL-6, IL-10 in thymus ↓ IL-10 and IFN-γ in the spleen	Wistar rat	1, 5, 30 mg/kg b.w. 36 days	[72]
↓ $CD3^+$, $CD4^+$, $CD8^+$, $CD56^+$ cells	BALB/c mice	40 mg/kg b.w. 48h	[71]
↓ $CD4^+$, $CD8^+$ cells in peripheral blood	BPC and SPC Sheep	3.07– 14.49 µg/kg feed winter time	[106]
ZEA 40 µM: Inhibit T cell-chemotaxis by CCL19 ↑ $CD4^+$ T cells induced by CCL19 chemotaxis ZEA 20 µM: ↑ CD8+ T cells induced by CCL21 chemotaxis ↓ expression of chemokine receptor CCR7 and CCR2	BALB/c mouse splenic lymphocytes	10, 20, 40 µM 48h	[107]

Table 3. Cont.

Effect (s)	Species/Cell Type	Dose/Time of ZEA Administration	References
↓ CD3⁺CD4⁺ T cells ↑ CD3⁺CD8⁺ T cells	Female Kunming Mice	20, 30 mg/kg b.w. 12 days	[108]
↓ CD21⁺B, CD2⁺T, CD4⁺CD8⁻ T ↑ CD8⁺CD4⁻ and TCRγδ⁺ T	Polish Large White female	0.1 mg/kg 42 days	[109]
↓ CD4⁺CD8⁺, CD4⁺, CD4⁺/CD8⁺ (2 mg/kg) ↑ CD8⁺ (3.2 mg/kg)	Landrace × York- shire × Duroc Piglets	1.1, 2, 3.2 mg/kg feed 18 days	[76]
↑ IL-1β and IL-6, ↓ IFN-γ cytoplasmic edema chromatin deformation splenic damages	Yorkshire × Lan- drace × Duroc Piglets	1.1, 2.0, 3.2 mg/kg feed 18 days	[110]
↓ IFN-γ, IL-10↓ proliferation	kidneys of piglets	0.8 mg/kg 4 weeks	[111]
↑ IL-2, ↓ IL-6	Isa Brown chicken splenic lymphocytes	0.1–25 µg/mL 48 h	[82]

Other examples concerning the effect of zearalenone on cellular immune response are illustrated in Table 3.

5. Effect of Zearalenone on Immune Organs

Zearalenone is responsible for the increase of reproductive organs' weight such as the uterus [112]. By contrast, the weight of the immune organs seems to be less affected by the exposure to ZEA as resulted from the literature data (Table 4), but the toxin has been responsible for immune organs atrophy and depletion as well as for other histopathological modifications in immune organs. ZEA caused also a decrease of B cell percentage in the spleen or swelling of red pulp [57,108,111].

Table 4. The effect of zearalenone on immune organs weight and structure.

Effect (s)	Species/Cell Type	Dose/Time of ZEA Administration	References
Thymic atrophy with histological and thymocyte phenotype changes and decrease in the B cell percentage in the spleen	Wistar rats	3.0 mg/kg b.w. 28 days	[57]
Atrophy of white pulp and swelling of red pulp	post-weanling gilts	2.0, 3.2 mg/kg feed 18 days	[110]
No effect on spleen and bursa of Fabricius weights	one-day-old broiler chicks	10–800 mg/kg feed 21 days	[113]
No effect on spleen and bursa of Fabricius weights	one-day-old broiler chicks	50–800 mg/kg feed 3 weeks	[114]
Enlargement of the spleen in males	Sprague Dawley rats	1.25, 3.75 mg/kg b.w. 8 weeks	[115]
No effect on spleen weight	Sprague Dawley rats	0.5, 0.9, 1.8, 3.6 mg/kg b.w. 4 weeks	[116]
No effect on spleen weight	BALB/c mice female, 7-weeks-old	5, 20 mg/kg b.w. 14 days	[38]
No effect on spleen weight	White Leghorn female chickens, 2-weeks-old	50, 200, 400, 800 mg/kg b.w. 7 days	[117]

Table 4. Cont.

Effect (s)	Species/Cell Type	Dose/Time of ZEA Administration	References
No macroscopic changes and no histopathologic effect on lymph nodes	32-day-old gilts	0.75 mg/kg feed 21 days	[81]
No effect on thymus and spleen weights No histopathologic changes	B6C3F1 weanling female mice	10 mg/kg feed 56 days	[77]
Decreased immune organ weight and lymphocyte counts, lymphoid atrophy and depletion in the spleen	BALB/c female mice	40, 80 mg ZEN/kg b.w. 28 days	[118]

6. Mechanisms of Action

Zearalenone and its metabolites are considered to be endocrine disruptors, due to the similarity between their chemical structure and that of the endogenous estrogen, 17-estradiol, which allow them to bind to estrogen receptors (ERs) [119]. ZEA can bind to ER-α and ER-β [120], being a partial antagonist for ER-β and complete agonist for ER-α [121]. Among ZEA metabolites, α-ZOL has the highest capacity to bind ERs, followed by ZEA and β-ZOL [122].

Yip and collaborators reported that ZEA binds to ERs which are presented in different target cells and tissues including the immune cells and is able to modulate their expression [123]. ER-α expression was found in macrophages, B cells, NK cells, CD4+T cells, CD8+T cells, while ER-β expression is presented in monocytes, macrophages, B cells or NK cells [124,125]. The ratio between the two receptors ER-α and ER-β and their density is different in various cells and tissues [126]. The expression of ER-α after ZEA exposure was increased in the pig jejunal explants [25], but a decrease in the expression of this receptor and an increase in that of ER-β in the colon of intoxicated mice was observed [61].

ERs are members of the nuclear hormone receptors family that acts as transcription factors [127] which interact with chromatin target sites by two different path-ways: One dependent of estrogen response element (ERE) and another ERE-independent through signal transduction via RAS/mitogen-activated protein kinase (MAPK) and phosphoinositide 3-kinase (PI3K/Akt) [127,128]. After activation, ERs translocate into the nucleus where they form complexes with co-regulatory proteins, transcription factors, at specific DNA sites leading to epigenetic modifications of chromatin and to the initiation of the transcription process [129]. Very recently, it was demonstrated that ZEA induces ER translocation in endometrial stroma cells [130], but this was not proved yet for immune cells.

5.1. Mechanisms Triggered by ZEA in Proliferation of the Immune Cell

As already presented in the previous sections, ZEA can induce opposite biological effects in various cells/tissues that could be related to the ratio between ER-α vs. ER-β and the density of ER receptors. For example, it was shown that the activation of ER-α is related mainly to cell proliferation, while the activation of ER-β rather inhibits cell proliferation when it is co-expressed with ER-α [131]. In intestinal pig explants, activation of ER-α following ZEA exposure was associated with an activation of pro-proliferative Wnt/β catenin signaling pathway and a down regulation of immunosuppressive TGF-β signaling [25] (Figure 2).

In other immune tissues, zearalenone is responsible for a decrease of cell proliferation and apoptosis [29,38] as previously described. According to a recent review of Zeng and collaborators concerning the capacity of zearalenone to induce cell proliferation or to determine cell death, at least three mechanisms are involved: (i) Alteration of the cell cycle as well as of the expressions of cell cycle regulating proteins; (ii) cell oxidative stress and (iii) cell apoptosis through ERs stress, ROS producing and mitochondrial signaling pathway [132]. These mechanisms are equally involved in apoptosis and cell death induced by zearalenone in immune cells. ZEA induced apoptosis in T lymphocytes, increase the ratio of Bax/Bcl-2 and promote the expression of cleaved caspase-3 and cleaved caspase-9, which indicates that the toxin activates the mitochondrial apoptosis pathway [133]. Similarly, an increased number of apoptotic cells were observed in the Peyer' patches of the 20 mg/kg b.w. ZEA-treated mice associated with a significantly increase of Bax gene expression and of the ratio of Bax:Bcl-2 [38].

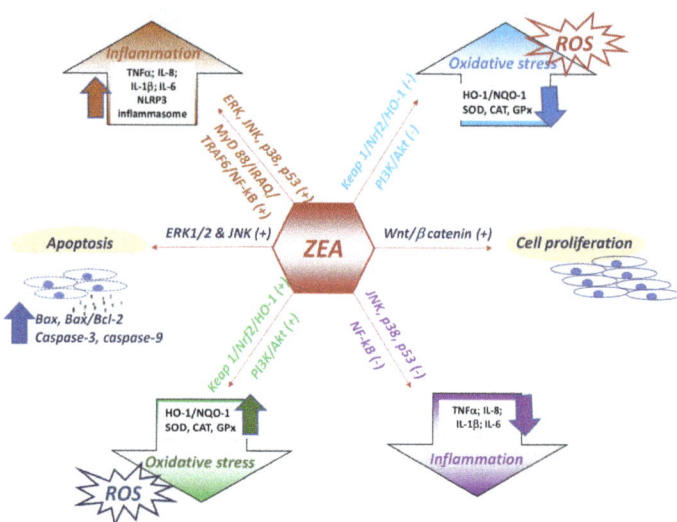

Figure 2. Suggested mechanisms involved by zearalenone in immune cells.

In mouse MODE-K intestinal epithelial cells exposed to zearalenone, the toxin increased the gene expression and protein synthesis of molecules involved in ERS-induced apoptosis pathway as: c-Jun N-terminal kinase (JNK), C/EBP homologous protein, GRP78, caspase-1 and the pro-apoptotic protein Bax, while decreasing the levels of the anti-apoptotic related protein Bcl-2 [35].

The apoptosis triggered by the exposure of T lymphocytes to ZEA was accompanied by the over activation of MAPKs as extracellular regulated protein kinases (ERK) and JNK [133]. ERK pathway is involved in cell proliferation, differentiation and survival [134], while JNK is involved in apoptosis, inflammation, cytokine production, and metabolism [135]. The over activation of MAPKs following ZEA action was shown also in another cell types [119], but the mechanisms responsible for MAPKs activation is still unclear. It was suggested that for ERK1/2 activation, an important role is played by G-protein-coupled protein homolog, GPR30 associated or not with the estrogen receptor (α or β) [136].

5.2. Mechanisms Triggered by ZEA in Inflammation and Oxidative Stress

Many studies have linked apoptosis induced by zearalenone to oxidative stress [137–139]. For example, an in vitro study on RAW264.7 macrophage cells showed that cellular apoptosis is induced by ZEA through ROS accumulation, leading to the activation of p53-mediated signaling pathways, JNK and p38 MAPK-kinases. ZEA is thought to activate JNK and p38 MAPK, which drive to changes in mitochondrial Bcl-2/BAX proteins, a decrease of mitochondrial membrane potential, and ultimately to ROS generation. Through a self-propagation mechanism, increased ROS stimulates again JNK/p38 phosphorylation in ZEA-contaminated cells [93]. p38 MAPK signaling activation by the oxidative stress produced via cytochrome P450 reductase was found to be the main pathway through which ZEA induces toxicity in IPEC-J2 intestinal epithelial cells. It was observed that ZEA increased the level of both gene and phosphorylated protein expression of *p38 MAPK* which led to the autophagy induction [140]. The fact that ZEA affects the immune response via MAPK-kinases modulation is also suggested by the results obtained by Pistol et al., in the spleen of piglets receiving a diet contaminated with 316 ppm of ZEA in which JNK pathway was responsible for the activation of the inflammatory response assessed by pro-inflammatory cytokines and other molecules involved in inflammatory processes (MMPs/TIMPs) [141] (Figure 2).

Nuclear factor erythroid 2–related factor 2 (Nrf2) is an essential regulator of antioxidant genes, and it is early activated in response to the oxidative stress [142]. Nrf2-mediated pathway is considered one of the mechanism responsible for the alteration of the antioxidant and inflammatory responses induced by ZEA at least at the intestinal level [28,143]. The activation of the Keap1–Nrf2 signaling pathway was observed after ZEA exposure and might contribute to the reduction of ZEA toxicity in immune cells and organs [141,142]. However, other studies have shown that zearalenone compromise the capacity of the organism to provide an adequate response to the oxidative stress, resulting in a downregulation of Keap1/Nrf2/HO-1 pathway [144] and of phosphoinositide 3-kinase (PI3K)/Akt signaling pathway related to Nrf-2 [145].

Oxidative stress and inflammation are tightly correlated, reactive oxygen species playing an important role in the progression of inflammatory disorders [146] which are mainly regulated by the nuclear transcription factor-κB (NF-κB) pathway, the NF-κB receptor playing an essential role as a mediator in the regulation of the innate and adaptive immune responses [110]. An increase of Nrf2 after ZEA exposure was correlated with a decrease of NF-κB and the experimentally induction of NF-κB [22,141] significantly increased ZEA-induced oxidative stress [104]. However, the mechanisms by which zearalenone can influence the expression of the genes involved in the inflammatory response is unclear, zearalenone acting both as pro- or anti-inflammatory molecule/agent.

Although the involvement of ERS in the mechanism of apoptosis vs. cell death induced by ZEA is well defined, their involvement in the pro- or anti-inflammatory activity of ZEA is less evident. The activation of both ER-α or ER-β receptors reduced the inflammation [147,148] and this is the reason for which the estrogens are used as therapeutic agents in inflammation associated with metabolic diseases [149]. However, ER-α or ER-β were not involved in the alteration of the innate immune response induced by ZEA [51].

Toll like receptors (TLRs) plays a role in the ZEA induced inflammation. Pre-stimulation of RAW264.7 macrophages with different TLR ligands led to a different activation of TLR signaling and consequently to a different modulation of pro- and anti-inflammatory cytokines [38]. Thus, priming of RAW264.7 macrophages with TLR4 and TLR9 for 12 h increase both expression and synthesis of IL-1β and decrease that of TNF-α, while the TLR2 priming resulted in increase of IL-1β, TNF-α and IL-10. Also, other studies showed that ZEA promotes a pro-inflammatory response in response to TLR ligand stimulation. Increased protein and mRNA expression of trans-membrane receptor TLR4 was observed in kidney of pregnant rats exposed to increased concentrations of zearalenone and was associated with an increase of NF-κB/p65 and pro- inflammatory cytokine level [150]. TLR4 plays an important role in initiating and accelerating of inflammation and it is a key element in the TLR4/MyD88 signaling pathway [151]. It can be assumed that TLR-4 role in ZEA induced inflammation is very important especially under simultaneously infectious disease and mycotoxin contamination. Indeed, using a microarray technology and the analyses of gene expression pattern it was observed that the exposure of IPEC-1 cells to 10μM of ZEA up-regulated the expression of several genes involved in the inflammatory response, while the co-exposure to both ZEA and *Escherichia coli*, up-regulated 33 genes [45]. Also, in the same cell line, co-exposure to ZEA and *E. coli* resulted in an increase of inflammatory response through an activation of the MyD88/IRAQ/TRAF6/NF-κB pathway via TLR4 [33]. In vivo studies demonstrated that at the level of the two important immune organs ZEA generate a biphasic inflammatory effect by triggering two different mechanisms. In the spleen of growing piglets fed diet contaminated with 316ppb of ZEA, 10% of the total up-regulated genes were genes involved in inflammation. The inflammatory mechanism involved by ZEA was the activation of JNK pathway [141]. Through mechanisms related also to MAPK-kinases pathways activation (ERK and p38), ZEA induced in activated neutrophiles the formation of neutrophil extracellular trap, consisting in extracellular chromatin filaments with a major role in inflammation [138]. By contrast, in the liver ZEA produced a dramatically decreased in gene expression coding for pro-inflammatory cytokines along with the decrease of NF-κB and p38 MAPK gene expression.

Recent studies have shown the involvement of inflammasome in the inflammation induced by ZEA. In vitro and in vivo exposure to ZEA activated the ROS-mediated NLRP3 inflammasome in mouse peritoneal macrophages and in the colon of ZEA exposed mice, which resulted in the caspase-1 dependent activation of the inflammatory cytokines IL-1ß and IL-18 [152]. NF-κB/p65 activation induced by ZEA also contribute to the activation of the NLRP3 inflammasome, inflammatory response and cell death caspase-1 dependent in insulinoma cell line [153]. However, in colon tissue of mice with dextran sulphate induced colitis ZEA was able to reduce the inflammatory reaction [154]. The immunosuppressive effect of ZEA is due to the inhibition of MAPK activity (TAK1/JNK/p38) and NF-κB [64].

The capacity of ZEA to interfere with the immune response is probably related to an alteration of the organism self-tolerance. For example, in pig spleen, ZEA can decrease the expression of FoxP3 gene, a master gene involved in the immune tolerance mechanisms that can be correlated with a potentiation of the inflammatory response [141]. This hypothesis is also sustained by a decrease of Treg cells after ZEA exposure with consequences on self-tolerance maintenance and control of the immune response [38].

In conclusion, despite an increasing number of studies concerning the mechanisms involved in immunotoxicity induced by ZEA, the available data are unsubstantial and needs further works. Nevertheless, the data presented here in showed that zearalenone and its metabolites are immunotoxic and altered the immune cell viability and proliferation, cell cycle as well as immune cells functionality such as inflammatory response and their capacity to synthesize active molecules. In this review, we have suggested the mechanisms responsible for the immunotoxic effects induced by ZEA. However, more studies are needed in the future, in order to validate the proposed mechanisms.

Author Contributions: D.E.M. and I.T.-conceptualization; C.V.B.-original draft preparation; I.T., D.E.M., C.V.B. and G.C.P. writing—review and editing. All authors have read and agreed to the published version of the manuscript.

Funding: This work was financed thought the projects 8PCCDI0473-PC1 and ADER 9.2.1. financed by Romanian Ministry of Education and Research and Ministry of Agriculture and Rural Development.

Institutional Review Board Statement: Not applicable.

Informed Consent Statement: Not applicable.

Data Availability Statement: Not applicable.

Conflicts of Interest: The authors declare no conflict of interest.

References

1. Bakker, M.G.; Brown, D.W.; Kelly, A.C.; Kim, H.-S.; Kurtzman, C.P.; Mccormick, S.P.; O'Donnell, K.L.; Proctor, R.H.; Vaughan, M.M.; Ward, T.J. Fusarium mycotoxins: A trans-disciplinary overview. *Can. J. Plant Pathol.* **2018**, *40*, 161–171. [CrossRef]
2. Rai, A.; Das, M.; Tripathi, A. Occurrence and toxicity of a fusarium mycotoxin, zearalenone. *Crit. Rev. Food Sci. Nutr.* **2020**, *60*, 2710–2729. [CrossRef] [PubMed]
3. Cavret, S.; Lecoeur, S. Fusariotoxin transfer in animal. *Food Chem. Toxicol.* **2006**, *44*, 444–453. [CrossRef] [PubMed]
4. Ünüsan, N. Systematic review of mycotoxins in food and feeds in Turkey. *Food Control* **2019**, *97*, 1–14. [CrossRef]
5. Aiko, V.; Mehta, A. Occurrence, detection and detoxification of mycotoxins. *J. Biosci.* **2015**, *40*, 943–954. [CrossRef] [PubMed]
6. Eriksen, G.S.; Pettersson, H.; Lindberg, J.E. Absorption, metabolism and excretion of 3-acetyl DON in pigs. *Arch. Tierernahr.* **2003**, *57*, 335–345. [CrossRef]
7. Kamle, M.; Mahato, D.K.; Devi, S.; Lee, K.E.; Kang, S.G.; Kumar, P. Fumonisins: Impact on Agriculture, Food, and Human Health and their Management Strategies. *Toxins* **2019**, *11*, 328. [CrossRef]
8. Rodríguez-Blanco, M.; Ramos, A.J.; Sanchis, V.; Marín, S. Mycotoxins occurrence and fungal populations in different types of silages for dairy cows in Spain. *Fungal Biol.* **2019**. [CrossRef]

9. Rogowska, A.; Pomastowski, P.; Sagandykova, G.; Buszewski, B. Zearalenone and its metabolites: Effect on human health, metabolism and neutralisation methods. *Toxicon* **2019**, *162*, 46–56. [CrossRef]
10. Maragos, C. Zearalenone occurrence and human exposure. *World Mycotoxin J.* **2010**, *3*. [CrossRef]
11. Złoch, M.; Rogowska, A.; Pomastowski, P.; Railean-Plugaru, V.; Walczak-Skierska, J.; Rudnicka, J.; Buszewski, B. Use of Lactobacillus paracasei strain for zearalenone binding and metabolization. *Toxicon* **2020**, *181*, 9–18. [CrossRef] [PubMed]
12. Jia, R.; Liu, W.; Zhao, L.; Cao, L.; Shen, Z. Low doses of individual and combined deoxynivalenol and zearalenone in naturally moldy diets impair intestinal functions via inducing inflammation and disrupting epithelial barrier in the intestine of piglets. *Toxicol. Lett.* **2020**, *333*, 159–169. [CrossRef] [PubMed]
13. Zhou, J.; Zhu, L.; Chen, J.; Wang, W.; Zhang, R.; Li, Y.; Zhang, Q.; Wang, W. Degradation mechanism for Zearalenone ring-cleavage by Zearalenone hydrolase RmZHD: A QM/MM study. *Sci. Total Environ.* **2020**, *709*, 135897. [CrossRef]
14. Kowalska, K.; Habrowska-Górczyńska, D.E.; Piastowska-Ciesielska, A.W. Zearalenone as an endocrine disruptor in humans. *Environ. Toxicol. Pharmacol.* **2016**, *48*, 141–149. [CrossRef]
15. Busk, Ø.L.; Ndossi, D.; Verhaegen, S.; Connolly, L.; Eriksen, G.; Ropstad, E.; Sørlie, M. Relative quantification of the proteomic changes associated with the mycotoxin zearalenone in the H295R steroidogenesis model. *Toxicon* **2011**, *58*, 533–542. [CrossRef] [PubMed]
16. Zinedine, A.; Soriano, J.M.; Moltó, J.C.; Mañes, J. Review on the toxicity, occurrence, metabolism, detoxification, regulations and intake of zearalenone: An oestrogenic mycotoxin. *Food Chem. Toxicol.* **2007**, *45*, 1–18. [CrossRef] [PubMed]
17. Rogowska, A.; Pomastowski, P.; Rafińska, K.; Railean-Plugaru, V.; Złoch, M.; Walczak, J.; Buszewski, B. A study of zearalenone biosorption and metabolisation by prokaryotic and eukaryotic cells. *Toxicon* **2019**, *169*, 81–90. [CrossRef] [PubMed]
18. Bennett, J.W.; Klich, M. Mycotoxins. *Clin. Microbiol. Rev.* **2003**, *16*, 497 LP–516. [CrossRef]
19. Marin, D.E.; Taranu, I.; Burlacu, R.; Manda, G.; Motiu, M.; Neagoe, I.; Dragomir, C.; Stancu, M.; Calin, L. Effects of zearalenone and its derivatives on porcine immune response. *Toxicol. Vitr.* **2011**, *25*, 1981–1988. [CrossRef]
20. Chang, S.; Su, Y.; Sun, Y.; Meng, X.; Shi, B.; Shan, A. Response of the nuclear receptors PXR and CAR and their target gene mRNA expression in female piglets exposed to zearalenone. *Toxicon* **2018**, *151*, 111–118. [CrossRef]
21. Pierron, A.; Alassane-Kpembi, I.; Oswald, I.P. Impact of mycotoxin on immune response and consequences for pig health. *Anim. Nutr.* **2016**, *2*, 63–68. [CrossRef]
22. Taranu, I.; Braicu, C.; Marin, D.E.; Pistol, G.C.; Motiu, M.; Balacescu, L.; Beridan Neagoe, I.; Burlacu, R. Exposure to zearalenone mycotoxin alters in vitro porcine intestinal epithelial cells by differential gene expression. *Toxicol. Lett.* **2015**, *232*, 310–325. [CrossRef] [PubMed]
23. Groschwitz, K.R.; Hogan, S.P. Intestinal barrier function: Molecular regulation and disease pathogenesis. *J. Allergy Clin. Immunol.* **2009**, *124*, 3–20. [CrossRef]
24. Vancamelbeke, M.; Vermeire, S. The intestinal barrier: A fundamental role in health and disease. *Expert Rev. Gastroenterol. Hepatol.* **2017**, *11*, 821–834. [CrossRef] [PubMed]
25. Lahjouji, T.; Bertaccini, A.; Neves, M.; Puel, S.; Oswald, I.P.; Soler, L. Acute Exposure to Zearalenone Disturbs Intestinal Homeostasis by Modulating the Wnt/β-Catenin Signaling Pathway. *Toxins* **2020**, *12*, 113. [CrossRef] [PubMed]
26. Lewczuk, B.; Przybylska-Gornowicz, B.; Gajęcka, M.; Targońska, K.; Ziółkowska, N.; Prusik, M.; Gajęcki, M. Histological structure of duodenum in gilts receiving low doses of zearalenone and deoxynivalenol in feed. *Exp. Toxicol. Pathol.* **2016**, *68*, 157–166. [CrossRef]
27. Gajęcka, M.; Tarasiuk, M.; Zielonka, Ł.; Dąbrowski, M.; Gajęcki, M. Risk assessment for changes in the metabolic profile and body weights of pre-pubertal gilts during long-term monotonic exposure to low doses of zearalenone (ZEN). *Res. Vet. Sci.* **2016**, *109*, 169–180. [CrossRef] [PubMed]
28. Liu, M.; Gao, R.; Meng, Q.; Zhang, Y.; Bi, C.; Shan, A. Toxic Effects of Maternal Zearalenone Exposure on Intestinal Oxidative Stress, Barrier Function, Immunological and Morphological Changes in Rats. *PLoS ONE* **2014**, *9*, 1–14. [CrossRef]
29. Zheng, W.-L.; Wang, B.-J.; Wang, L.; Shan, Y.-P.; Zou, H.; Song, R.-L.; Wang, T.; Gu, J.-H.; Yuan, Y.; Liu, X.-Z.; et al. ROS-Mediated Cell Cycle Arrest and Apoptosis Induced by Zearalenone in Mouse Sertoli Cells via ER Stress and the ATP/AMPK Pathway. *Toxins* **2018**, *10*, 24. [CrossRef]
30. Johansson, M.E.V.; Hansson, G.C. Mucus and the Goblet Cell. *Dig. Dis.* **2013**, *31*, 305–309. [CrossRef]
31. Wang, X.; Yu, H.; Fang, H.; Zhao, Y.; Jin, Y.; Shen, J.; Zhou, C.; Zhou, Y.; Fu, Y.; Wang, J.; et al. Transcriptional profiling of zearalenone-induced inhibition of IPEC-J2 cell proliferation. *Toxicon* **2019**, *172*, 8–14. [CrossRef]
32. Marin, D.; Motiu, M.; Taranu, I. Food Contaminant Zearalenone and Its Metabolites Affect Cytokine Synthesis and Intestinal Epithelial Integrity of Porcine Cells. *Toxins* **2015**, *7*, 1979–1988. [CrossRef] [PubMed]
33. Taranu, I.; Marin, D.E.; Pistol, G.C.; Motiu, M.; Pelinescu, D. Induction of pro-inflammatory gene expression by Escherichia coli and mycotoxin zearalenone contamination and protection by a Lactobacillus mixture in porcine IPEC-1 cells. *Toxicon* **2015**, *97*, 53–63. [CrossRef] [PubMed]
34. Fan, W.; Lv, Y.; Ren, S.; Shao, M.; Shen, T.; Huang, K.; Zhou, J.; Yan, L.; Song, S. Zearalenone (ZEA)-induced intestinal inflammation is mediated by the NLRP3 inflammasome. *Chemosphere* **2018**, *190*, 272–279. [CrossRef] [PubMed]
35. Long, M.; Chen, X.; Wang, N.; Wang, M.; Pan, J.; Tong, J.; Li, P.; Yang, S.; He, J. Proanthocyanidins Protect Epithelial Cells from Zearalenone-Induced Apoptosis via Inhibition of Endoplasmic Reticulum Stress-Induced Apoptosis Pathways in Mouse Small Intestines. *Molecules* **2018**, *23*, 1508. [CrossRef]

36. Ben Salem, I.; Prola, A.; Boussabbeh, M.; Guilbert, A.; Bacha, H.; Abid-Essefi, S.; Lemaire, C. Crocin and Quercetin protect HCT116 and HEK293 cells from Zearalenone-induced apoptosis by reducing endoplasmic reticulum stress. *Cell Stress Chaperones* **2015**, *20*, 927–938. [CrossRef]
37. Obremski, K.; Gonkowski, S.; Wojtacha, P. Zearalenone-induced changes in the lymphoid tissue and mucosal nerve fibers in the porcine ileum. *Pol. J. Vet. Sci.* **2015**, *18*, 357–365. [CrossRef]
38. Islam, M.R.; Kim, J.W.; Roh, Y.-S.; Kim, J.-H.; Han, K.M.; Kwon, H.-J.; Lim, C.W.; Kim, B. Evaluation of immunomodulatory effects of zearalenone in mice. *J. Immunotoxicol.* **2017**, *14*, 125–136. [CrossRef]
39. Kato, L.M.; Kawamoto, S.; Maruya, M.; Fagarasan, S. Gut TFH and IgA: Key players for regulation of bacterial communities and immune homeostasis. *Immunol. Cell Biol.* **2014**, *92*, 49–56. [CrossRef]
40. Okumura, R.; Takeda, K. Maintenance of intestinal homeostasis by mucosal barriers. *Inflamm. Regen.* **2018**, *38*, 5. [CrossRef]
41. Wang, X.; Yu, H.; Shan, A.; Jin, Y.; Fang, H.; Zhao, Y.; Shen, J.; Zhou, C.; Zhou, Y.; Fu, Y.; et al. Toxic effects of Zearalenone on intestinal microflora and intestinal mucosal immunity in mice. *Food Agric. Immunol.* **2018**, *29*, 1002–1011. [CrossRef]
42. Linden, S.K.; Sutton, P.; Karlsson, N.G.; Korolik, V.; McGuckin, M.A. Mucins in the mucosal barrier to infection. *Mucosal Immunol.* **2008**, *1*, 183–197. [CrossRef] [PubMed]
43. Wan, L.-Y.M.; Allen, K.J.; Turner, P.C.; El-Nezami, H. Modulation of Mucin mRNA (MUC5AC and MUC5B) Expression and Protein Production and Secretion in Caco-2/HT29-MTX Co-cultures Following Exposure to Individual and Combined Fusarium Mycotoxins. *Toxicol. Sci.* **2014**, *139*, 83–98. [CrossRef]
44. Wan, M.L.-Y.; Woo, C.-S.J.; Allen, K.J.; Turner, P.C.; El-Nezami, H. Modulation of Porcine β-Defensins 1 and 2 upon Individual and Combined Fusarium Toxin Exposure in a Swine Jejunal Epithelial Cell Line. *Appl. Environ. Microbiol.* **2013**, *79*, 2225–2232. [CrossRef] [PubMed]
45. Braicu, C.; Selicean, S.; Cojocneanu-Petric, R.; Lajos, R.; Balacescu, O.; Taranu, I.; Marin, D.E.; Motiu, M.; Jurj, A.; Achimas-Cadariu, P.; et al. Evaluation of cellular and molecular impact of zearalenone and Escherichia coli co-exposure on IPEC-1 cells using microarray technology. *BMC Genom.* **2016**, *17*, 576. [CrossRef] [PubMed]
46. Benthem de Grave, X.; Saltzmann, J.; Laurain, J.; Rodriguez, M.A.; Molist, F.; Dänicke, S.; Santos, R.R. Transmission of Zearalenone, Deoxynivalenol, and Their Derivatives from Sows to Piglets during Lactation. *Toxins* **2021**, *13*, 37. [CrossRef] [PubMed]
47. Medzhitov, R.; Janeway, C.J. Innate immune recognition: Mechanisms and pathways. *Immunol. Rev.* **2000**, *173*, 89–97. [CrossRef]
48. Shaw, A.C.; Joshi, S.; Greenwood, H.; Panda, A.; Lord, J.M. Aging of the innate immune system. *Curr. Opin. Immunol.* **2010**, *22*, 507–513. [CrossRef]
49. Edreva, A. Generation and scavenging of reactive oxygen species in chloroplasts: a submolecular approach. *Agric. Ecosyst. Environ.* **2005**, *106*, 119–133. [CrossRef]
50. Chen, X.; Song, M.; Zhang, B.; Zhang, Y. Reactive Oxygen Species Regulate T Cell Immune Response in the Tumor Microenvironment. *Oxid. Med. Cell. Longev.* **2016**, *2016*, 1580967. [CrossRef]
51. Wang, J.; Wei, Z.; Han, Z.; Liu, Z.; Zhu, X.; Li, X.; Wang, K.; Yang, Z. Zearalenone Induces Estrogen-Receptor-Independent Neutrophil Extracellular Trap Release in Vitro. *J. Agric. Food Chem.* **2019**, *67*. [CrossRef]
52. Marin, D.E.; Taranu, I.; Burlacu, R.; Tudor, D.S. Effects of zearalenone and its derivatives on the innate immune response of swine. *Toxicon* **2010**, *56*, 956–963. [CrossRef]
53. Murata, H.; Sultana, P.; Shimada, N.; Yoshioka, M. Structure-activity relationships among zearalenone and its derivatives based on bovine neutrophil chemiluminescence. *Vet. Hum. Toxicol.* **2003**, *45*, 18—20.
54. Borutova, R.; Faix, S.; Placha, I.; Gresakova, L.; Cobanova, K.; Leng, L. Effects of deoxynivalenol and zearalenone on oxidative stress and blood phagocytic activity in broilers. *Arch. Anim. Nutr.* **2008**, *62*, 303–312. [CrossRef]
55. Solhaug, A.; Karlsøen, L.M.; Holme, J.A.; Kristoffersen, A.B.; Eriksen, G.S. Immunomodulatory effects of individual and combined mycotoxins in the THP-1 cell line. *Toxicol. Vitr.* **2016**, *36*, 120–132. [CrossRef]
56. Chen, F.; Li, Q.; Zhang, Z.; Lin, P.; Lei, L.; Wang, A.; Jin, Y. Endoplasmic Reticulum Stress Cooperates in Zearalenone-Induced Cell Death of RAW 264.7 Macrophages. *Int. J. Mol. Sci.* **2015**, *16*, 19780–19795. [CrossRef] [PubMed]
57. Hueza, I.; Raspantini, P.; Raspantini, L.; Latorre, A.; Górniak, S. Zearalenone, an Estrogenic Mycotoxin, Is an Immunotoxic Compound. *Toxins* **2014**, *6*, 1080–1095. [CrossRef]
58. Skiepko, N.; Przybylska-Gornowicz, B.; Gajęcka, M.; Gajęcki, M.; Lewczuk, B. Effects of Deoxynivalenol and Zearalenone on the Histology and Ultrastructure of Pig Liver. *Toxins* **2020**, *12*, 463. [CrossRef]
59. Oswald, I.I.; Bouhet, S.; Marin, D.E.; Pinton, P.P.; Taranu, I. Mycotoxin effects on the pig immune system. *Feed Compd.* **2003**, *9*, 16–20.
60. Peveri, P.; Walz, A.; Dewald, B.; Baggiolini, M. A novel neutrophil-activating factor produced by human mononuclear phagocytes. *J. Exp. Med.* **1988**, *167*, 1547–1559. [CrossRef]
61. Ding, J.; Yeh, C.-R.; Sun, Y.; Lin, C.; Chou, J.; Ou, Z.; Chang, C.; Qi, J.; Yeh, S. Estrogen receptor β promotes renal cell carcinoma progression via regulating LncRNA HOTAIR-miR-138/200c/204/217 associated CeRNA network. *Oncogene* **2018**, *37*, 5037–5053. [CrossRef]
62. Ruh, M.F.; Bi, Y.; Cox, L.; Berk, D.; Howlett, A.C.; Bellone, C.J. Effect of environmental estrogens on IL-1beta promoter activity in a macrophage cell line. *Endocrine* **1998**, *9*, 207–211. [CrossRef]

63. Seyed Toutounchi, N.; Hogenkamp, A.; Varasteh, S.; van't Land, B.; Garssen, J.; Kraneveld, A.D.; Folkerts, G.; Braber, S. Fusarium Mycotoxins Disrupt the Barrier and Induce IL-6 Release in a Human Placental Epithelium Cell Line. *Toxins* **2019**, *11*, 665. [CrossRef]
64. Pistol, G.C.; Gras, M.A.; Marin, D.E.; Israel-Roming, F.; Stancu, M.; Taranu, I. Natural feed contaminant zearalenone decreases the expressions of important pro- and anti-inflammatory mediators and mitogen-activated protein kinase/NF-κB signalling molecules in pigs. *Br. J. Nutr.* **2014**, *111*, 452–464. [CrossRef]
65. Abbès, S.; Salah-Abbès, J.B.; Sharafi, H.; Noghabi, K.A.; Oueslati, R. Interaction of Lactobacillus plantarum MON03 with Tunisian Montmorillonite clay and ability of the composite to immobilize Zearalenone in vitro and counteract immunotoxicity in vivo. *Immunopharmacol. Immunotoxicol.* **2012**, *34*, 944–950. [CrossRef]
66. Salah-Abbès, J.; Abbes, S.; Houas, Z.; Abdel-Wahhab, P.M.; Oueslati, R. Zearalenone induces immunotoxicity in mice: Possible protective effects of Radish extract (Raphanus Sativus). *J. Pharm. Pharmacol.* **2008**, *60*, 761–770. [CrossRef] [PubMed]
67. Ben Salah-Abbès, J.; Belgacem, H.; Ezzdini, K.; Abdel-Wahhab, M.A.; Abbès, S. Zearalenone nephrotoxicity: DNA fragmentation, apoptotic gene expression and oxidative stress protected by Lactobacillus plantarum MON03. *Toxicon* **2020**, *175*, 28–35. [CrossRef]
68. Del Fabbro, L.; Jesse, C.R.; de Gomes, M.G.; Borges Filho, C.; Donato, F.; Souza, L.C.; Goes, A.R.; Furian, A.F.; Boeira, S.P. The flavonoid chrysin protects against zearalenone induced reproductive toxicity in male mice. *Toxicon* **2019**, *165*, 13–21. [CrossRef] [PubMed]
69. Virk, P.; Al-mukhaizeem, N.A.R.; Bin Morebah, S.H.; Fouad, D.; Elobeid, M. Protective effect of resveratrol against toxicity induced by the mycotoxin, zearalenone in a rat model. *Food Chem. Toxicol.* **2020**, *146*, 111840. [CrossRef]
70. Yin, S.; Zhang, Y.; Gao, R.; Cheng, B.; Shan, A. The immunomodulatory effects induced by dietary Zearalenone in pregnant rats. *Immunopharmacol. Immunotoxicol.* **2014**, *36*, 187–194. [CrossRef] [PubMed]
71. Abbès, S.; Salah-Abbès, J.B.; Ouanes, Z.; Houas, Z.; Othman, O.; Bacha, H.; Abdel-Wahhab, M.A.; Oueslati, R. Preventive role of phyllosilicate clay on the Immunological and Biochemical toxicity of zearalenone in Balb/c mice. *Int. Immunopharmacol.* **2006**, *6*, 1251–1258. [CrossRef]
72. Choi, B.-K.; Cho, J.-H.; Jeong, S.-H.; Shin, H.-S.; Son, S.-W.; Yeo, Y.-K.; Kang, H.-G. Zearalenone affects immune-related parameters in lymphoid organs and serum of rats vaccinated with porcine parvovirus vaccine. *Toxicol. Res.* **2012**, *28*, 279–288. [CrossRef]
73. Wu, F.; Cui, J.; Yang, X.; Liu, S.; Han, S.; Chen, B. Effects of zearalenone on genital organ development, serum immunoglobulin, antioxidant capacity, sex hormones and liver function of prepubertal gilts. *Toxicon* **2021**, *189*, 39–44. [CrossRef]
74. Reddy, K.; Lee, W.; Lee, S.; Jeong, J.; Kim, D.; Kim, M.; Lee, H.; Oh, Y.; Jo, H. Effects of dietary deoxynivalenol and zearalenone on the organ pro-inflammatory gene expressions and serum immunoglobulins of pigs. *J. Anim. Sci.* **2017**, *95*, 203. [CrossRef]
75. Ren, Z.H.; Zhou, R.; Deng, J.L.; Zuo, Z.C.; Peng, X.; Wang, Y.C.; Wang, Y.; Yu, S.M.; Shen, L.H.; Cui, H.M.; et al. Effects of the Fusarium toxin zearalenone (ZEA) and/or deoxynivalenol (DON) on the serum IgA, IgG and IgM levels in mice. *Food Agric. Immunol.* **2014**, *25*, 600–606. [CrossRef]
76. Yang, L.; Yang, W.; Feng, Q.; Huang, L.; Zhang, G.; Liu, F.; Jiang, S.; Yang, Z. Effects of purified zearalenone on selected immunological measurements of blood in post-weaning gilts. *Anim. Nutr.* **2016**, *2*, 142–148. [CrossRef]
77. Forsell, J.H.; Witt, M.F.; Tai, J.-H.; Jensen, R.; Pestka, J.J. Effects of 8-week exposure of the B6C3F1 mouse to dietary deoxynivalenol (vomitoxin) and zearalenone. *Food Chem. Toxicol.* **1986**, *24*, 213–219. [CrossRef]
78. Jakovac-Strajn, B.; Vengušt, A.; Pestevšek, U. Effects of a deoxynivalenol-contaminated diet on the reproductive performance and immunoglobulin concentrations in pigs. *Vet. Rec.* **2009**, *165*, 713–718. [CrossRef]
79. Pestka, J.J.; Tai, J.-H.; Witt, M.F.; Dixon, D.E.; Forsell, J.H. Suppression of immune response in the B6C3F1 mouse after dietary exposure to the fusarium mycotoxins deoxynivalenol (vomitoxin) and zearalenone. *Food Chem. Toxicol.* **1987**, *25*, 297–304. [CrossRef]
80. Antonissen, G.; Martel, A.; Pasmans, F.; Ducatelle, R.; Verbrugghe, E.; Vandenbroucke, V.; Li, S.; Haesebrouck, F.; Van Immerseel, F.; Croubels, S. The Impact of Fusarium Mycotoxins on Human and Animal Host Susceptibility to Infectious Diseases. *Toxins* **2014**, *6*. [CrossRef] [PubMed]
81. Teixeira, L.C.; Montiani-Ferreira, F.; Locatelli-Dittrich, R.; Santin, E.; Alberton, G.C. Effects of zearalenone in prepubertal gilts. *Pesqui. Veterinária Bras.* **2011**, *31*, 656–662. [CrossRef]
82. Wang, Y.C.; Deng, J.L.; Xu, S.W.; Peng, X.; Zuo, Z.C.; Cui, H.M.; Wang, Y.; Ren, Z.H. Effects of Zearalenone on IL-2, IL-6, and IFN-? mRNA Levels in the Splenic Lymphocytes of Chickens. *Sci. World J.* **2012**, *2012*, 567327. [CrossRef]
83. Berek, L.; Petri, I.B.; Mesterházy, Á.; Téren, J.; Molnár, J. Effects of mycotoxins on human immune functions in vitro. *Toxicol. Vitr.* **2001**, *15*, 25–30. [CrossRef]
84. Committee, E.S. Scientific opinion on genotoxicity testing strategies applicable to food and feed safety assessment. *EFSA J.* **2011**, *9*, 2379. [CrossRef]
85. Forsell, J.H.; Kateley, J.R.; Yoshizawa, T.; Pestka, J.J. Inhibition of mitogen-induced blastogenesis in human lymphocytes by T-2 toxin and its metabolites. *Appl. Environ. Microbiol.* **1985**, *49*, 1523 LP–1526. [CrossRef]
86. Forsell, J.H.; Pestka, J.J. Relation of 8-ketotrichothecene and zearalenone analog structure to inhibition of mitogen-induced human lymphocyte blastogenesis. *Appl. Environ. Microbiol.* **1985**, *50*, 1304 LP–1307. [CrossRef]
87. Vlata, Z.; Porichis, F.; Tzanakakis, G.; Tsatsakis, A.; Krambovitis, E. A study of zearalenone cytotoxicity on human peripheral blood mononuclear cells. *Toxicol. Lett.* **2006**, *165*, 274–281. [CrossRef] [PubMed]

88. Zhang, K.; Tan, X.; Li, Y.; Liang, G.; Ning, Z.; Ma, Y.; Li, Y. Transcriptional profiling analysis of Zearalenone-induced inhibition proliferation on mouse thymic epithelial cell line 1. *Ecotoxicol. Environ. Saf.* **2018**, *153*, 135–141. [CrossRef]
89. Zheng, W.; Fan, W.; Feng, N.; Lu, N.; Zou, H.; Gu, J.; Yuan, Y.; Liu, X.; Bai, J.; Bian, J.; et al. The Role of miRNAs in Zearalenone-Promotion of TM3 Cell Proliferation. *Int. J. Environ. Res. Public Health* **2019**, *16*, 1517. [CrossRef] [PubMed]
90. Swamy, H.V.L.N.; Smith, T.K.; Karrow, N.A.; Boermans, H.J. Effects of feeding blends of grains naturally contaminated with Fusarium mycotoxins on growth and immunological parameters of broiler chickens1. *Poult. Sci.* **2004**, *83*, 533–543. [CrossRef] [PubMed]
91. Delves, P.J.; Martin, S.J.; Burton, D.R.; Roitt, I.M. *Roitt's Essential Immunology*, 13th ed.; Wiley-Blackwell: London, UK, 2017; ISBN 978-1-118-41577-1.
92. Roitt, I. *Roitt's Essential Immunology*; Blackwell Publishing: London, UK, 2006.
93. Yu, J.-Y.; Zheng, Z.-H.; Son, Y.-O.; Shi, X.; Jang, Y.-O.; Lee, J.-C. Mycotoxin zearalenone induces AIF- and ROS-mediated cell death through p53- and MAPK-dependent signaling pathways in RAW264.7 macrophages. *Toxicol. Vitr.* **2011**, *25*, 1654–1663. [CrossRef]
94. Yang, L.-J.; Zhou, M.; Huang, L.-B.; Yang, W.-R.; Yang, Z.-B.; Jiang, S.-Z.; Ge, J.-S. Zearalenone-Promoted Follicle Growth through Modulation of Wnt-1/β-Catenin Signaling Pathway and Expression of Estrogen Receptor Genes in Ovaries of Postweaning Piglets. *J. Agric. Food Chem.* **2018**, *66*, 7899–7906. [CrossRef]
95. Song, T.; Yang, W.; Huang, L.; Yang, Z.; Jiang, S. Zearalenone exposure affects the Wnt/β-catenin signaling pathway and related genes of porcine endometrial epithelial cells in vitro. *Asian-Australas J. Anim. Sci.* **2020**. [CrossRef]
96. Chen, F.; Wen, X.; Lin, P.; Chen, H.; Wang, A.; Jin, Y. HERP depletion inhibits zearalenone-induced apoptosis through autophagy activation in mouse ovarian granulosa cells. *Toxicol. Lett.* **2019**, *301*, 1–10. [CrossRef] [PubMed]
97. Zhang, G.-L.; Song, J.-L.; Zhou, Y.; Zhang, R.-Q.; Cheng, S.-F.; Sun, X.-F.; Qin, G.-Q.; Shen, W.; Li, L. Differentiation of sow and mouse ovarian granulosa cells exposed to zearalenone in vitro using RNA-seq gene expression. *Toxicol. Appl. Pharmacol.* **2018**, *350*, 78–90. [CrossRef] [PubMed]
98. Zhang, R.Q.; Sun, X.F.; Wu, R.Y.; Cheng, S.F.; Zhang, G.L.; Zhai, Q.Y.; Liu, X.L.; Zhao, Y.; Shen, W.; Li, L. Zearalenone exposure elevated the expression of tumorigenesis genes in mouse ovarian granulosa cells. *Toxicol. Appl. Pharmacol.* **2018**, *356*, 191–203. [CrossRef]
99. Cortinovis, C.; Caloni, F.; Schreiber, N.B.; Spicer, L.J. Effects of fumonisin B1 alone and combined with deoxynivalenol or zearalenone on porcine granulosa cell proliferation and steroid production. *Theriogenology* **2014**, *81*, 1042–1049. [CrossRef] [PubMed]
100. Pan, P.; Ma, F.; Wu, K.; Yu, Y.; Li, Y.; Li, Z.; Chen, X.; Huang, T.; Wang, Y.; Ge, R. Maternal exposure to zearalenone in masculinization window affects the fetal Leydig cell development in rat male fetus. *Environ. Pollut.* **2020**, *263*, 114357. [CrossRef]
101. Wang, S.; Ren, X.; Hu, X.; Zhou, L.; Zhang, C.; Zhang, M. Cadmium-induced apoptosis through reactive oxygen species-mediated mitochondrial oxidative stress and the JNK signaling pathway in TM3 cells, a model of mouse Leydig cells. *Toxicol. Appl. Pharmacol.* **2019**, *368*, 37–48. [CrossRef]
102. Cai, G.; Si, M.; Li, X.; Zou, H.; Gu, J.; Yuan, Y.; Liu, X.; Liu, Z.; Bian, J. Zearalenone induces apoptosis of rat Sertoli cells through Fas-Fas ligand and mitochondrial pathway. *Environ. Toxicol.* **2019**, *34*, 424–433. [CrossRef]
103. Márton, É.; Varga, A.; Széles, L.; Göczi, L.; Penyige, A.; Nagy, B.; Szilágyi, M. The Cell-Free Expression of MiR200 Family Members Correlates with Estrogen Sensitivity in Human Epithelial Ovarian Cells. *Int. J. Mol. Sci.* **2020**, *21*, 9725. [CrossRef]
104. Kowalska, K.; Habrowska-Górczyńska, D.E.; Domińska, K.; Urbanek, K.A.; Piastowska-Ciesielska, A.W. ERβ and NFκB—Modulators of Zearalenone-Induced Oxidative Stress in Human Prostate Cancer Cells. *Toxins* **2020**, *12*, 199. [CrossRef] [PubMed]
105. Dąbrowski, M.; Obremski, K.; Gajęcka, M.; Gajęcki, M.; Zielonka, Ł. Changes in the Subpopulations of Porcine Peripheral Blood Lymphocytes Induced by Exposure to Low Doses of Zearalenone (ZEN) and Deoxynivalenol (DON). *Molecules* **2016**, *21*, 557. [CrossRef]
106. Kostro, K.; Gajęcka, M.; Lisiecka, U.; Majer-Dziedzic, B.; Obremski, K.; Zielonka, Ł.; Gajęcki, M. Subpopulation of lymphocytes CD4 + and CD8 + in peripheral blood of sheep with zearalenone mycotoxicosis. *Bull. Vet. Inst. Pulawy* **2011**, *55*, 241–246.
107. Cai, G.; Pan, S.; Feng, N.; Zou, H.; Gu, J.; Yuan, Y.; Liu, X.; Liu, Z.; Bian, J. Zearalenone inhibits T cell chemotaxis by inhibiting cell adhesion and migration related proteins. *Ecotoxicol. Environ. Saf.* **2019**, *175*, 263–271. [CrossRef] [PubMed]
108. Ren, Z.H.; Deng, H.D.; Wang, Y.C.; Deng, J.L.; Zuo, Z.C.; Wang, Y.; Peng, X.; Cui, H.M.; Fang, J.; Yu, S.M.; et al. The Fusarium toxin zearalenone and deoxynivalenol affect murine splenic antioxidant functions, interferon levels, and T-cell subsets. *Environ. Toxicol. Pharmacol.* **2016**, *41*, 195–200. [CrossRef]
109. Obremski, K.; Wojtacha, P.; Podlasz, P.; Żmigrodzka, M. The influence of experimental administration of low zearalenone doses on the expression of Th1 and Th2 cytokines and on selected subpopulations of lymphocytes in intestinal lymph nodes. *Pol. J. Vet. Sci.* **2015**, *18*, 489–497. [CrossRef]
110. Chen, P.; Liu, T.; Jiang, S.; Yang, Z.; Huang, L.; Liu, F. Effects of purified zearalenone on selected immunological and histopathologic measurements of spleen in post-weanling gilts. *Anim. Nutr.* **2017**, *3*, 212–218. [CrossRef] [PubMed]
111. Reddy, K.E.; Lee, W.; Jeong, J.Y.; Lee, Y.; Lee, H.-J.; Kim, M.S.; Kim, D.-W.; Yu, D.; Cho, A.; Oh, Y.K.; et al. Effects of deoxynivalenol- and zearalenone-contaminated feed on the gene expression profiles in the kidneys of piglets. *Asian-Australas. J. Anim. Sci.* **2018**, *31*, 138–148. [CrossRef] [PubMed]
112. Minervini, F.; Dell'Aquila, M.E. Zearalenone and Reproductive Function in Farm Animals. *Int. J. Mol. Sci.* **2008**, *9*, 2570–2584. [CrossRef]

113. Chi, M.S.; Mirocha, C.J.; Kurtz, H.J.; Weaver, G.A.; Bates, F.; Robison, T.; Shimoda, W. Effect of Dietary Zearalenone on Growing Broiler Chicks1,2. *Poult. Sci.* **1980**, *59*, 531–536. [CrossRef]
114. Allen, N.K.; Mirocha, C.J.; Weaver, G.; Aakhus-Allen A, S.; Bates, F. Effects of Dietary Zearalenone on Finishing Broiler Chickens and Young Turkey Poults1,2. *Poult. Sci.* **1981**, *60*, 124–131. [CrossRef]
115. Kiessling, K.-H. The Effect of Zearalenone on Growth Rate, Organ Weight and Muscle Fibre Composition in Growing Rats. *Acta Pharmacol. Toxicol. (Cph.)* **1982**, *51*, 154–158. [CrossRef]
116. Denli, M.; Blandon, J.C.; Salado, S.; Guynot, M.E.; Pérez, J.F. Effect of dietary zearalenone on the performance, reproduction tract and serum biochemistry in young rats. *J. Appl. Anim. Res.* **2017**, *45*, 619–622. [CrossRef]
117. Chi, M.S.; Mirocha, C.J.; Weaver, G.A.; Kurtz, H.J. Effect of zearalenone on female White Leghorn chickens. *Appl. Environ. Microbiol.* **1980**, *39*, 1026–1030. [CrossRef]
118. Salah-Abbès, J.; Abbes, S.; Abdel-Wahhab, P.M.; Oueslati, R. Immunotoxicity of zearalenone in Balb/c mice in a high subchronic dosing study counteracted by Raphanus sativus extract. *Immunopharmacol. Immunotoxicol.* **2010**, *32*, 628–636. [CrossRef] [PubMed]
119. Parveen, M.; Zhu, Y.; Kiyama, R. Expression profiling of the genes responding to zearalenone and its analogues using estrogen-responsive genes. *FEBS Lett.* **2009**, *583*, 2377–2384. [CrossRef] [PubMed]
120. Shier, W.T.; Shier, A.C.; Xie, W.; Mirocha, C.J. Structure-activity relationships for human estrogenic activity in zearalenone mycotoxins. *Toxicon* **2001**, *39*, 1435–1438. [CrossRef]
121. Kuiper, G.G.J.M.; Lemmen, J.G.; Carlsson, B.; Corton, J.C.; Safe, S.H.; van der Saag, P.T.; van der Burg, B.; Gustafsson, J.-A. Interaction of Estrogenic Chemicals and Phytoestrogens with Estrogen Receptor β. *Endocrinology* **1998**, *139*, 4252–4263. [CrossRef]
122. Frizzell, C.; Ndossi, D.; Verhaegen, S.; Dahl, E.; Eriksen, G.; Sørlie, M.; Ropstad, E.; Muller, M.; Elliott, C.T.; Connolly, L. Endocrine disrupting effects of zearalenone, alpha- and beta-zearalenol at the level of nuclear receptor binding and steroidogenesis. *Toxicol. Lett.* **2011**, *206*, 210–217. [CrossRef] [PubMed]
123. Yip, K.Y.; Wan, M.L.Y.; Wong, A.S.T.; Korach, K.S.; El-Nezami, H. Combined low-dose zearalenone and aflatoxin B1 on cell growth and cell-cycle progression in breast cancer MCF-7 cells. *Toxicol. Lett.* **2017**, *281*, 139–151. [CrossRef]
124. Curran, E.M.; Berghaus, L.J.; Vernetti, N.J.; Saporita, A.J.; Lubahn, D.B.; Estes, D.M. Natural Killer Cells Express Estrogen Receptor-α and Estrogen Receptor-β and Can Respond to Estrogen Via a Non-Estrogen Receptor-α-Mediated Pathway. *Cell. Immunol.* **2001**, *214*, 12–20. [CrossRef] [PubMed]
125. Lang, T.J. Estrogen as an immunomodulator. *Clin. Immunol.* **2004**, *113*, 224–230. [CrossRef] [PubMed]
126. Böttner, M.; Thelen, P.; Jarry, H. Estrogen receptor beta: Tissue distribution and the still largely enigmatic physiological function. *J. Steroid Biochem. Mol. Biol.* **2014**, *139*, 245–251. [CrossRef]
127. Yaşar, P.; Ayaz, G.; Muyan, M. Estradiol-Estrogen Receptor α Mediates the Expression of the CXXC5 Gene through the Estrogen Response Element-Dependent Signaling Pathway. *Sci. Rep.* **2016**, *6*, 37808. [CrossRef]
128. Ferraiuolo, R.-M.; Tubman, J.; Sinha, I.; Hamm, C.; Porter, L.A. The cyclin-like protein, SPY1, regulates the ERα and ERK1/2 pathways promoting tamoxifen resistance. *Oncotarget* **2017**, *8*, 23337–23352. [CrossRef]
129. Kovats, S. Estrogen receptors regulate innate immune cells and signaling pathways. *Cell. Immunol.* **2015**, *294*, 63–69. [CrossRef]
130. Yao, S.; Wei, W.; Cao, R.; Lu, L.; Liang, S.; Xiong, M.; Zhang, C.; Liang, X.; Ma, Y. Resveratrol alleviates zea-induced decidualization disturbance in human endometrial stromal cells. *Ecotoxicol. Environ. Saf.* **2021**, *207*, 111511. [CrossRef]
131. Paterni, I.; Granchi, C.; Katzenellenbogen, J.A.; Minutolo, F. Estrogen receptors alpha (ERα) and beta (ERβ): Subtype-selective ligands and clinical potential. *Steroids* **2014**, *90*, 13–29. [CrossRef]
132. Zheng, W.; Wang, B.; Li, X.; Wang, T.; Zou, H.; Gu, J.; Yuan, Y.; Liu, X.; Bai, J.; Bian, J.; et al. Zearalenone Promotes Cell Proliferation or Causes Cell Death? *Toxins* **2018**, *10*, 184. [CrossRef]
133. Cai, G.; Sun, K.; Xia, S.; Feng, Z.; Zou, H.; Gu, J.; Yuan, Y.; Zhu, J.; Liu, Z.; Bian, J. Decrease in immune function and the role of mitogen-activated protein kinase (MAPK) overactivation in apoptosis during T lymphocytes activation induced by zearalenone, deoxynivalenol, and their combinations. *Chemosphere* **2020**, *255*, 126999. [CrossRef]
134. Guo, Y.; Pan, W.; Liu, S.; Shen, Z.; Xu, Y.; Hu, L. ERK/MAPK signalling pathway and tumorigenesis (Review). *Exp. Ther. Med.* **2020**, *19*, 1997–2007. [CrossRef]
135. Weston, C.R.; Davis, R.J. The JNK signal transduction pathway. *Curr. Opin. Cell Biol.* **2007**, *19*, 142–149. [CrossRef]
136. Filardo, E.J.; Quinn, J.A.; Bland, K.I.; Frackelton, A.R., Jr. Estrogen-Induced Activation of Erk-1 and Erk-2 Requires the G Protein-Coupled Receptor Homolog, GPR30, and Occurs via Trans-Activation of the Epidermal Growth Factor Receptor through Release of HB-EGF. *Mol. Endocrinol.* **2000**, *14*, 1649–1660. [CrossRef]
137. Marin, D.E.; Pistol, G.C.; Neagoe, I.V.; Calin, L.; Taranu, I. Effects of zearalenone on oxidative stress and inflammation in weanling piglets. *Food Chem. Toxicol.* **2013**, *58*, 408–415. [CrossRef]
138. Wang, Y.-L.; Zhou, X.-Q.; Jiang, W.-D.; Wu, P.; Liu, Y.; Jiang, J.; Wang, S.-W.; Kuang, S.-Y.; Tang, L.; Feng, L. Effects of Dietary Zearalenone on Oxidative Stress, Cell Apoptosis, and Tight Junction in the Intestine of Juvenile Grass Carp (Ctenopharyngodon idella). *Toxins* **2019**, *11*, 333. [CrossRef]
139. da Silva, E.O.; Bracarense, A.P.F.L.; Oswald, I.P. Mycotoxins and oxidative stress: Where are we? *World Mycotoxin J.* **2018**, *11*, 113–134. [CrossRef]
140. Shen, T.; Miao, Y.; Ding, C.; Fan, W.; Liu, S.; Lv, Y.; Gao, X.; De Boevre, M.; Yan, L.; Okoth, S.; et al. Activation of the p38/MAPK pathway regulates autophagy in response to the CYPOR-dependent oxidative stress induced by zearalenone in porcine intestinal epithelial cells. *Food Chem. Toxicol.* **2019**, *131*, 110527. [CrossRef]

141. Pistol, G.C.; Braicu, C.; Motiu, M.; Gras, M.A.; Marin, D.E.; Stancu, M.; Calin, L.; Israel-Roming, F.; Berindan-Neagoe, I.; Taranu, I. Zearalenone Mycotoxin Affects Immune Mediators, MAPK Signalling Molecules, Nuclear Receptors and Genome-Wide Gene Expression in Pig Spleen. *PLoS One* **2015**, *10*, e0127503. [CrossRef]
142. da Costa, R.M.; Rodrigues, D.; Pereira, C.A.; Silva, J.F.; Alves, J.V.; Lobato, N.S.; Tostes, R.C. Nrf2 as a Potential Mediator of Cardiovascular Risk in Metabolic Diseases. *Front. Pharmacol.* **2019**, *10*, 382. [CrossRef]
143. Kozieł, M.J.; Kowalska, K.; Piastowska-Ciesielska, A.W. Nrf2: A main responsive element in cells to mycotoxin-induced toxicity. *Arch. Toxicol.* **2021**. [CrossRef]
144. Wu, K.; Liu, X.; Fang, M.; Wu, Y.; Gong, Z. Zearalenone induces oxidative damage involving Keap1/Nrf2/HO-1 pathway in hepatic L02 cells. *Mol. Cell. Toxicol.* **2014**, *10*, 451–457. [CrossRef]
145. Rajendran, P.; Ammar, R.B.; Al-Saeedi, F.J.; Mohamed, M.E.; ElNaggar, M.A.; Al-Ramadan, S.Y.; Bekhet, G.M.; Soliman, A.M. Kaempferol Inhibits Zearalenone-Induced Oxidative Stress and Apoptosis via the PI3K/Akt-Mediated Nrf2 Signaling Pathway: In Vitro and In Vivo Studies. *Int. J. Mol. Sci.* **2021**, *22*.
146. Mittal, M.; Siddiqui, M.R.; Tran, K.; Reddy, S.P.; Malik, A.B. Reactive Oxygen Species in Inflammation and Tissue Injury. *Antioxid. Redox Signal.* **2013**, *20*, 1126–1167. [CrossRef] [PubMed]
147. de Rivero Vaccari, J.P.; Patel, H.H.; Brand III, F.J.; Perez-Pinzon, M.A.; Bramlett, H.M.; Raval, A.P. Estrogen receptor beta signaling alters cellular inflammasomes activity after global cerebral ischemia in reproductively senescence female rats. *J. Neurochem.* **2016**, *136*, 492–496. [CrossRef] [PubMed]
148. Vegeto, E.; Cuzzocrea, S.; Crisafulli, C.; Mazzon, E.; Sala, A.; Krust, A.; Maggi, A. Estrogen Receptor-α as a Drug Target Candidate for Preventing Lung Inflammation. *Endocrinology* **2010**, *151*, 174–184. [CrossRef] [PubMed]
149. Monteiro, R.; Teixeira, D.; Calhau, C. Estrogen Signaling in Metabolic Inflammation. *Mediators Inflamm.* **2014**, *2014*, 615917. [CrossRef]
150. Jia, Z.; Liu, M.; Qu, Z.; Zhang, Y.; Yin, S.; Shan, A. Toxic effects of zearalenone on oxidative stress, inflammatory cytokines, biochemical and pathological changes induced by this toxin in the kidney of pregnant rats. *Environ. Toxicol. Pharmacol.* **2014**, *37*, 580–591. [CrossRef] [PubMed]
151. Xu, H.; Hao, S.; Gan, F.; Wang, H.; Xu, J.; Liu, D.; Huang, K. In vitro immune toxicity of ochratoxin A in porcine alveolar macrophages: A role for the ROS-relative TLR4/MyD88 signaling pathway. *Chem. Biol. Interact.* **2017**, *272*, 107–116. [CrossRef]
152. Fan, W.; Shen, T.; Ding, Q.; Lv, Y.; Li, L.; Huang, K.; Yan, L.; Song, S. Zearalenone induces ROS-mediated mitochondrial damage in porcine IPEC-J2 cells. *J. Biochem. Mol. Toxicol.* **2017**, *31*, e21944. [CrossRef]
153. Wang, X.; Jiang, L.; Shi, L.; Yao, K.; Sun, X.; Yang, G.; Jiang, L.; Zhang, C.; Wang, N.; Zhang, H.; et al. Zearalenone induces NLRP3-dependent pyroptosis via activation of NF-κB modulated by autophagy in INS-1 cells. *Toxicology* **2019**, *428*, 152304. [CrossRef] [PubMed]
154. Ding, C.; Fan, W.; Shen, T.; Huang, K.; Song, S.; Yan, L. Zearalenone can relieve dextran sulfate sodium-induced inflammatory reaction. *J. Biochem. Mol. Toxicol.* **2019**, *33*, e22236. [CrossRef] [PubMed]

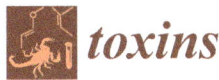

Article

Combined Effect of Deoxynivalenol (DON) and Porcine Circovirus Type 2 (Pcv2) on Inflammatory Cytokine mRNA Expression

Chao Gu [1,†], Xiuge Gao [1,†], Dawei Guo [1], Jiacai Wang [2], Qinghua Wu [3,4], Eugenie Nepovimova [3], Wenda Wu [1,3,*] and Kamil Kuca [3,5,*]

[1] MOE Joint International Research Laboratory of Animal Health and Food Safety, Engineering Center of Innovative Veterinary Drugs, College of Veterinary Medicine, Nanjing Agricultural University, Nanjing 210095, China; guchao0990@163.com (C.G.); vetgao@njau.edu.cn (X.G.); gdawei0123@njau.edu.cn (D.G.)
[2] Shandong Vocational Animal Science and Veterinary College, 88 Shengli East Street, Weifang 261061, China; sdmyjcw@163.com
[3] Department of Chemistry, Faculty of Science, University of Hradec Králové, Rokitanského 62, 500 03 Hradec Kralove, Czech Republic; wqh212@yangtzeu.edu.cn (Q.W.); eugenie.nepovimova@uhk.cz (E.N.)
[4] College of Life Science, Yangtze University, Jingzhou 434025, China
[5] Biomedical Research Center, University Hospital Hradec Kralove, 500 03 Hradec Kralove, Czech Republic
* Correspondence: wuwenda@njau.edu.cn (W.W.); kamil.kuca@uhk.cz (K.K.)
† Chao Gu and Xiuge Gao contributed equally to this work.

Abstract: A host's immune system can be invaded by mycotoxin deoxynivalenol (DON) poisoning and porcine circovirus type 2 (PCV2) infections, which affect the host's natural immune function. Pro-inflammatory cytokines, IL-1β and IL-6, are important regulators in the process of natural immune response, which participate in inflammatory response and enhance immune-mediated tissue damage. Preliminary studies have shown that DON promotes PCV2 infection by activating the MAPK signaling pathway. Here, we explored whether the mRNA expression of IL-1β and IL-6, induced by the combination of DON and PCV2, would depend on the MAPK signaling pathway. Specific pharmacological antagonists U0126, SP600125 and SB203580, were used to inhibit the activities of ERK, JNK and p38 in the MAPK signaling pathway, respectively. Then, the mRNA expression of IL-1β and IL-6 in PK-15 cells was detected to explore the effect of the MAPK signaling pathway on IL-1β and IL-6 mRNA induced by DON and PCV2. The results showed that PK-15 cells treated with DON or PCV2 induced the mRNA expression of IL-1β and IL-6 in a time- and dose-dependent manner. The combination of DON and PCV2 has an additive effect on inducing the mRNA expression of IL-1β and IL-6. Additionally, both DON and PCV2 could induce the mRNA expression of IL-1β and IL-6 via the ERK and the p38 MAPK signal pathways, while PCV2 could induce it via the JNK signal pathway. Taken together, our results suggest that MAPKs play a contributory role in IL-1β and IL-6 mRNA expression when induced by both DON and PCV2.

Keywords: deoxynivalenol; PCV2; IL-1β; IL-6; MAPK

Key Contribution: This study demonstrates that the MAPK pathway can up-regulate mRNA levels of IL-1β and IL-6 in PK-15 cells after DON and/or PCV2 treatment, leading to changes in inflammation and immune function. These data provide a new perspective to advance the understanding of the mechanisms of DON poisoning and PCV2 infection, as well as providing new ideas for the prevention and control of both DON and PCV2.

1. Introduction

Trichothecene mycotoxins, the secondary metabolites produced by fungi such as *Fusarium* and *Trichothecium*, are widely distributed across the world [1]. Since these toxins have been linked to human and animal toxicoses, their presence in global food commodities and feedstuffs is a matter of considerable public health concern [2]. Deoxynivalenol (DON, Vomitoxin), the most abundant trichothecene mycotoxin associated with *Fusarium* head blight (FHB), can survive processing and persist into the food chain. In humans and animals, DON has been associated with a series of adverse effects including anorexia, vomiting, growth retardation, diarrhea, neuroendocrine changes, gastrointestinal inflammation, and immunosuppression [3]. The immuno-toxic effects induced by DON is of particular concern from the perspective of human and animal health. According to the timing and dose of exposure, DON has the potential to elicit either an immunosuppressive response or immune stress [4]. Our previous studies indicate that exposure to DON induces the overexpression of proinflammatory cytokines, such as IL-1β and IL-6, in the plasma and organs of mouse [5,6].

Cytokines are a class of small molecular proteins with a size of 5-20kDa. They play a role in a wide range of biological activities and in a variety of life activities inside the body [7]. The expression of proinflammatory cytokines is aberrantly upregulated for the activation of the innate immune system, leading to immune stress, which can cause physiological and immune function impairment [8]. A large number of studies have shown that proinflammatory cytokines including IL-1β and IL-6 can cause anorexia, daily weight decrease, a decrease in immunity causing inflammation, and an increased likelihood of other diseases occurring [9,10]. This is similar to DON causing animal refusal, malnutrition, and secondary infection with other pathogens [11]. In addition to the capacity of DON to upregulate proinflammatory cytokines in vivo, some studies have found that DON also increased the mRNA and protein expression of IL-1β and IL-6 in human peripheral blood mononuclear cells, human monocyte cell lines and mouse macrophage cell lines [12–14]. DON may target phagocytes to produce immunotoxicity.

Porcine circovirus (PCV), first discovered in 1974 as a contaminant of a continuous porcine kidney cell line (PK-15), is classified in the genus *Circovirus* of the family *Circoviridae* [15]. Two genotypes of PCV have been identified. PCV type 1 (PCV1) is known to be nonpathogenic to pigs. PCV type 2 (PCV2) is a DNA virus that can severely damage the respiratory, digestive and nervous systems of pigs of all ages, among which piglets are the most sensitive [16,17]. Pigs infected with PCV2 have multi-system inflammation, indicating disordered expression of proinflammatory cytokines. Some studies have reported that PCV2 infects porcine alveolar macrophages (PAM) to activate NF-κB and induce IL-1β overexpression [18,19]. Another study showed that the expression of IL-1β and IL-6 mRNA in piglets suffering from postweaning multisystemic wasting syndrome (PMWS), caused by PCV2, was significantly up-regulated [20]. However, the reasons why PCV2 infection causes the production and/or secretion of cytokines and the imbalance of cytokines are not completely clear, and the regulatory mechanism involved is still unclear.

As an important signal pathway that transfers signals from the cell surface to the nucleus, the mitogen-activated protein kinase (MAPK) pathway includes extracellular signal regulated protein kinase 1 and 2 (ERK 1/2), p54 and p46 c-Jun N-terminal kinase 1 and 2 (JNK 1/2), and p38 [21]. After being subjected to extracellular stimuli such as toxins and pathogens, MAPK can be sequentially activated and contribute to various pathological and physiological processes such as inflammatory response, stress adaptation, cell growth and differentiation [22]. The MAPK pathway is also closely related to DON poisoning and PCV2 infection [23,24]. However, the role of MAPK signaling pathway in the induction of proinflammatory cytokines such as IL-1β and IL-6 by DON and PCV2 in PK-15 cell remains unclear and requires further study.

In this study, we evaluated the effect of MAPK on the expression of IL-1β and IL-6 cytokines that mRNA induced by DON and PCV2. We found that the MAPK pathway can up-regulate mRNA levels of relative cytokine in PK-15 cells after DON and/or PCV2 treatment, leading to changes in inflammation and immune function. Our findings will provide a new perspective to advance the understanding of the mechanisms of DON poisoning and PCV2 infection, as well as providing new ideas for the prevention and control of both DON and PCV2.

2. Results

2.1. DON Exposure Induces Elevations in IL-1β and IL-6 mRNA

DON-induced PK-15 cells IL-1β mRNA were elevated at 2 h, reached peak concentrations at 12 h and returned to basal level at 24 h post-exposure (Figure 1A). IL-6 mRNA was upregulated and reached peak concentrations at 6 h, and were still markedly raised at 24 h, but returned to basal level at 48 h post-exposure (Figure 1B).

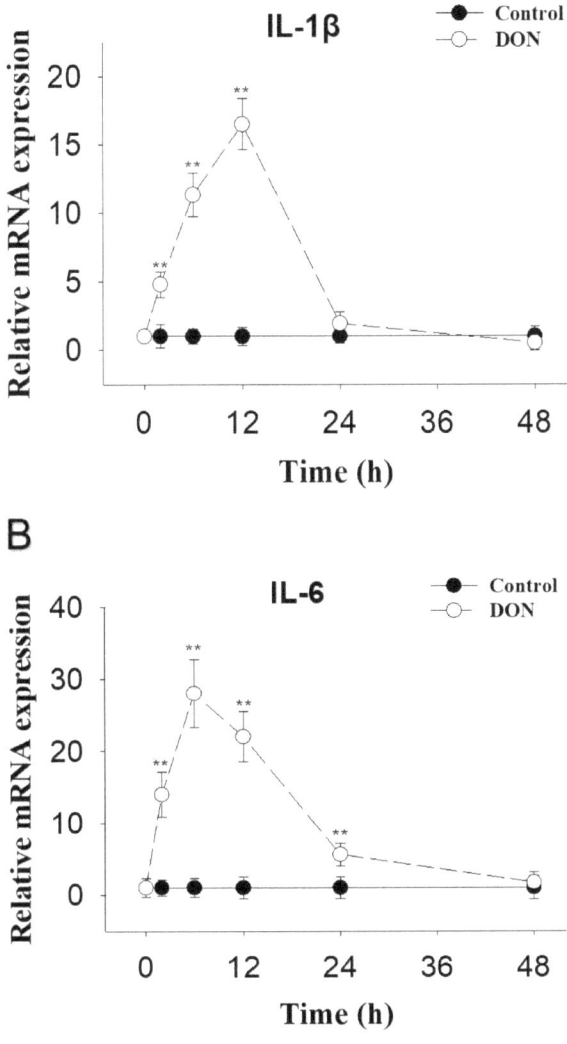

Figure 1. DON-induced cytokine IL-1β and IL-6 mRNA upregulation in PK-15 cells. qRT-PCR were performed to analyze the mRNA expression of IL-1β (**A**) and IL-6 (**B**). Data are mean ± SEM (n = 3). Symbol ** $p < 0.01$.

DON in 0.5, 1, 1.5 and 2 µg/mL upregulation PK-15 cells IL-1β mRNA by 3-, 5-, 10- and 13-fold at 12 h, respectively (Figure 2A). IL-6 mRNA expression was elevated by 6-, 17-, 22- and 28-fold (Figure 2B).

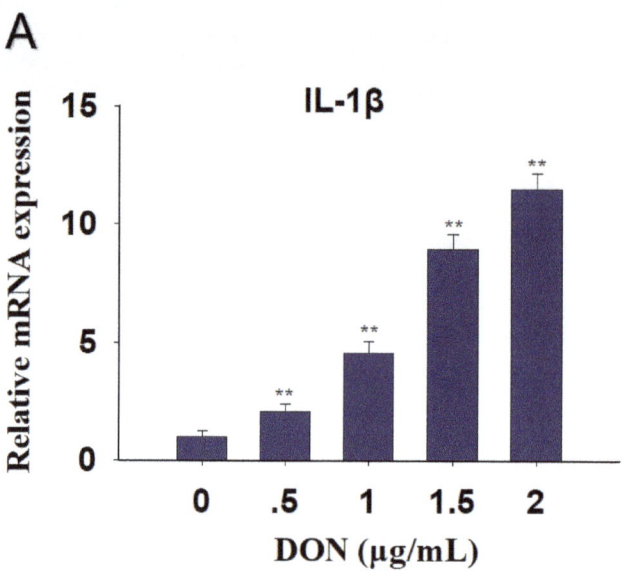

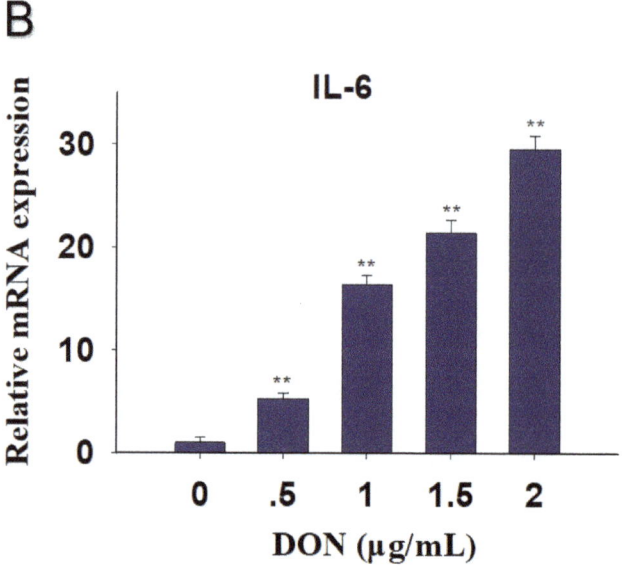

Figure 2. Different concentrations of DON-induced cytokine IL-1β and IL-6 mRNA upregulation in PK-15 cells. qRT-PCR were performed to analyze the mRNA expression of IL-1β (**A**) and IL-6 (**B**). Data are mean ± SEM (n = 3). Symbol ** $p < 0.01$.

2.2. PCV2 Infection Induces Elevations in IL-1β and IL-6 mRNA

PCV2-induced PK-15 cells IL-1β mRNA were elevated at 6 h, reached peak concentrations at 12 h, and were still markedly raised at 48 h post-exposure (Figure 3A). IL-6 mRNA was upregulated at 12 h, reached peak concentrations at 24 h, and was still markedly raised at 48 h post-exposure (Figure 3B).

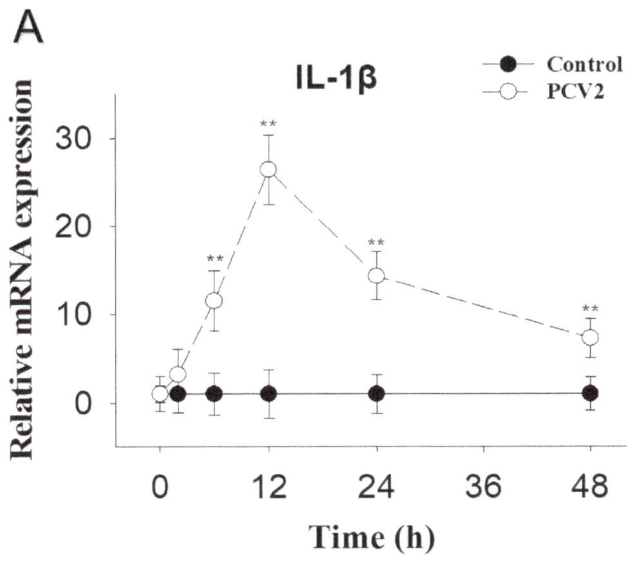

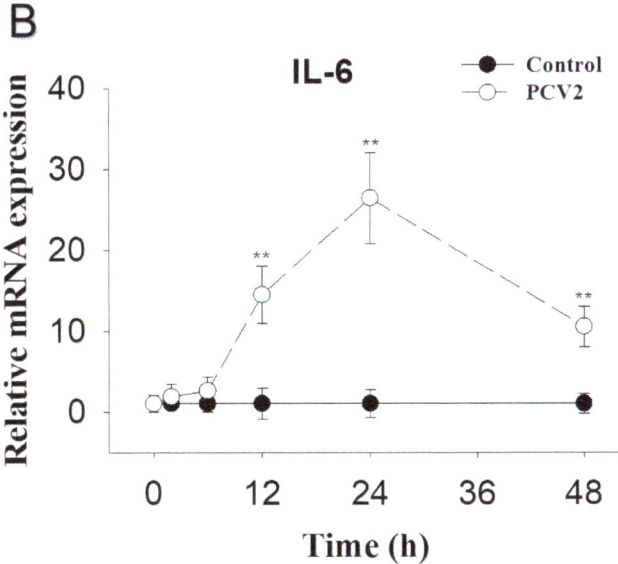

Figure 3. PCV2-induced cytokine IL-1β and IL-6 mRNA upregulation in PK-15 Cells. qRT-PCR were performed to analyze the mRNA expression of IL-1β (**A**) and IL-6 (**B**). Data are mean ± SEM (n = 3). Symbol ** $p < 0.01$.

PCV2 in 0.1, 0.5 and 1 MOI upregulation PK-15 cells IL-1β mRNA by 6-, 14-, and 19-fold at 12h, respectively, while 0.05 MOI had no effect (Figure 4A). IL-6 mRNA expression was elevated by 3-, 6-, 9- and 14-fold, respectively (Figure 4B).

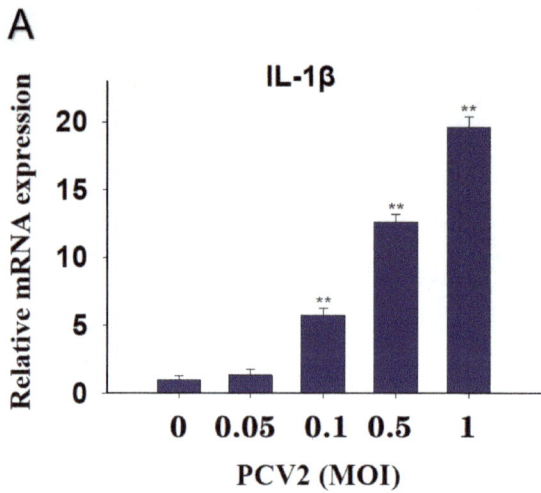

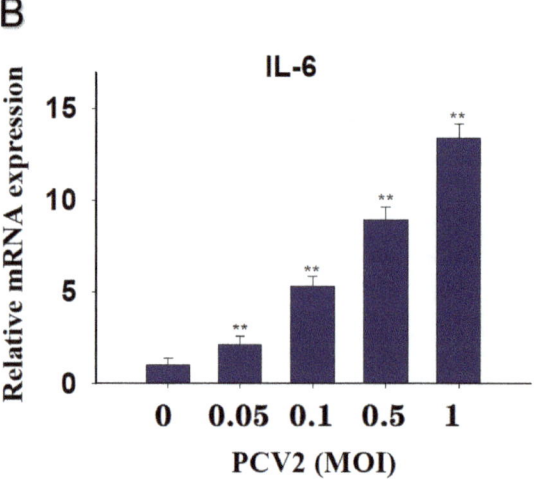

Figure 4. Different MOI of PCV2 induced cytokine IL-1β and IL-6 mRNA upregulation in PK-15 Cells. qRT-PCR were performed to analyze the mRNA expression of IL-1β (**A**) and IL-6 (**B**). Data are mean ± SEM (n = 3). Symbol ** $p < 0.01$.

2.3. Combined Effect of DON and PCV2 Induces the Expression of IL-1β and IL-6 mRNA

IL-1β mRNA expression was elevated by DON (10-fold), PCV2 (20-fold) and the combined effect of DON and PCV2 (45-fold) (Figure 5A). As for IL-6, the mRNA expression was markedly increased by DON (28-fold), PCV2 (10-fold) and the combined effect of DON and PCV2 (56-fold) (Figure 5B).

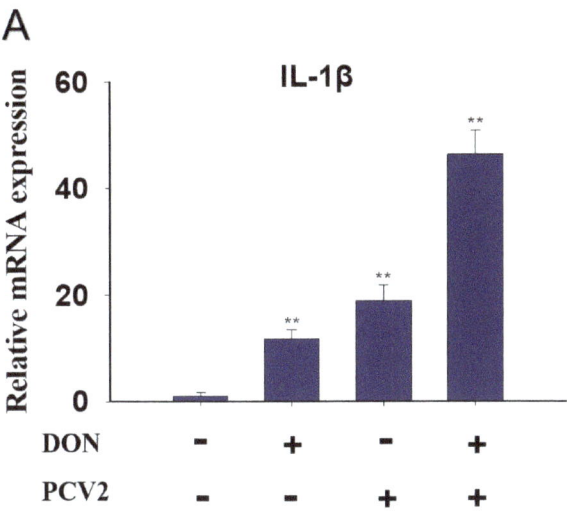

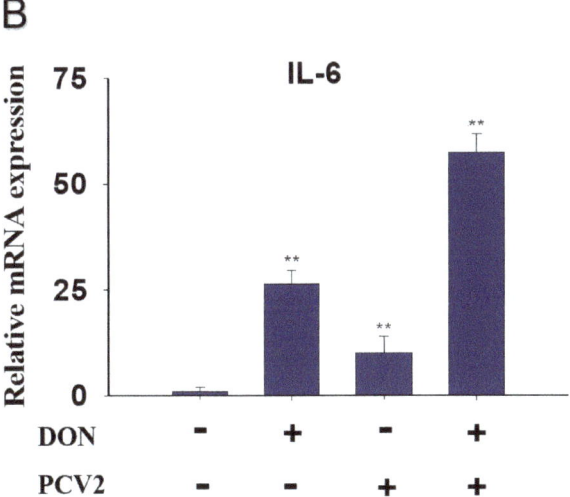

Figure 5. Combined effect of DON and PCV2 induced cytokine IL-1β and IL-6 mRNA upregulation in PK-15 Cells. qRT-PCR were performed to analyze the mRNA expression of IL-1β (**A**) and IL-6 (**B**). Data are mean ± SEM (n = 3). Symbol ** $p < 0.01$.

2.4. DON and PCV2 Induce the Expression of IL-1β and IL-6 mRNA via ERK Signaling Pathway

To explore whether the ERK signaling pathway participated in the DON and PCV2-induced IL-1β and IL-6 mRNA expression, the inhibitor of p-ERK, U0126, was supplied. The data showed that U0126 decreased IL-1β mRNA expression in the DON group from 12-fold to 5-fold, in the PCV2 group from 20-fold to 10-fold, and in the DON+PCV2 group from 41-fold to 22-fold (Figure 6A). U0126 decreased IL-6 mRNA expression in the DON group from 25-fold to 10-fold, in the PCV2 group from 13-fold to 8-fold, and in the DON+PCV2 group from 52-fold to 22-fold (Figure 6B).

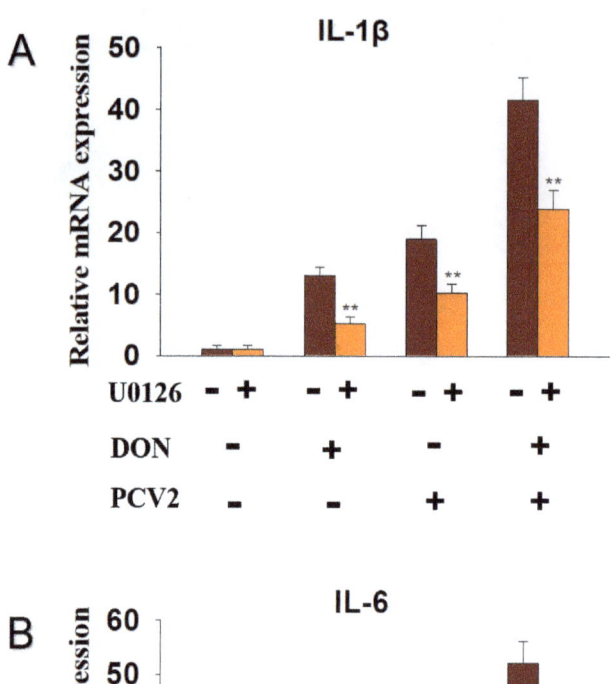

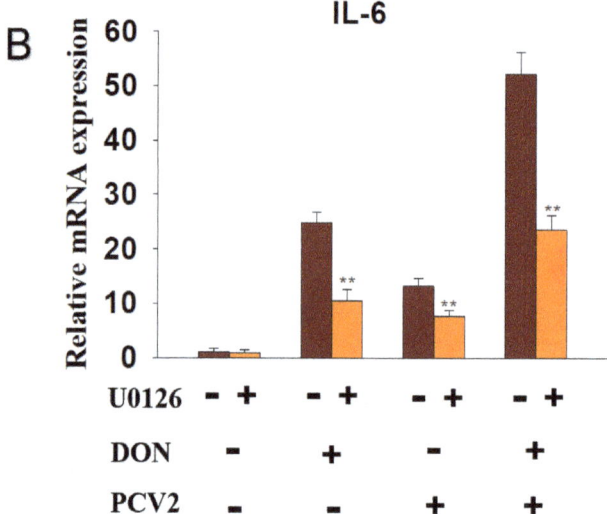

Figure 6. ERK participated in DON and PCV2-induced cytokine IL-1β and IL-6 mRNA upregulation in PK-15 cells. qRT-PCR were performed to analyze the mRNA expression of IL-1β (**A**) and IL-6 (**B**). Data are mean ± SEM (n = 3). Symbol ** $p < 0.01$.

2.5. PCV2 Induces the Expression of IL-1β and IL-6 mRNA via JNK Signaling Pathway

To explore whether JNK signaling pathway participated in the DON and PCV2-induced IL-1β and IL-6 mRNA expression, the inhibitor of p-JNK, SP600125, was supplied. The data showed that SP600125 decreased IL-1β mRNA expression in the PCV2 group from 20-fold to 11-fold and in the DON+PCV2 group from 41-fold to 28-fold, while the DON group had no effect (Figure 7A). SP600125 decreased IL-6 mRNA expression in the PCV2 group from 12-fold to 7-fold and in the DON+PCV2 group from 52-fold to 30-fold, while the DON group had no effect (Figure 7B).

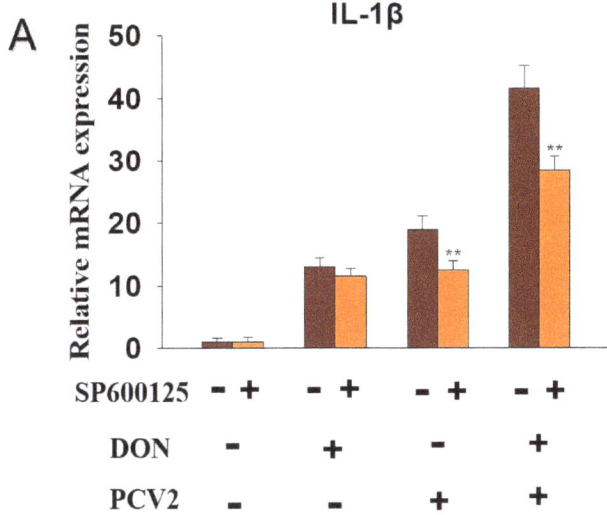

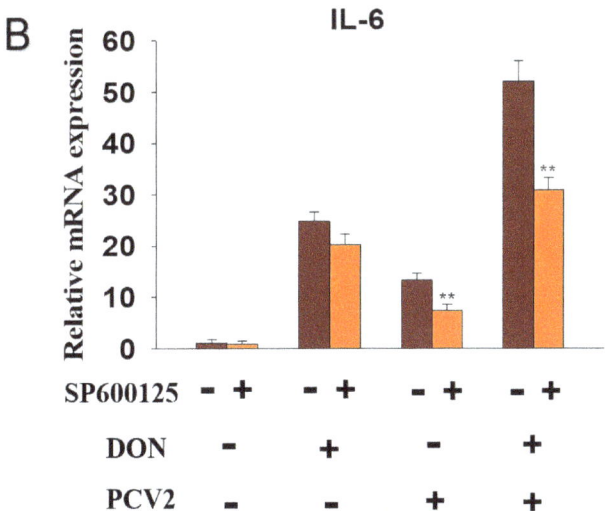

Figure 7. JNK participated in PCV2-induced cytokine IL-1β and IL-6 mRNA upregulation in PK-15 Cells. qRT-PCR were performed to analyze the mRNA expression of IL-1β (**A**) and IL-6 (**B**). Data are mean ± SEM (n = 3). Symbol ** $p < 0.01$.

2.6. DON and PCV2 Induce the Expression of IL-1β and IL-6 mRNA via p38 Signaling Pathway

To explore whether ERK signaling pathway participated in the DON and PCV2-induced IL-1β and IL-6 mRNA expression, the inhibitor of p-p38, SB203580, was supplied. The data showed that SB203580 decreased IL-1β mRNA expression in the DON group from 13-fold to 5-fold, in the PCV2 group from 19-fold to 9-fold, and in the DON+PCV2 group from 41-fold to 18-fold (Figure 8A). SB203580 decreased IL-6 mRNA expression in the DON group from 24-fold to 11-fold, in the PCV2 group from 12-fold to 5-fold, and in the DON+PCV2 group from 52-fold to 20-fold (Figure 8B).

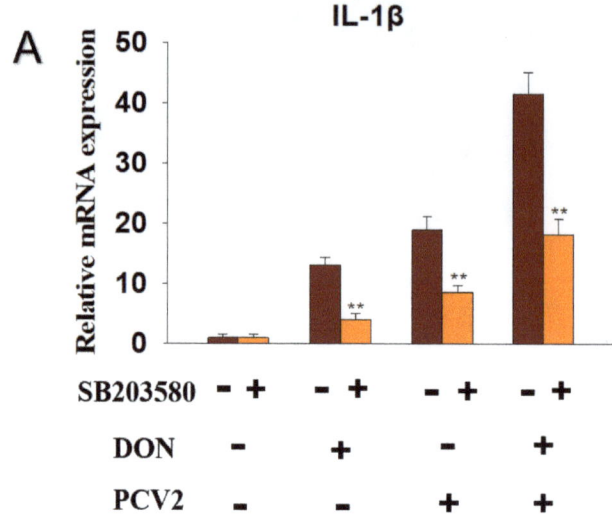
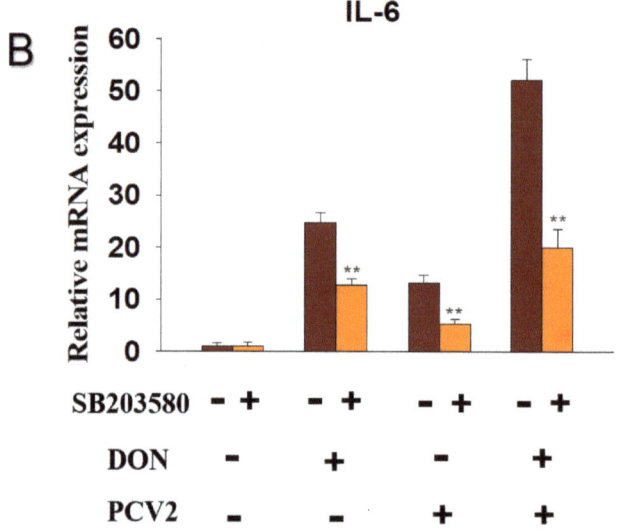

Figure 8. p38 participated in DON and PCV2-induced cytokine IL-1β and IL-6 mRNA upregulation in PK-15 cells. qRT-PCR were performed to analyze the mRNA expression of IL-1β (**A**) and IL-6 (**B**). Data are mean ± SEM (n = 3). Symbol ** $p < 0.01$.

3. Discussion

Mycotoxins are widespread in the environment and coexist alongside other pathogens such as virus and bacteria. To a certain extent, mycotoxins enhance the pathogenicity of other pathogens [25–28]. DON has the potential to evoke a wide spectrum of pathophysiological effects that are partly attributable to a ribo-toxic stress-mediated cytokine storm [29]. With respect to PCV2 infection, the immune injury is always accompanied by a change in proinflammatory cytokine expression, including IL-1β and IL-6 [30]. In this study, we focused on the role of the MAPK signaling pathway in the mRNA expression of IL-1β and IL-6, induced by DON and PCV2. Several key findings were evident and demonstrate that (1) DON and PCV2 induced the mRNA expression of IL-1β and IL-6 in a time- and dose-dependent manner, respectively. (2) The combination of DON and PCV2 has an additive effect on the induction of the mRNA expression of IL-1β and IL-6 in the PK-15 cell. (3) DON induced the mRNA expression of IL-1β and IL-6 via the ERK and p38 MAPK signaling pathways and (4) PCV2 induced the mRNA expression of IL-1β and IL-6 via the ERK, JNK and p38 MAPK signaling pathways.

The dose response of DON-induced IL-1β and IL-6 mRNA expression suggested that the mRNA expression of these two cytokines increased after PK-15 cells were challenged with different concentrations of DON at 0.5, 1, 1.5, and 2 µg/mL. Furthermore, the kinetics of IL-1β and IL-6 mRNA responses to DON indicated that upregulation of these genes was maximal at 12 h and 6 h, respectively. These findings are consistent with several in vitro studies by Pestka and co-workers [31,32]. For instance, from 100 to 1000 ng/mL of DON significantly increased production of IL-6 from 3 h to 24 h in U-937 cells [31]. Robustly elevated IL-1β and IL-6 intracellular protein and mRNA expression was also observed in peripheral blood mono-nuclear cells treated with DON at 500 ng/mL [32]. DON's in vitro effects on IL-1β and IL-6 can be reproduced in a mouse, a commonly used model of the human immune system. DON has the capacity to induce IL-1β and IL-6 mRNAs not only in the plasma, but also in organs such as the spleen, liver, lung, kidney, small intestine and brain [33,34]. Eventually, both cytokines were returned to basal levels in this study. A possible reason for the decreased cytokines response might be mRNA degradation caused by reduced MAPK activation [35,36].

Similarly, PCV2 was shown to induce the expression of IL-1β and IL-6 at the transcriptional level in PK-15 cells through time- and dose-dependent manners. Consistent with this finding, PCV2 was reported to increase IL-1β production in porcine alveolar macrophages, and the changes in cytokine expression are related to the TLR-MyD88-NF-κB signaling pathway [19]. In PK-15 cells, PCV2 was reported to elevate IL-6 production via suppressor of cytokine signaling 3 [37]. In addition to in vitro studies, the levels of IL-1β and IL-6 in both serum and spleen were significantly upregulated after PCV2 infection in the mouse [30]. Proinflammatory cytokines are important factors for the elimination of invading pathogens [38]. Excessive release of proinflammatory cytokines can lead to undesired tissue lesions and decrease the body's immunity to other pathogen infections [39]. Therefore, controlling the inflammatory response is crucial. However, environmental factors, such as toxins, can interfere with this control.

This is the first report to demonstrate that co-treatment with DON and PCV2 in PK-15 cells can enhance the up-regulation effect of IL-1β and IL-6 mRNA with an additive effect. The possible reason may be related to the ability of the mycotoxin to promote virus replication, leading to an increase in cytokines expression. Qian et al indicated that mycotoxin ochratoxin A had the capacity to induce PCV2 replication promotion in PK-15 cells [40]. The molecular mechanisms of this effect are associated with ochratoxin A-induced autophagy involving in AKT/mTOR and ERK1/2 MAPK signaling pathway [41]. DON significantly promoted the replication of porcine epidemic diarrhea virus in IPEC-J2 cells, along with the induction of a complete autophagy triggered by p38 MAPK signaling pathway [42]. Our preliminary data also indicate that DON promotes PCV2 infection by activating the MAPK signaling pathway. However, the underlying mechanism of this effect still requires further research to substantiate such findings.

The results presented here demonstrate that ERK and p38 MAPK participate in DON-induced IL-1β and IL-6 mRNA up-regulation in PK-15 cells. PCV2, however, induced IL-1β and IL-6 mRNA up-regulation via the ERK, JNK and p38 MAPK signaling pathways. Some studies have found that the expression of cytokine genes is caused by DON-mediated rRNA perforation and the induction of damage-related molecular patterns (DAMPs) by ribosomal-related stress kinases [43,44]. The latter can activate members of the MAPK family, which mediate transcription factor activation and mRNA stabilization, and lead to an increased expression of the pro-inflammatory gene mRNA and ultimately, protein [14]. He and co-workers found that the ability of DON to change the translation and expression of inflammation-related genes is mainly driven by selective transcription and mRNA stabilization through ERK and p38 MAPK signaling pathways [13]. On the other hand, studies have also shown that activation of the ERK, JNK and p38 MAPK signaling pathways contribute to the promotion PCV2 infection [30,37]. These viewpoints are consistent with the findings in our study.

4. Conclusions

Treatment of PK-15 cells with DON or PCV2 can induce the expression of IL-1β and IL-6 mRNA; this is both time-dependent and dose-dependent. Furthermore, the combined effect of DON and PCV2 could increase the expression of IL-1β and IL-6 mRNA. The expression of IL-1β and IL-6 mRNA induced by DON is dependent on the ERK and p38 MAPK signaling pathways, while the expression of IL-1β and IL-6 mRNA induced by PCV2 depends on the ERK, JNK, and p38 MAPK signaling pathways.

5. Materials and Methods

5.1. Toxin and Virus

Deoxynivalenol (DON) were purchased from Sigma-Aldrich (Shanghai, China). PCV2 strains were kindly donated by the Laboratory of Infectious Disease, Department of Prevention Veterinary Medicine, Nanjing Agricultural University. It was isolated and sequenced from the kidneys of piglets, naturally infected with multiple system failure syndrome of weaned piglets, and stored at $-80\ °C$.

5.2. Cell Cultures and Virus Cultures

Porcine kidney cell (PK-15) cell line (without PCV contamination) was kindly donated by the Laboratory of Internal Veterinary Medicine, Department of Clinical Veterinary Medicine, Nanjing Agricultural University. All cells were cultured in DMEM (Gibco, Shanghai, China) medium with 10% newborn calf serum (Gibco, Shanghai, China) and 1% penicillin, at 37 °C and 5% carbon dioxide.

PCV2 was amplified using PK-15 cells. The cytopathic effect (CPE) was observed and PCV2 was detected by the indirect immunofluorescence assay in inoculated PK-15 cells. The viral titers were determined to be $10^{6.1}$ TCID50/0.1 mL, using the Reed–Muench assay.

5.3. Experimental Design

Three specific inhibitors U0126, SP600125 and SB203580 (MedChemExpress, Shanghai, China) were added in the PK-15 cells to block ERK, JNK and p38 MAPK signaling pathways, respectively. Then, PK-15 cells were treated with DON or PCV2. Total cell RNA was extracted, then an ultra-micro nucleic acid protein analyzer was used to determine OD260/OD280 value and detect RNA quality. qRT-PCR was used to detect the expression of IL-1β and IL-6 mRNA.

5.4. Quantative Real-Time PCR (qRT-PCR) Analysis

Total RNA was isolated from PK-15 cells using TRIzol Reagent (Takara, Dalian, China). cDNA was obtained by reverse transcription using a cDNA transcription kit (Takara, Dalian, China). qRT-PCR was performed using SYBR Premix Ex Taq™ (Takara, Dalian, China) and the primers are shown as IL-1β (F: 5′-TACCTCTTGGAGGCACAAAGG-3′ and R:5′-CTTCCTTGGCAGGTTCAGGT A-3′), IL-6 (F: 5′-AGCAAGGAGGTACTGGCAGA-3′ and R: 5′-CAGGGTCTGGATCAGTGCTT-3′) and GAPDH (F: 5′-CGTCAAGCTCATTTCCTGGT-3′ and R: 5′-TGGGATGGAAACTGGAAGTC-3′). Fold changes in cytokines were determined using $2^{(-\Delta\Delta Ct)}$ method and gene expression levels were normalized to GAPDH [45]. qRT-PCR was performed using the ABI PRISM 7900HT Real-Time PCR System.

5.5. Statistical Analyses

Statistical analyses were performed using GraphPad Prism 8.0 Software (GraphPad Software, Inc., San Diego, CA, USA). Data for each assay were analyzed with one-way analysis of variance (ANOVA) or two-way ANOVA. Data were expressed as the mean ± SEM. Statistical significance was set at $p < 0.05$.

Author Contributions: Conceptualization, W.W. and K.K.; methodology, W.W.; software, X.G. and Q.W.; validation, C.G., W.W. and X.G.; formal analysis, W.W.; investigation, C.G.; re-sources, C.G.; data curation, C.G.; writing—original draft preparation, C.G.; writing—review and editing, X.G. and D.G.; visu-alization, J.W. and E.N.; supervision, W.W.; project administration, W.W. and K.K.; funding acquisition, W.W. and K.K. All authors have read and agreed to the published version of the manuscript.

Funding: This work was supported by China-CEEC Joint University Education Project (202010), the long-term organization development plan (University Hospital, Hradec Kralove, Czech Re-public), National Key R & D Program (2016YFD0501207, 2016YFD0501009), NSFC (31972741, 31572576), China Postdoctoral Science Foundation (2016T90477), PAPD. The authors would like also to acknowledge the funding received from UHK VT2019-2012 and from the Ministry of Health of the Czech Republic (FN HK 00179906).

Institutional Review Board Statement: Not applicable.

Informed Consent Statement: Not applicable.

Data Availability Statement: The data presented in this study are available upon request to the corresponding author.

Acknowledgments: We would like to acknowledge the donations in kind from Ping Jiang.

Conflicts of Interest: The authors declare no conflict of interest.

References

1. Polak-Śliwińska, M.; Paszczyk, B. Trichothecenes in Food and Feed, Relevance to Human and Animal Health and Methods of Detection: A Systematic Review. *Molecules* **2021**, *26*, 454. [CrossRef] [PubMed]
2. Yang, C.; Song, G.; Lim, W. Effects of mycotoxin-contaminated feed on farm animals. *J. Hazard. Mater.* **2020**, *389*, 122087. [CrossRef]
3. Yao, Y.; Long, M. The biological detoxification of deoxynivalenol: A review. *Food Chem. Toxicol.* **2020**, *145*, 111649. [CrossRef] [PubMed]
4. Peng, Z.; Chen, L.; Xiao, J.; Zhou, X.; Nüssler, A.K.; Liu, L.; Liu, J.; Yang, W. Review of mechanisms of deoxynivalenol-induced anorexia: The role of gut microbiota. *J. Appl. Toxicol.* **2017**, *37*, 1021–1029. [CrossRef]
5. Wu, W.; Zhang, H. Role of tumor necrosis factor-α and interleukin-1β in anorexia induction following oral exposure to the trichothecene deoxynivalenol (vomitoxin) in the mouse. *J. Toxicol. Sci.* **2014**, *39*, 875–886. [CrossRef] [PubMed]
6. Wu, Q.; Yue, J.; Zhang, H.; Kuca, K.; Wu, W. Anorexic responses to trichothecene deoxynivalenol and its congeners correspond to secretion of tumor necrosis factor-α and interleukin-1β. *Environ. Toxicol. Pharmacol.* **2020**, *77*, 103871. [CrossRef]
7. Carty, M.; Guy, C.; Bowie, A.G. Detection of Viral Infections by Innate Immunity. *Biochem. Pharmacol.* **2021**, *183*, 114316. [CrossRef]
8. Riahi, I.; Marquis, V.; Pérez-Vendrell, A.M.; Brufau, J.; Esteve-Garcia, E.; Ramos, A.J. Effects of Deoxynivalenol-Contaminated Diets on Metabolic and Immunological Parameters in Broiler Chickens. *Animals* **2021**, *11*, 147. [CrossRef]
9. Plata-Salaman, C.R. Immunomodulators and feeding regulation: A humoral link between the immune and nervous systems. *Brain Behav. Immun.* **1989**, *3*, 193–213. [CrossRef]
10. Dantzer, R.; Kelley, K.W. Twenty years of research on cytokine-induced sickness behavior. *Brain Behav. Immun.* **2007**, *21*, 153–160. [CrossRef]
11. McCusker, R.H.; Kelley, K.W. Immune-neural connections: How the immune system's response to infectious agents influences behavior. *J. Exp. Biol.* **2013**, *216*, 84–98. [CrossRef]
12. Chung, Y.J.; Yang, G.H.; Islam, Z.; Pestka, J.J. Up-regulation of macrophage inflammatory protein-2 and complement 3A receptor by the trichothecenes deoxynivalenol and satratoxin G. *Toxicology* **2003**, *186*, 51–65. [CrossRef]
13. He, K.; Pan, X.; Zhou, H.R.; Pestka, J.J. Modulation of inflammatory gene expression by the ribotoxin deoxynivalenol involves coordinate regulation of the transcriptome and translatome. *Toxicol. Sci.* **2013**, *131*, 153–163. [CrossRef] [PubMed]
14. Wong, S.S.; Zhou, H.R.; Marin-Martinez, M.L.; Brooks, K.; Pestka, J.J. Modulation of IL-1beta, IL-6 and TNF-alpha secretion and mRNA expression by the trichothecene vomitoxin in the RAW 264.7 murine macrophage cell line. *Food Chem. Toxicol.* **1998**, *36*, 409–419. [CrossRef]

15. Meng, X.J. Porcine circovirus type 2 (PCV2): Pathogenesis and interaction with the immune system. *Annu Rev. Anim. Biosci.* **2013**, *1*, 43–64. [CrossRef] [PubMed]
16. Zhai, S.L.; Lu, S.S.; Wei, W.K.; Lv, D.H.; Wen, X.H.; Zhai, Q.; Chen, Q.L.; Sun, Y.W.; Xi, Y. Reservoirs of Porcine Circoviruses: A Mini Review. *Front. Vet. Sci.* **2019**, *6*, 319. [CrossRef]
17. Segalés, J. Porcine circovirus type 2 (PCV2) infections: Clinical signs, pathology and laboratory diagnosis. *Virus Res.* **2012**, *164*, 10–19. [CrossRef]
18. Yang, S.; Liu, B.; Yin, S.; Shang, Y.; Zhang, X.; Khan, M.U.Z.; Liu, X.; Cai, J. Porcine Circovirus Type 2 Induces Single Immunoglobulin Interleukin-1 Related Receptor (SIGIRR) Downregulation to Promote Interleukin-1β Upregulation in Porcine Alveolar Macrophage. *Viruses* **2019**, *11*, 1021. [CrossRef] [PubMed]
19. Han, J.; Zhang, S.; Zhang, Y.; Chen, M.; Lv, Y. Porcine circovirus type 2 increases interleukin-1beta and interleukin-10 production via the MyD88-NF-kappa B signaling pathway in porcine alveolar macrophages in vitro. *J. Vet. Sci.* **2017**, *18*, 183–191. [CrossRef]
20. Sipos, W.; Duvigneau, J.C.; Willheim, M.; Schilcher, F.; Hartl, R.T.; Hofbauer, G.; Exel, B.; Pietschmann, P.; Schmoll, F. Systemic cytokine profile in feeder pigs suffering from natural postweaning multisystemic wasting syndrome (PMWS) as determined by semiquantitative RT-PCR and flow cytometric intracellular cytokine detection. *Vet. Immunol. Immunopathol.* **2004**, *99*, 63–71. [CrossRef]
21. Sui, X.; Kong, N.; Ye, L.; Han, W.; Zhou, J.; Zhang, Q.; He, C.; Pan, H. p38 and JNK MAPK pathways control the balance of apoptosis and autophagy in response to chemotherapeutic agents. *Cancer Lett.* **2014**, *344*, 174–179. [CrossRef]
22. He, Y.; She, H.; Zhang, T.; Xu, H.; Cheng, L.; Yepes, M.; Zhao, Y.; Mao, Z. p38 MAPK inhibits autophagy and promotes microglial inflammatory responses by phosphorylating ULK1. *J. Cell Biol.* **2018**, *217*, 315–328. [CrossRef] [PubMed]
23. Wu, W.; He, K.; Zhou, H.R.; Berthiller, F.; Adam, G.; Sugita-Konishi, Y.; Watanabe, M.; Krantis, A.; Durst, T.; Zhang, H.; et al. Effects of oral exposure to naturally-occurring and synthetic deoxynivalenol congeners on proinflammatory cytokine and chemokine mRNA expression in the mouse. *Toxicol. Appl. Pharmacol.* **2014**, *278*, 107–115. [CrossRef] [PubMed]
24. Wei, L.; Zhu, Z.; Wang, J.; Liu, J. JNK and p38 mitogen-activated protein kinase pathways contribute to porcine circovirus type 2 infection. *J. Virol.* **2009**, *83*, 6039–6047. [CrossRef] [PubMed]
25. Memiş, E.Y.; Yalçın, S.S. Human milk mycotoxin contamination: Smoking exposure and breastfeeding problems. *J. Matern. Fetal Neonatal Med.* **2021**, *34*, 31–40. [CrossRef] [PubMed]
26. Cai, G.; Sun, K.; Xia, S.; Feng, Z.; Zou, H.; Gu, J.; Yuan, Y.; Zhu, J.; Liu, Z.; Bian, J. Decrease in immune function and the role of mitogen-activated protein kinase (MAPK) overactivation in apoptosis during T lymphocytes activation induced by zearalenone, deoxynivalenol, and their combinations. *Chemosphere* **2020**, *255*, 126999. [CrossRef]
27. Pierron, A.; Mimoun, S.; Murate, L.S.; Loiseau, N.; Lippi, Y.; Bracarense, A.P.; Schatzmayr, G.; He, J.W.; Zhou, T.; Moll, W.D.; et al. Microbial biotransformation of DON: Molecular basis for reduced toxicity. *Sci. Rep.* **2016**, *6*, 29105. [CrossRef]
28. Awad, W.; Ghareeb, K.; Böhm, J.; Zentek, J. The toxicological impacts of the Fusarium mycotoxin, deoxynivalenol, in poultry flocks with special reference to immunotoxicity. *Toxins* **2013**, *5*, 912–925. [CrossRef]
29. Pestka, J. Toxicological mechanisms and potential health effects of deoxynivalenol and nivalenol. *World Mycotoxin J.* **2010**, *3*, 323–347. [CrossRef]
30. Hai-Lan, C.; Hong-Lian, T.; Jian, Y.; Manling, S.; Heyu, F.; Na, K.; Wenyue, H.; Si-Yu, C.; Ying-Yi, W.; Ting-Jun, H. Inhibitory effect of polysaccharide of Sargassum weizhouense on PCV2 induced inflammation in mice by suppressing histone acetylation. *Biomed. Pharmacother.* **2019**, *112*, 108741. [CrossRef]
31. Sugita-Konishi, Y.; Pestka, J. Differential upregulation of TNF-alpha, IL-6, and IL-8 production by deoxynivalenol (vomitoxin) and other 8-ketotrichothecenes in a human macrophage model. *J. Toxicol. Environ. Health A* **2001**, *64*, 619–636. [CrossRef] [PubMed]
32. Islam, Z.; Gray, J.S.; Pestka, J.J. p38 Mitogen-activated protein kinase mediates IL-8 induction by the ribotoxin deoxynivalenol in human monocytes. *Toxicol. Appl. Pharmacol.* **2006**, *213*, 235–244. [CrossRef] [PubMed]
33. Amuzie, C.J.; Harkema, J.R.; Pestka, J. Tissue distribution and proinflammatory cytokine induction by the trichothecene deoxynivalenol in the mouse: Comparison of nasal vs. oral exposure. *Toxicology* **2008**, *248*, 39–44. [CrossRef]
34. Amuzie, C.J.; Shinozuka, J.; Pestka, J. Induction of suppressors of cytokine signaling by the trichothecene deoxynivalenol in the mouse. *Toxicol. Sci.* **2009**, *111*, 277–287. [CrossRef] [PubMed]
35. Chung, Y.J.; Zhou, H.R.; Pestka, J. Transcriptional and posttranscriptional roles for p38 mitogen-activated protein kinase in upregulation of TNF-alpha expression by deoxynivalenol (vomitoxin). *Toxicol. Appl. Pharmacol.* **2003**, *193*, 188–201. [CrossRef]
36. Gray, J.S.; Pestka, J. Transcriptional regulation of deoxynivalenol-induced IL-8 expression in human monocytes. *Toxicol. Sci.* **2007**, *99*, 502–511. [CrossRef] [PubMed]
37. Zhu, X.; Bai, J.; Liu, P.; Wang, X.; Jiang, P. Suppressor of cytokine signaling 3 plays an important role in porcine circovirus type 2 subclinical infection by downregulating proinflammatory responses. *Sci. Rep.* **2016**, *6*, 32538. [CrossRef]
38. Chen, H.L.; Tan, H.L.; Yang, J.; Wei, Y.Y.; Hu, T.J. Sargassum polysaccharide inhibits inflammatory response in PCV2 infected-RAW264.7 cells by regulating histone acetylation. *Carbohydr. Polym.* **2018**, *200*, 633–640. [CrossRef]
39. Yang, J.; Tan, H.L.; Gu, L.Y.; Song, M.L.; Wu, Y.Y.; Peng, J.B.; Lan, Z.B.; Wei, Y.Y.; Hu, T.J. Sophora subprosrate polysaccharide inhibited cytokine/chemokine secretion via suppression of histone acetylation modification and NF-κb activation in PCV2 infected swine alveolar macrophage. *Int. J. Biol. Macromol.* **2017**, *104 Pt A*, 900–908. [CrossRef]
40. Qian, G.; Liu, D.; Hu, J.; Gan, F.; Hou, L.; Chen, X.; Huang, K. Ochratoxin A-induced autophagy in vitro and in vivo promotes porcine circovirus type 2 replication. *Cell Death Dis.* **2017**, *8*, e2909. [CrossRef]

41. Qian, G.; Liu, D.; Hou, L.; Hamid, M.; Chen, X.; Gan, F.; Song, S.; Huang, K. Ochratoxin A induces cytoprotective autophagy via blocking AKT/mTOR signaling pathway in PK-15 cells. *Food Chem. Toxicol.* **2018**, *122*, 120–131. [CrossRef] [PubMed]
42. Liu, D.; Ge, L.; Wang, Q.; Su, J.; Chen, X.; Wang, C.; Huang, K. Low-level contamination of deoxynivalenol: A threat from environmental toxins to porcine epidemic diarrhea virus infection. *Environ. Int.* **2020**, *143*, 105949. [CrossRef]
43. Bae, H.K.; Pestka, J. Deoxynivalenol induces p38 interaction with the ribosome in monocytes and macrophages. *Toxicol. Sci.* **2008**, *105*, 59–66. [CrossRef]
44. Bae, H.K.; Gray, J.S.; Li, M.; Vines, L.; Kim, J.; Pestka, J. Hematopoietic cell kinase associates with the 40S ribosomal subunit and mediates the ribotoxic stress response to deoxynivalenol in mononuclear phagocytes. *Toxicol. Sci.* **2010**, *115*, 444–452. [CrossRef] [PubMed]
45. Livak, K.J.; Schmittgen, T.D. Analysis of relative gene expression data using real-time quantitative PCR and the 2(-Delta Delta C(T)) Method. *Methods* **2001**, *25*, 402–408. [CrossRef] [PubMed]

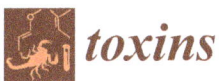

Article

Mycotoxin Zearalenone Attenuates Innate Immune Responses and Suppresses NLRP3 Inflammasome Activation in LPS-Activated Macrophages

Po-Yen Lee [1,2], Ching-Chih Liu [1,3], Shu-Chi Wang [4], Kai-Yin Chen [1], Tzu-Chieh Lin [1,5], Po-Len Liu [6], Chien-Chih Chiu [7], I-Chen Chen [1,8,9], Yu-Hung Lai [1,2,10], Wei-Chung Cheng [11,12], Wei-Ju Chung [1], Hsin-Chih Yeh [13,14], Chi-Han Huang [1], Chia-Cheng Su [1,15,16], Shu-Pin Huang [13,17,18] and Chia-Yang Li [1,19,*]

1. Graduate Institute of Medicine, College of Medicine, Kaohsiung Medical University, Kaohsiung 80708, Taiwan; maco69@gmail.com (P.-Y.L.); retina.liu@gmail.com (C.-C.L.); joice715@gmail.com (K.-Y.C.); 990327kmuh@gmail.com (T.-C.L.); yljane.chen@gmail.com (I.-C.C.); yuhung.lai@gmail.com (Y.-H.L.); chung.wj69@gmail.com (W.-J.C.); cheryl60286@gmail.com (C.-H.H.); s940854@gmail.com (C.-C.S.)
2. Department of Ophthalmology, Kaohsiung Medical University Hospital, Kaohsiung Medical University, Kaohsiung 80708, Taiwan
3. Department of Ophthalmology, Chi Mei Medical Center, Tainan 71004, Taiwan
4. Department of Medical Laboratory Science and Biotechnology, Kaohsiung Medical University, Kaohsiung 80708, Taiwan; shuchiwang@kmu.edu.tw
5. Department of Internal Medicine, Division of Cardiology, Kaohsiung Medical University, Kaohsiung 80708, Taiwan
6. Department of Respiratory Therapy, College of Medicine, Kaohsiung Medical University, Kaohsiung 80708, Taiwan; kisa@kmu.edu.tw
7. Department of Biotechnology, Kaohsiung Medical University, Kaohsiung 80708, Taiwan; cchiu@kmu.edu.tw
8. Department of Pediatrics, Kaohsiung Medical University Hospital, Kaohsiung 80756, Taiwan
9. Department of Pediatrics, School of Medicine, College of Medicine, Kaohsiung Medical University, Kaohsiung 80708, Taiwan
10. Department of Ophthalmology, School of Medicine, College of Medicine, Kaohsiung Medical University, Kaohsiung 80708, Taiwan
11. Research Center for Tumor Medical Science, Graduate Institute of Biomedical Sciences, China Medical University, Taichung 40402, Taiwan; cwc0702@gmail.com
12. Ph.D. Program for Cancer Biology and Drug Discovery, China Medical University and Academia Sinica, Taichung 40402, Taiwan
13. Department of Urology, School of Medicine, College of Medicine, Kaohsiung Medical University, Kaohsiung 80708, Taiwan; patrick1201.tw@yahoo.com.tw (H.-C.Y.); shpihu73@gmail.com (S.-P.H.)
14. Department of Urology, Kaohsiung Municipal Ta-Tung Hospital, Kaohsiung 80145, Taiwan
15. Department of Surgery, Division of Urology, Chi-Mei Medical Center, Tainan 71004, Taiwan
16. Department of Senior Citizen Service Management, Chia Nan University of Pharmacy and Science, Tainan 71710, Taiwan
17. Department of Urology, Kaohsiung Medical University Hospital, Kaohsiung Medical University, Kaohsiung 80708, Taiwan
18. Graduate Institute of Clinical Medicine, College of Medicine, Kaohsiung Medical University, Kaohsiung 80708, Taiwan
19. Department of Medical Research, Kaohsiung Medical University Hospital, Kaohsiung 80756, Taiwan
* Correspondence: chiayangli@kmu.edu.tw

Citation: Lee, P.-Y.; Liu, C.-C.; Wang, S.-C.; Chen, K.-Y.; Lin, T.-C.; Liu, P.-L.; Chiu, C.-C.; Chen, I.-C.; Lai, Y.-H.; Cheng, W.-C.; et al. Mycotoxin Zearalenone Attenuates Innate Immune Responses and Suppresses NLRP3 Inflammasome Activation in LPS-Activated Macrophages. *Toxins* **2021**, *13*, 593. https://doi.org/10.3390/toxins13090593

Received: 27 July 2021
Accepted: 22 August 2021
Published: 25 August 2021

Publisher's Note: MDPI stays neutral with regard to jurisdictional claims in published maps and institutional affiliations.

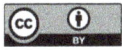

Copyright: © 2021 by the authors. Licensee MDPI, Basel, Switzerland. This article is an open access article distributed under the terms and conditions of the Creative Commons Attribution (CC BY) license (https:// creativecommons.org/licenses/by/ 4.0/).

Abstract: Zearalenone (ZEA) is a mycotoxin that has several adverse effects on most mammalian species. However, the effects of ZEA on macrophage-mediated innate immunity during infection have not been examined. In the present study, bacterial lipopolysaccharides (LPS) were used to induce the activation of macrophages and evaluate the effects of ZEA on the inflammatory responses and inflammation-associated signaling pathways. The experimental results indicated that ZEA suppressed LPS-activated inflammatory responses by macrophages including attenuating the production of proinflammatory mediators (nitric oxide (NO) and prostaglandin E_2 (PGE_2)), decreased the secretion of proinflammatory cytokines (tumor necrosis factor (TNF)-α, interleukin (IL)-1β and

IL-6), inhibited the activation of c-Jun amino-terminal kinase (JNK), p38 and nuclear factor-κB (NF-κB) signaling pathways, and repressed the nucleotide-binding and oligomerization domain (NOD)-, leucine-rich repeat (LRR)- and pyrin domain-containing protein 3 (NLRP3) inflammasome activation. These results indicated that mycotoxin ZEA attenuates macrophage-mediated innate immunity upon LPS stimulation, suggesting that the intake of mycotoxin ZEA-contaminated food might result in decreasing innate immunity, which has a higher risk of adverse effects during infection.

Keywords: zearalenone; mycotoxin; innate immunity; NLRP3 inflammasome; macrophages

Key Contribution: The present study determined that ZEA attenuates innate immune responses, inhibits the activation of JNK, p38 and NF-κB signaling pathways, and suppresses NLRP3 inflammasome activation in LPS-activated macrophages.

1. Introduction

Zearalenone (ZEA), a non-steroidal estrogenic mycotoxin, is produced by several species of Fusarium fungi that widely contaminate many cereal crops including wheat, corn, sorghum, oats, and barley, and subsequently produce ZEA at low temperatures and high humidity environments [1]. The European Food Safety Authority (EFSA) established a tolerable daily intake (TDI) for ZEA at 0.25 µg/kg body weight in 2011 [2]. While ZEA exhibits low acute toxicity (oral LD_{50} > 2000 mg/kg body weight [3]), long-term exposure to ZEA has several harmful effects due to its toxicity and high estrogenic activity including immunotoxic [4], hepatotoxic [5], and genotoxic [6] effects; however, the effect of ZEA on regulation of immune responses has not been well evaluated.

The innate immunity acts as the first line of defense against pathogen infection, and macrophages are antigen-presenting cells in the innate immune system that can phagocytose bacteria and produce both proinflammatory cytokines (e.g., tumor necrosis factor-α (TNF-α), interleukin (IL)-1β and IL-6), and mediators (e.g., nitric oxide (NO) and cyclooxygenase-2 (COX-2, a key enzyme in the synthesis of prostaglandins)) [7]. Moreover, macrophages can also present antigens to T cells and act as effectors for the induction of adaptive immune responses. Macrophages recognize pathogen-associated molecular patterns (e.g., lipopolysaccharide (LPS)) and damage-associated molecular patterns (e.g., adenosine triphosphate (ATP) and nigericin) by pathogen recognition receptors (e.g., toll-like receptors (TLRs)) and subsequently activate the downstream mitogen-activated protein kinases (MAPKs, such as the c-Jun amino-terminal kinase (JNK), the extracellular signal-regulated protein kinase (ERK), the p38 MAP kinase (p38)) and transcription factors (e.g., nuclear factor-κB (NF-κB)) to regulate immune responses against pathogen infection [8,9].

Inflammasomes are cytosolic protein complexes that modulate caspase-1 activation in innate immune responses and subsequently process both IL-1β and IL-18 maturation and secretion [10]. Nucleotide-binding and oligomerization domain (NOD)-, leucine-rich repeat (LRR)- and pyrin domain-containing protein 3 (NLRP3) inflammasome, the best-characterized inflammasome, can be activated by many stimuli, including extracellular adenosine triphosphate (ATP), pore-forming toxins, mitochondrial reactive oxygen species (ROS), potassium efflux, and destabilized lysosomes [11]. The activation of NLRP3 inflammasomes are central to elicit innate immune responses and are crucial for host immune response to bacterial [12], fungal [13], and viral infections [14,15]. Defects of inflammasome activation have been demonstrated to increased bacterial burden in systemic organs like the liver, lung, and spleen [16].

Although several reports have indicated that ZEA has either stimulating or suppressing effects on innate immunity [17,18], the cellular mechanisms activated by ZEA in triggering innate immune responses in macrophages during pathogen infection are not yet well understood. The present study investigated the effects of ZEA on the activities of innate immune responses during pathogen infection by macrophages in vitro and ex vivo.

LPS was used as stimulus to mimic bacterial infection, which can trigger innate immune responses by macrophages. The secretions of proinflammatory cytokines and mediators, NLRP3 inflammasome activation, and the activities of both MAPKs and NF-κB signaling pathways were examined.

2. Results

2.1. ZEA Attenuates Inducible Nitric Oxide Synthase (iNOS) and COX-2 Expressions of and Inhibits NO and Prostaglandin E2 (PGE_2) Productions by LPS-Activated Macrophages

In response to pathogen infection, NO is an important proinflammatory mediator secreted by activated macrophages, which are produced by enzyme iNOS [19]. The levels of NO and iNOS are associated with COX-2 expression, which is an essential enzyme converting arachidonic acid to PGE_2, one of the main pro-inflammatory factors [20,21]. LPS was used as a stimulus to mimic bacterial infection for macrophage activation. The effect of mycotoxin ZEA on the secretion of NO and PGE_2 was determined using Griess reaction and enzyme-linked immunosorbent assay (ELISA) respectively, while the expression of iNOS and COX-2 was determined by quantitative polymerase chain reaction (qPCR) and Western blot. The experimental results pointed out that ZEA suppressed the iNOS and COX-2 expressions in both mRNA and protein levels (Figure 1A–E), inhibited the production of NO (Figure 1F), and reduced the secretion of PGE_2 (Figure 1G) in LPS-activated J774A.1 cells. To exclude the potential cytotoxic effect of ZEA on LPS-activated inflammatory responses by macrophages, the effect of ZEA on the cell viability was detected by 3-[4,5-dimethylthiazol-2-yl]-2,5 diphenyl tetrazolium bromide (MTT) assay. The results pointed out that the doses of ZEA $\leq$ 50 μM did not affect the viability of LPS-activated J774.1 cells (Figure 1H), indicating that ZEA exhibited inhibitory effects on LPS-activated inflammatory responses by macrophages.

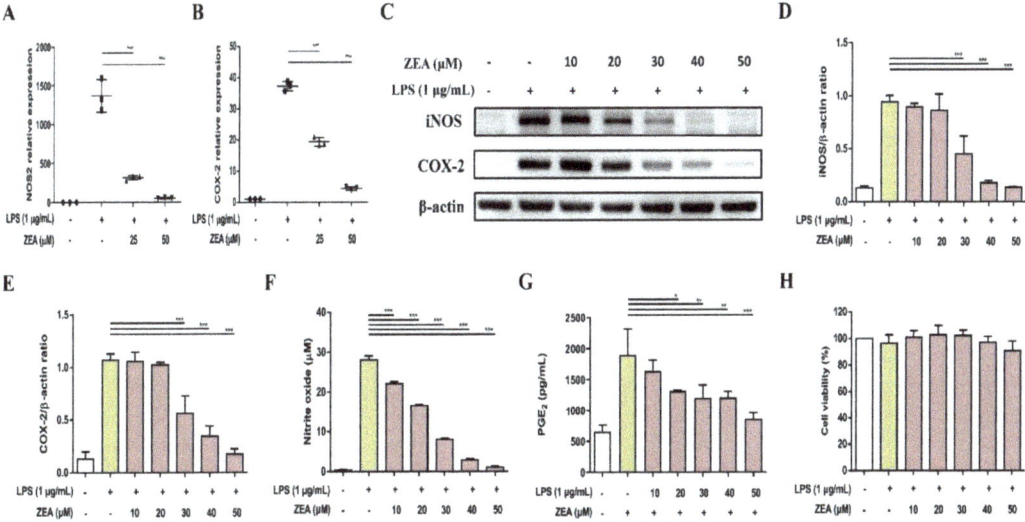

Figure 1. The effect of ZEA on the inflammatory mediator productions by LPS-activated macrophages. J774A.1 cells were pre-treated with ZEA for 1 h, and then treated with 1 μg/mL LPS for 6 (for qPCR) and 24 h (for Griess reaction, Western blot, ELISA and MTT assay). (**A,B**) The gene expression of *NOS2* and *COX-2* was measured using qPCR (n = 5). The expression of iNOS and COX-2 was detected by Western blot. The representative images are shown in (**C**), and the quantified results from three independent experiments in (**D,E**). (**F**) The levels of NO production were analyzed using Griess reaction (**G**) The secretion of PGE_2 was analyzed by ELISA. (**H**) Cell viability was examined using MTT assay. Data from three separate experiments are presented as mean ± standard deviation (SD). Statistical significances are presented as * $p < 0.05$; ** $p < 0.01$; *** $p < 0.001$.

2.2. ZEA Suppresses the Expression and Production of TNF-α and IL-6 by LPS-Activated Macrophages

Both TNF-α and IL-6 are critical proinflammatory cytokines against pathogen infection, and a lack of TNF-α and IL-6 results in higher mortality and more susceptibility to bacterial infection [22,23]. To examine whether ZEA affects LPS-activated TNF-α and IL-6 production by macrophages, J774A.1 cells were pretreated with ZEA for 1 h, and then treated with 1 μg/mL LPS for 6 or 24 h. The secretion of TNF-α and IL-6 was analyzed by ELISA and the gene expression of *TNF-α* and *IL-6* was measured by qPCR. The experimental results indicated that ZEA significantly attenuated the secretion of TNF-α and IL-6 by LPS-activated macrophages (Figure 2A,B). In addition, ZEA also suppressed the expression of *TNF-α* and *IL-6* by LPS-activated J774A.1 cells (Figure 2C,D).

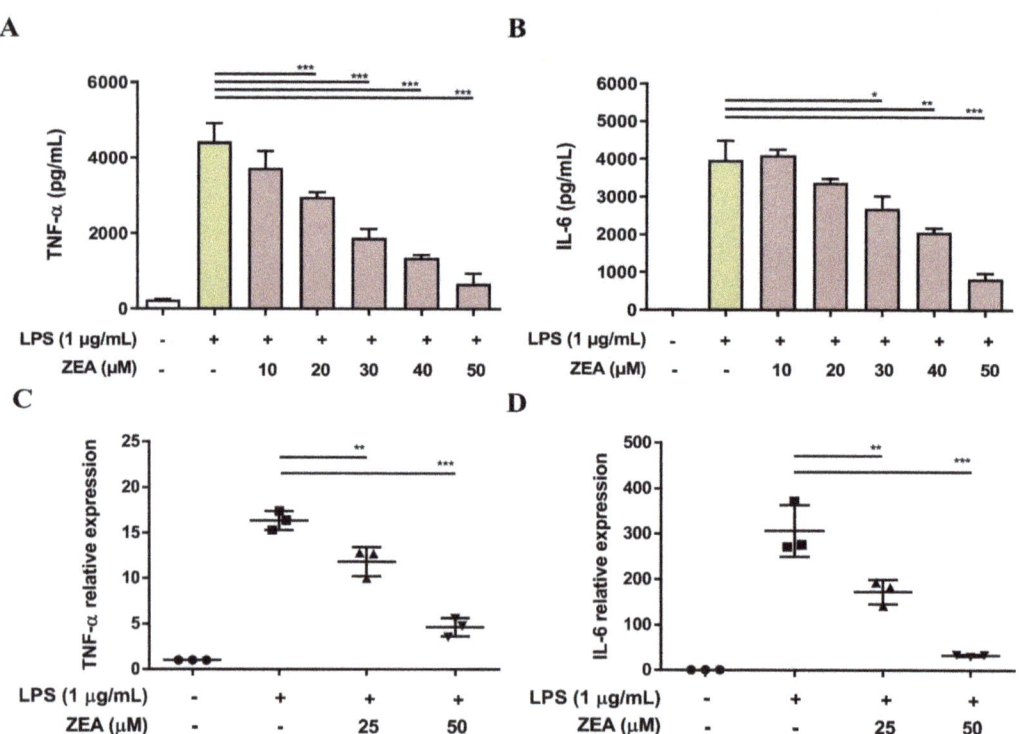

Figure 2. The effect of ZEA on the secretion of proinflammatory cytokines by LPS-activated macrophages. J774A.1 cells were pre-treated with ZEA for 1 h, and then treated with 1 μg/mL LPS for 6 (for qPCR) and 24 h (for ELISA). (**A,B**) The secretion of TNF-α and IL-6 was determined using ELISA. Data from three separate experiments are presented as mean ± SD. (**C,D**) The gene expression of *TNF-α* and *IL-6* was measured by qPCR (n = 5). Statistical significances are presented as * $p < 0.05$; ** $p < 0.01$; *** $p < 0.001$.

2.3. ZEA Inhibits the Activation of MAPKs and NF-κB Signaling Pathways by LPS-Activated Macrophages

MAPKs and NF-κB signaling are two critical pathways downstream of TLRs that drive inflammatory responses during infection [24]. To examine whether ZEA affects LPS-activated MAPKs and NF-κB signaling pathways by macrophages, J774A.1 cells were pretreated with ZEA for 1 h, and then treated with 1 μg/mL LPS for 2 or 24 h. These activations were measured by Western blot and promoter reporter assay respectively. As shown in Figure 3A–D, ZEA significantly attenuated the phosphorylation of JNK and p38 by LPS-activated macrophages, but not ERK. Moreover, ZEA was found to significantly decrease the promoter reporter activity of NF-κB by LPS-activated macrophages (Figure 3E).

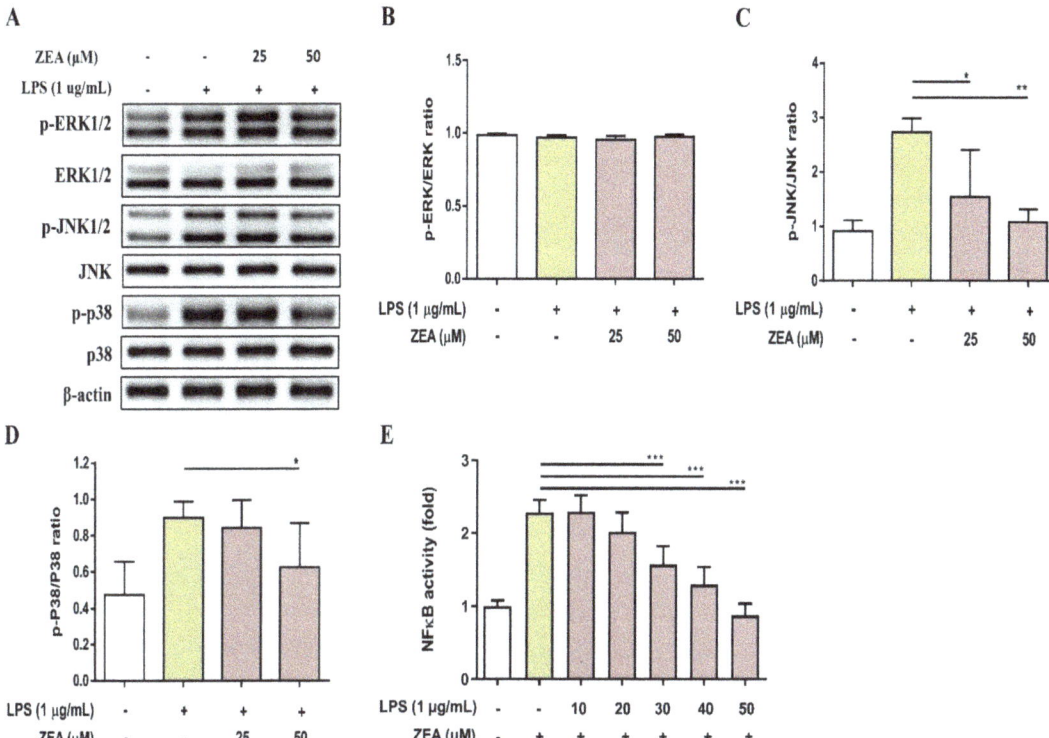

Figure 3. The effect of ZEA on the expression of MAPK signaling cascades-associated protein and the promoter activity of NF-κB by LPS-activated macrophages. J774A.1 cells were pretreated with ZEA for 1 h, and then treated with 1 μg/mL LPS for 2 h. The phosphorylation and expression of ERK, JNK and p38 were detected by Western blot. The expression of β-actin was used as loading control. The representative images are shown in (**A**), and the quantified results from three independent experiments shown in (**B–D**). (**E**) J-blue cells were pretreated with ZEA for 1 h, and then treated with 1 μg/mL LPS for 24 h. The level of secreted embryonic alkaline phosphatase (SEAP) was examined. Data from three separate experiments are presented as mean ± SD. Statistical significances are presented as * $p < 0.05$; ** $p < 0.01$; *** $p < 0.001$.

2.4. ZEA Inhibits IL-1β Secretion and Suppresses NLRP3 Inflammasome Activation by LPS/ATP- and LPS/nigericin-Activated Macrophages

The activation of NLRP3 inflammasome by microbial stimuli plays a critical role in regulating IL-1β and IL-18 secretion during infection [25]. To examine whether ZEA affects the activation of NLRP3 inflammasome by LPS/ATP- and LPS/nigericin-activated macrophages, J774A.1 cells were pretreated with ZEA for 1 h, and then treated with 1 μg/mL LPS for 5 h following 5 mM ATP or 10 μM nigericin treatments for 30 min. IL-1β secretion, NLRP3 inflammasome-associated protein expressions, and ASC and caspase-1 colocalization were analyzed by ELISA, Western blot, and immunofluorescence staining. Our experimental results showed that ZEA significantly suppressed IL-1β secretion of by LPS/ATP- and LPS/nigericin-activated macrophages (Figure 4A,B). ZEA also inhibited the expression of NLRP3, the cleavage of pro-caspase-1 to cleaved caspase-1 and the cleavage of pro-IL-1β to cleaved IL-1β by LPS/ATP-activated macrophages (Figure 4C). Moreover, ZEA inhibited ASC and caspase-1 colocalization in LPS/ATP- and LPS/nigericin-activated macrophages (Figure 5), indicating the ZEA inhibited the NLRP3 inflammasome assembly.

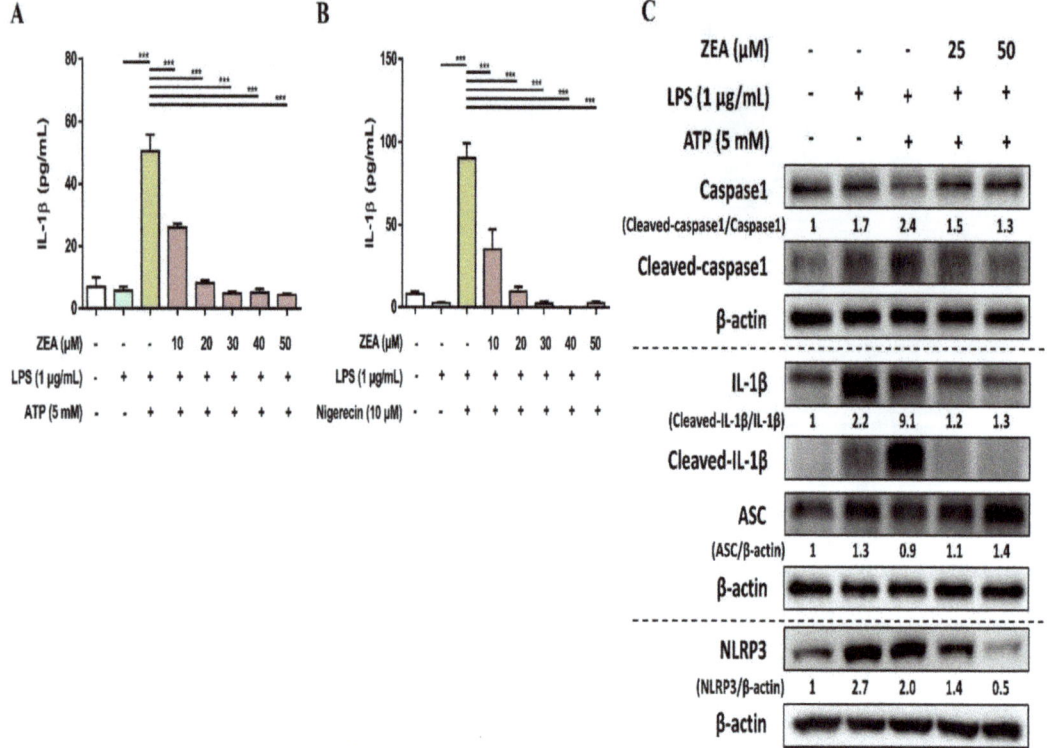

Figure 4. The effect of ZEA on the activation of NLRP3 inflammasome by LPS-activated macrophages. J774A.1 cells were pretreated with ZEA for 1 h, and then treated with 1 μg/mL LPS for 5 h following 5 mM ATP or 10 μM nigericin treatments for 30 min. (**A**,**B**) The secretion of IL-1β was analyzed by ELISA. Data from three separate experiments are presented as mean ± SD. NLRP3 inflammasome-associated protein expressions were determined by Western blot. A representative image of three independent experiments is shown in (**C**). Statistical significances are presented as *** $p < 0.001$.

2.5. ZEA Suppresses Proinflammatory Cytokine Secretions by LPS-Activated Human Macrophages

To examine whether ZEA affects LPS-activated proinflammatory cytokine secretions by human macrophages, THP-1 cells were induced to undergo macrophage differentiation by phorbol 12-myristate 13-acetate (PMA) for 24 h and then pretreated with ZEA for 1 h following 1 μg/mL LPS treatment for 24 h. The secretion of TNF-α and IL-6 was analyzed by ELISA. Cell viability was measured by MTT assay. As shown in Figure 6A,B, ZEA suppressed LPS-activated TNF-α and IL-6 secretions by human macrophages. In addition, the doses of ZEA ≤ 50 μM did not affect cell viability in LPS-activated human macrophages, indicating that inhibitory effects of ZEA on the production of TNF-α and IL-6 by LPS-activated human macrophages were not caused by dying effects (Figure 6C). For the NLRP3 inflammasome-derived IL-1β secretion, the cells were pretreated with ZEA for 1 h, and then treated with 1 μg/mL LPS for 5 h following ATP (5 mM) or nigericin (10 μM) treatments for 30 min. The secretion of IL-1β was detected using ELISA. Our experimental results indicated that ZEA decreased LPS/ATP- and LPS/nigericin-activated IL-1β secretion by human macrophages (Figure 6D,E).

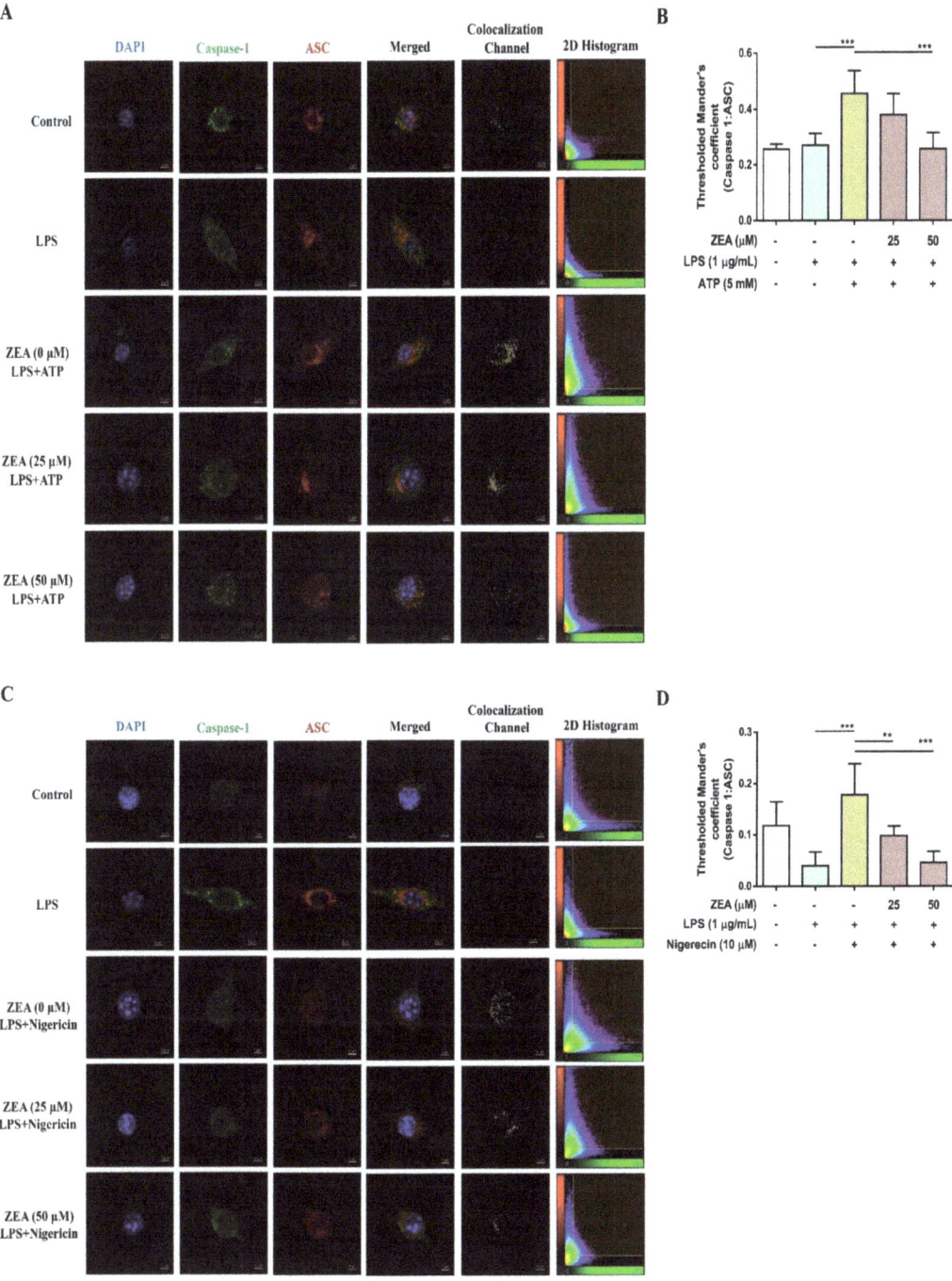

Figure 5. The effect of ZEA on the formation of NLRP3 inflammasome by LPS-activated macrophages. J774A.1 cells were pretreated with ZEA for 1 h, and then treated with 1 μg/mL LPS for 5 h following ATP (5 mM) or nigericin (10 μM) treatments

for 30 min. (**A,C**) Representative images of colocalization of caspase-1 (green) with ASC (red) were shown. DAPI was used as a nuclear counterstain. (**B,D**) The formation of ASC speck was quantified using the colocalization of caspase-1 and ASC signals in the threshold of 2D histogram (in the panel **A,C**) by Mander's coefficient. Data from three separate experiments are presented as mean ± SD. Statistical significances are presented as ** $p < 0.01$; *** $p < 0.001$.

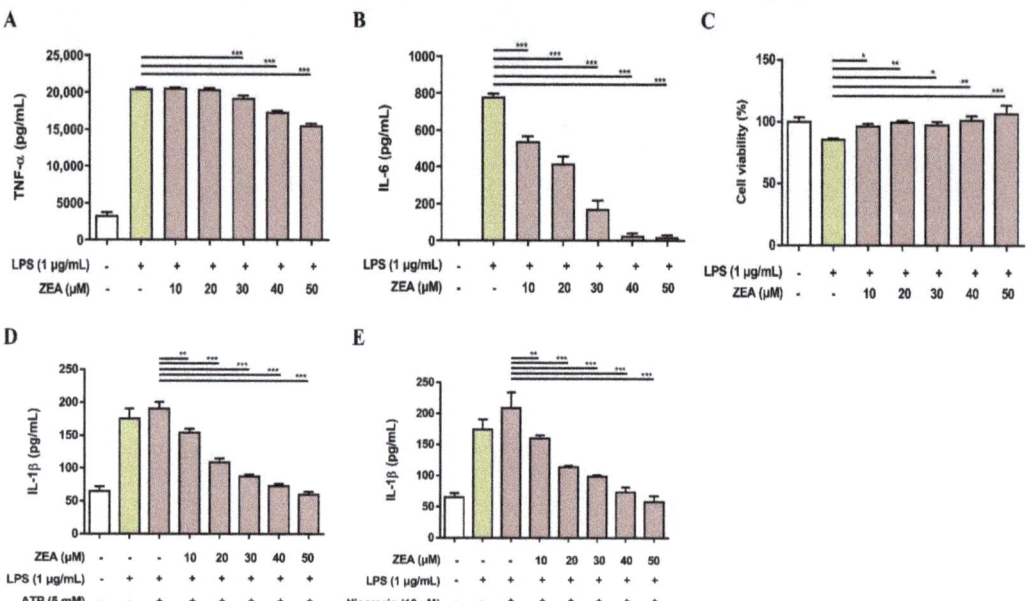

Figure 6. The effect of ZEA on the proinflammatory cytokine production by LPS-activated human monocyte-derived macrophages. THP-1 cells were stimulated with 50 ng/mL PMA for 24 h to induce macrophage differentiation. Afterwards, cells were pretreated with ZEA for 1 h following 1 μg/mL LPS treatment for 24 h. The secretion of (**A**) TNF-α and (**B**) IL-6 was detected by ELISA. (**C**) Cell viability was measured using MTT assay. (**D,E**) Human monocyte-derived macrophages were pretreated with ZEA for 1 h, and then treated with 1 μg/mL LPS for 5 h following ATP (5 mM) or nigericin (10 μM) treatments for 30 min. The secretion of IL-1β was examined using ELISA. Data from three separate experiments are presented as mean ± SD. Statistical significances are presented as * $p < 0.05$; ** $p < 0.01$; *** $p < 0.001$.

2.6. ZEA Reduces the Secretion of Proinflammatory Mediator and Cytokines by LPS-Activated Murine Peritoneal and Bone Marrow-Derived Macrophages (BMDMs)

To validate the above cell line results, the inhibitory effects of ZEA on LPS-activated inflammatory responses were further tested using primary cells. Both murine peritoneal macrophages and BMDMs were pretreated with ZEA for 1 h, and then treated with 1 μg/mL LPS for 24 h. The level of NO production was detected using Griess reaction and the secretions of TNF-α and IL-6 were analyzed by ELISA. Cell viability was measured by MTT assay. For the detection of IL-1β secretion, the cells were pretreated with ZEA for 1 h, and then treated with 1 μg/mL LPS for 5 h following ATP (5 mM) or nigericin (10 μM) treatments for 30 min. The levels of IL-1β production were detected using ELISA. As shown in Figure 7, ZEA suppressed LPS-induced NO, TNF-α, IL-6, IL-1β in murine peritoneal macrophages, while the inhibitory doses of ZEA ≤ 40 μM had no cytotoxic effect but 50 μM ZEA revealed cell toxicity. On the other hand, the results also demonstrated that ZEA decreased LPS-induced NO, TNF-α, IL-6, IL-1β in BMDMs. The inhibitory doses of ZEA ≤ 40 μM had no cytotoxic effect but 50 μM ZEA also revealed cell toxicity (Figure 8).

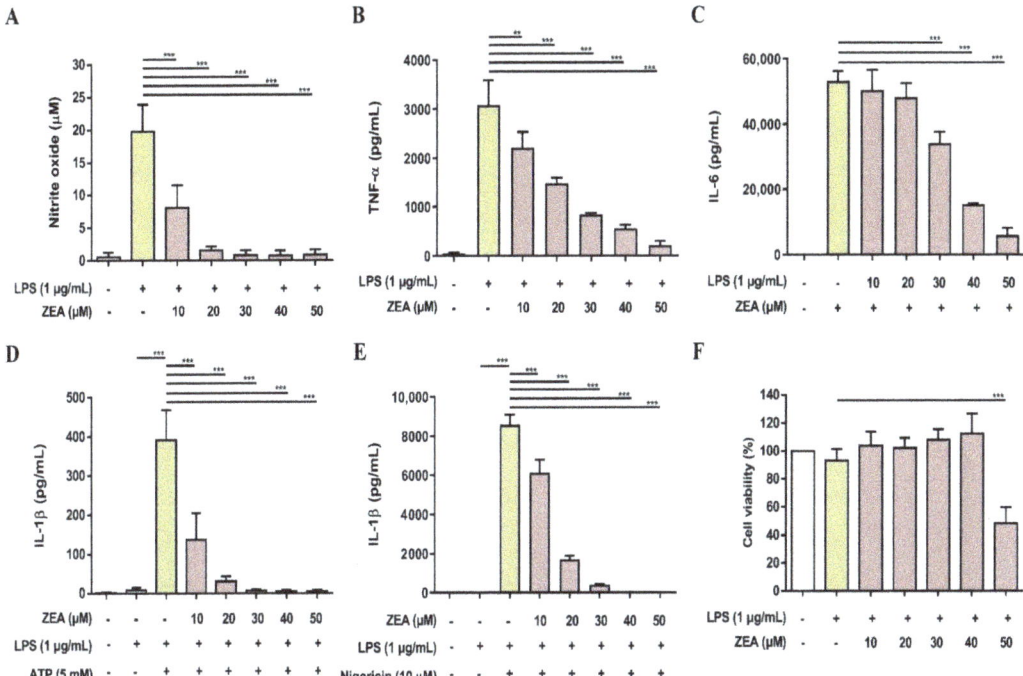

Figure 7. The effect of ZEA on the production of NO and proinflammatory cytokines by LPS-activated murine peritoneal macrophages. The cells were pretreated with ZEA for 1 h, and then treated with 1 µg/mL LPS for 24 h. (**A**) The levels of NO production were analyzed using Griess reaction. Secretions of (**B**) TNF-α and (**C**) IL-6 were detected by ELISA. (**D**,**E**) Murine peritoneal macrophages were pretreated with ZEA for 1 h, and then treated with 1 µg/mL LPS for 5 h following 5 mM ATP or 10 µM nigericin treatments for 30 min. The secretion of IL-1β was examined by ELISA. (**F**) Cell viability was detected using MTT assay. Data from three separate experiments are presented as mean ± SD. Statistical significances are presented as ** $p < 0.01$; *** $p < 0.001$.

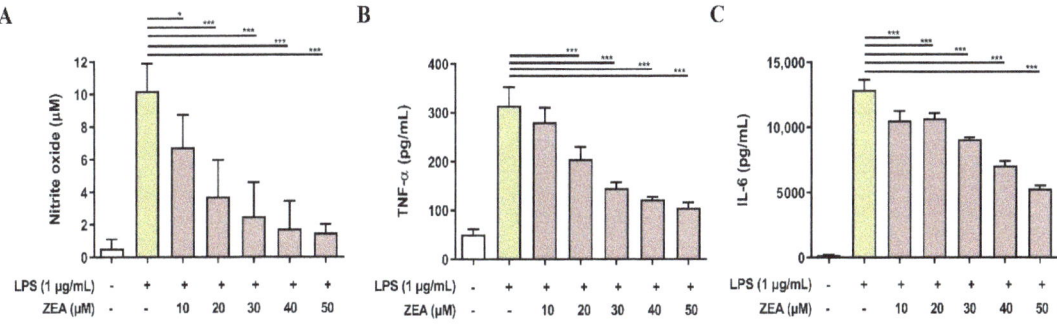

Figure 8. *Cont.*

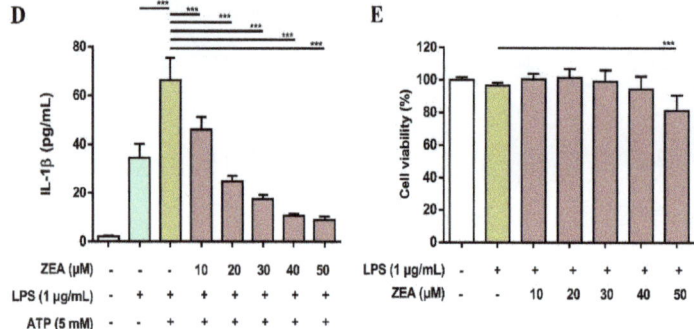

Figure 8. The effect of ZEA on the production of NO and proinflammatory cytokines by LPS-activated BMDMs. The cells were pretreated with ZEA for 1 h, and then treated with 1 μg/mL LPS for 24 h. (**A**) The levels of NO production were analyzed using Griess reaction. Secretions of (**B**) TNF-α and (**C**) IL-6 were detected by ELISA. (**D**) BMDMs were pretreated with ZEA Figure 1. h, and then treated with 1 μg/mL LPS for 5 h following 5 mM ATP for 30 min. The secretion of IL-1β was examined by ELISA. (**E**) Cell viability was detected using MTT assay. Data from three separate experiments are presented as mean ± SD. Statistical significances are presented as * $p < 0.05$; *** $p < 0.001$.

3. Discussion

The innate immune system has evolved to protect the host from pathogen infection and macrophages are effector cells of the innate immunity that respond to pathogen infection by initiating phagocytosis and the synthesis and release of pro-inflammatory cytokines [26]. People with a weak immunity have a higher risk of experiencing frequent infections and high mortality rate [27]. Mycotoxins are toxic secondary metabolites produced by fungi and found in many agricultural commodities that have unlike toxic effects according to the toxin and concentration and result in immunostimulatory or immunosuppressive effects [18]. ZEA has been known to have toxic effects on reproduction and fertility [28] and induce an estrogenic activity [4], but the effect of ZEA on immunoregulation has not been well investigated. In the present study, the immunoregulatory effects of ZEA on macrophages under LPS stimulation were examined.

During infection, activated macrophages secrete proinflammatory cytokines (e.g., TNF-α, IL-1β and IL-6) and inflammatory mediators (e.g., NO and PGE$_2$) to regulate inflammatory responses against pathogens. A previous study showed that ZEA decreases the iNOS expression and NO production by bovine aortic endothelial cells, resulting in vessel dysfunction [29]. Marin et al. also pointed out that ZEA reveals antagonistic effects on inflammation by decreasing IL-1β and TNF-α expressions in a human hepatocellular carcinoma cell line, HepG2 [30]; additionally, daily intake of ZEA also decreases the serum level of TNF-α in mice [31]. Our experimental results indicated that ZEA attenuates the activities of macrophage upon LPS stimulation, including decreasing NO and PGE$_2$ productions and suppressing TNF-α and IL-6 secretions by LPS-activated macrophages. Taken together, these results indicate that ZEA suppresses the LPS-activated immune response in macrophages by decreasing proinflammatory mediator and cytokine productions.

TLR4 stimulation by LPS triggers downstream signaling cascades including MAPKs and NF-κB pathways that are critical in the development of the immune system and regulation of inflammatory and acute immune responses [9]. A previous study indicated that the administration of a ZEA-contaminated diet in weaned pigs for 18 days affects the gene expression of immune regulators, MAPKs, and NF-κB in spleen cells [32]. They found that ZEA increases pro-inflammatory cytokine expression and synthesis, including TNF-α, IL-1β, IL-6 and IL-8, and promotes JNK pathway activation, whereas the activation of p-38MAPK and NF-κB is decreased [32]. In addition, Pistol et al. pointed out that ZEA is a potential hepatotoxin, which reduces NF-κB1 and TAK1/p38α MAPK gene expressions and decreases the production of TNF-α, IL-1β, IL-6, IL-8, and IFN-γ in the liver of the experimentally intoxicated piglets [33]. In the present study, the experimental results indicated that ZEA inhibited the phosphorylation of JNK and p38 and attenuated the activation of NF-κB by LPS-activated macrophages, suggesting that ZEA suppresses the LPS-activated immune response in macrophages through attenuating the JNK, p38, and NF-κB signaling pathways.

NLRP3 is a critical intracellular Nod-like receptor that is involved in the recognition of microbial or danger signals and mediates NLRP3 inflammasome assembly, resulting in the maturation and secretion of the pro-inflammatory cytokines, IL-1β and IL-18 [11]. In the present study, the NLRP3 inflammasome activation in macrophages was induced by LPS/ATP and LPS/nigericin, thereby inducing the secretion of IL-1β, enhancing the expression of cleaved caspase-1 and cleaved IL-1β, and increasing the colocalization of ASC and caspase-1, whereas ZEA significantly attenuated the activation of NLRP3 inflammasome by LPS/ATP- and LPS/nigericin-activated macrophages through decreasing the secretion of IL-1β, suppressing the expression of cleaved caspase-1 and cleaved IL-1β, and reducing the colocalization of ASC and caspase-1. These results suggest that ZEA might diminish the activation of NLRP3 inflammasome in macrophages during bacterial infection.

4. Conclusions

These experimental results demonstrated that mycotoxin ZEA attenuates innate immune responses by decreasing the production of proinflammatory mediators (NO and PGE_2) and cytokines (TNF-α, IL-1β and IL-6) by LPS-activated macrophages and inhibiting LPS-activated signaling cascades, including JNK, p38 and NF-κB signaling pathways. Moreover, mycotoxin ZEA also suppresses NLRP3 inflammasome activation by LPS-activated macrophages. Since people with a weak immunity have a higher risk of experiencing frequent infections and severe symptoms, these results suggest that an intake of mycotoxin ZEA-contaminated food might result in decreasing innate immunity, which poses a higher risk of adverse effects during infection.

5. Materials and Methods

5.1. Animals

Female C57BL/6 mice (six- to eight-week-old) were obtained from National Lab Animal Center (Taipei, Taiwan) and were kept in pathogen-free facility. All animal handling and experiments were permitted by the Institutional Animal Care and Use Committee at Kaohsiung Medical University (Permit Number: 108101; Period of Protocol: Valid from 1 August 2020 to 31 July 2023).

5.2. Cell Culture

The murine macrophage cell line (J774A.1), murine fibroblast cell line (L-929), and human THP-1 monocytic cell line were purchased from Bioresource Collection and Research Center (Hsinchu, Taiwan) and cultured in the complete RPMI-1640 medium (Corning, Corning, NY, USA), contained with heat-inactivated fetal bovine serum (10%, Corning), penicillin (100 U/mL, Corning), and streptomycin (100 U/mL, Corning) in a humidified chamber (Binder, Tuttlingen, Germany) at 37 °C. For the differentiation of the THP-1 monocyte into macrophage, the cells were treated with phorbol 12-myristate 13-acetate (PMA, 50 ng/mL) for 24 h at 37 °C in 5% CO_2.

5.3. Peritoneal Macrophags and BMDMs Preparation

The isolation of thioglycollate-elicited peritoneal macrophages was done following the method of Hung et al. [34] as described previously. Murine bone marrow cells were isolated by the method of Liu et al. [35] as described previously and macrophage differentiation was induced by treating L929 cell-conditioned medium (contained granulocyte-macrophage colony-stimulating factor) for a week following previous studies [36,37].

5.4. Cell Viability Assay

The cells (1×10^5) was seeded on a 96-well plate with 200 µL RPMI-1640 medium in each well, and the plate was incubated overnight. Afterwards, cells were pre-treated with 0 ~ 50 µM ZEA (purity ≥ 98%, ChemFaces, Wuhan, Hubei, China) for 1 h following 1 µg/mL LPS treatment (from *E. coli* O111:B4, Sigma Aldrich, St. Louis, MO, USA) for 24 h. Afterwards, the cells were incubated with MTT reagent (5 mg/mL, Sigma Aldrich) for 4 h at 37 °C, followed by 10 min of incubation with stop solution (100 µL isopropanol/0.04 M HCl). The absorbance at 570 nm was detected using a microplate reader (Epoch 2, BioTek Instruments Inc., Winoosky, VT, USA).

5.5. NO Production Assay

The NO assay was followed previously with slight modification [34]. The cells (1×10^5) was seeded on a 96-well plate with 200 µL RPMI-1640 medium overnight. Afterwards, the cells were pre-treated with 0 ~ 50 µM ZEA for 1 h following 1 µg/mL LPS treatment for 24 h. The cell supernatant was harvested and analyzed using Griess reagent (Sigma Aldrich). The absorbance at 540 nm was detected using a microplate reader. The quantity of nitrite was calculated from a sodium nitrite standard curve.

5.6. Western Blot Analysis

J774 A.1 macrophage cells (5×10^5 cells/well) were seeded in 6-well plates overnight. Afterwards, the cells were pre-treated with 0 ~ 50 µM ZEA for 1 h following 1 µg/mL LPS treatment for 2 or 24 h. For the detection of NLRP3 inflammasome-associated protein expression, the cells were pre-treated with different doses (25 and 50 µM) of ZEA for 1 h, and then treated with 1 µg/mL LPS for 5 h following 5 mM ATP treatment for 30 min. After treatments, the cells were washed twice with cold PBS and harvested using RIPA buffer, contained with protease inhibitors (Sigma Aldrich) and phosphatase inhibitors (Fivephoton Biochemicals, San Diego, CA, USA). The protein concentration was quantified by BCA protein assay (Thermo Scientific, Rockford, IL, USA), and equal amounts of proteins were separated by sodium dodecyl sulfate-polyacrylamide gel electrophoresis (SDS-PAGE), and then transferred onto a polyvinylidene fluoride (PVDF) membrane. Afterwards, the PVDF membrane was blocked by 5% non-fat milk/Tris-buffered saline containing 0.05% Tween-20 (TBST), incubated with primary antibodies (Supplemental Table S1), washed by TBST for three times, and then incubated with horseradish-conjugated secondary antibody (Santa Cruz). Then, the PVDF membrane was incubated with ECL chemiluminescence substrate (Thermo Fisher Scientific), and the signals were captured and quantified using a gel imaging system (Bio-Rad Laboratories Inc., Hercules, CA, USA).

5.7. qPCR

The total RNA of J774A.1 cells was extracted using TRIzol reagent and cDNA was generated by SuperScript VILO cDNA synthesis kit (Thermo Fisher Scientific, Rockford, IL, USA). Afterwards, qPCR was performed using SYBR Green PCR Master Mix (Thermo Fisher Scientific) by StepOne Plus Real-Time PCR system (Thermo Fisher Scientific). The primer sequences used in the present study were as follows: *NOS2* forward (F), 5'-GTTCTCAGCCCAACAATACAAGA-3' and reverse (R), 5'-GTGGACGGGTCGATGTCAC-3'; *COX2* F, 5'-CAAATCCTTGCTGTTCCCACCCAT-3' and R, 5'-GTGCACTGTGTTTGGA-GTGGGTTT-3'; *TNF-α* F, 5'-CAGGCGGTGCCTATGTCTC-3' and R, 5'-CGATCACCCCGA-AGTTCAGTAG-3'; *IL-6* F, 5'-CTGCAAGAGACTTCCATCCAG-3' and R, 5'-GTGGTATAGA-CAGGTCTGTTGG-3'; *18S rRNA* F, 5'-CGACGACCCATTCGAACGTCT-3' and R, 5'-CTCT-CCGGAATCGAACCCTGA-3'. Experimental Ct values were normalized to *18S rRNA* and relative mRNA expression calculated versus untreated control sample.

5.8. ELISA

The cells (1×10^5) were seeded on 96-well plates and incubated overnight. Subsequently, the cells were pre-treated with 0 ~ 50 µM of ZEA for 1 h following 1 µg/mL LPS treatment for 24 h. The levels of the TNF-α, IL-6 and PGE$_2$ secreted in the cell culture supernatants were analyzed by ELISA kits (Thermo Fisher Scientific) following the manufacturer's instructions. For the IL-1β secretion, were pretreated with ZEA for 1 h, and then treated with 1 μg/mL LPS for 5 h following 5 mM ATP or 10 μM nigericin treatments for 30 min.

5.9. NF-κB Promoter Reporter Assay

J-blue is a J774A.1 subline that stably expresses an NF-kB-inducible SEAP as described previously [34]. The cells were grown in a 96-well plate at a density of 1×10^5 cells/well and incubated overnight. Subsequently, the cells were pre-treated with 0 ~ 50 μM ZEA for 1 h following 1 μg/mL LPS treatment for 24 h. Briefly, Culture supernatant (20 μL) was mixed with QUANTI-blue medium (200 μL, InvivoGen, San Diego, CA, USA), incubated for 45 min at 37 °C, and then the absorbance at 655 nm was detected using a microplate reader.

5.10. Immunofluorescence Staining

J774A.1 cells (1×10^5 cells/well) were seeded on 8-well μ-Slide overnight (ibidi GmbH, Munich, Germany). Afterwards, the cells were pre-treated with various concentrations (25 and 50 μM) of ZEA for 1 h, and then treated with 1 μg/mL LPS for 5 h following 5 mM ATP or 10 μM nigericin treatments for 30 min. The cells were washed briefly with PBS and fixed by 4% paraformaldehyde, permeabilized by 0.1% Triton-X 100, incubated with primary antibodies (Supplemental Table S1), washed by PBS, incubated with the secondary antibodies, and then stained nuclei by DAPI (Invitrogen, Carlsbad, CA, USA). The cells were examined using a confocal laser microscope (Leica, Exton, PA, USA) and the images were further analyzed by the Imaris 8 Image Analysis Software (Oxford Instruments, Oxford, UK).

5.11. Statistical Analysis

Data from three separate experiments were presented as mean ± SD and the significant differences were evaluated by one-way ANOVA followed by Tukey post-hoc test using GraphPad Prism software version 9 (GraphPad Software, San Diego, CA). Statistical significances are presented as * $p < 0.05$; ** $p < 0.01$; *** $p < 0.001$.

Supplementary Materials: The following are available online at https://www.mdpi.com/article/10.3390/toxins13090593/s1, Table S1: List of primary antibodies used in this study.

Author Contributions: Conceptualization, P.-Y.L. and C.-Y.L.; methodology, P.-Y.L. and C.-Y.L.; formal analysis, P.-Y.L., C.-C.L., S.-C.W., K.-Y.C., T.-C.L., I.-C.C., Y.-H.L., W.-J.C., H.-C.Y., C.-H.H. and C.-C.S.; investigation, P.-Y.L. and C.-Y.L; resources, P.-L.L., C.-C.C., W.-C.C., S.-P.H.; data curation, P.-Y.L. and C.-Y.L.; writing—original draft preparation, P.-Y.L.; writing—review and editing, C.-Y.L.; funding acquisition, W.-C.C., S.-P.H. and C.-Y.L. All authors have read and agreed to the published version of the manuscript.

Funding: This study was supported by grants from the Ministry of Science and Technology, Taiwan, R.O.C. (grant No. MOST 108-2314-B-037-079-MY3, MOST 109-2622-E-039-004-CC2, MOST 109-2628-E-039-001-MY3, MOST 109-2327-B-039-002 and MOST 109-2320-B-037-007-MY3), Kaohsiung Medical University Chung-Ho Memorial Hospital (grant No. KMUH105-5M55) and China Medical University, Taiwan, R.O.C. (grant No. CMU107-S-24, CMU108-Z-02, CMU108-S-22 and CMU109-MF-61).

Institutional Review Board Statement: All animal handling and experiments were permitted by the Institutional Animal Care and Use Committee at Kaohsiung Medical University (Permit Number: 108101; Period of Protocol: Valid from 1 August 2020 to 31 July 2023).

Informed Consent Statement: Not applicable.

Data Availability Statement: Data will be provided on request.

Conflicts of Interest: The authors declare no conflict of interest.

References

1. Zheng, W.; Feng, N.; Wang, Y.; Noll, L.; Xu, S.; Liu, X.; Lu, N.; Zou, H.; Gu, J.; Yuan, Y.; et al. Effects of zearalenone and its derivatives on the synthesis and secretion of mammalian sex steroid hormones: A review. *Food Chem. Toxicol.* **2019**, *126*, 262–276. [CrossRef]
2. Mally, A.; Solfrizzo, M.; Degen, G.H. Biomonitoring of the mycotoxin Zearalenone: Current state-of-the art and application to human exposure assessment. *Arch. Toxicol.* **2016**, *90*, 1281–1292. [CrossRef] [PubMed]
3. Ropejko, K.; Twaruzek, M. Zearalenone and Its Metabolites-General Overview, Occurrence, and Toxicity. *Toxins* **2021**, *13*, 35. [CrossRef] [PubMed]
4. Hueza, I.M.; Raspantini, P.C.; Raspantini, L.E.; Latorre, A.O.; Gorniak, S.L. Zearalenone, an estrogenic mycotoxin, is an immunotoxic compound. *Toxins* **2014**, *6*, 1080–1095. [CrossRef] [PubMed]
5. Sun, L.H.; Lei, M.Y.; Zhang, N.Y.; Zhao, L.; Krumm, C.S.; Qi, D.S. Hepatotoxic effects of mycotoxin combinations in mice. *Food Chem. Toxicol.* **2014**, *74*, 289–293. [CrossRef] [PubMed]
6. El-Makawy, A.; Hassanane, M.S.; Abd Alla, E.S. Genotoxic evaluation for the estrogenic mycotoxin zearalenone. *Reprod. Nutr. Dev.* **2001**, *41*, 79–89. [CrossRef] [PubMed]
7. Hirayama, D.; Iida, T.; Nakase, H. The Phagocytic Function of Macrophage-Enforcing Innate Immunity and Tissue Homeostasis. *Int. J. Mol. Sci.* **2017**, *19*, 92. [CrossRef] [PubMed]
8. Nyati, K.K.; Masuda, K.; Zaman, M.M.; Dubey, P.K.; Millrine, D.; Chalise, J.P.; Higa, M.; Li, S.; Standley, D.M.; Saito, K.; et al. TLR4-induced NF-kappaB and MAPK signaling regulate the IL-6 mRNA stabilizing protein Arid5a. *Nucleic Acids Res.* **2017**, *45*, 2687–2703. [CrossRef]
9. Peroval, M.Y.; Boyd, A.C.; Young, J.R.; Smith, A.L. A critical role for MAPK signalling pathways in the transcriptional regulation of toll like receptors. *PLoS ONE* **2013**, *8*, e51243. [CrossRef]
10. Franchi, L.; Eigenbrod, T.; Munoz-Planillo, R.; Nunez, G. The inflammasome: A caspase-1-activation platform that regulates immune responses and disease pathogenesis. *Nat. Immunol.* **2009**, *10*, 241–247. [CrossRef]
11. Kelley, N.; Jeltema, D.; Duan, Y.; He, Y. The NLRP3 Inflammasome: An Overview of Mechanisms of Activation and Regulation. *Int. J. Mol. Sci.* **2019**, *20*, 3328. [CrossRef]
12. Zhong, Y.; Lu, Y.; Yang, X.; Tang, Y.; Zhao, K.; Yuan, C.; Zhong, X. The roles of NLRP3 inflammasome in bacterial infection. *Mol. Immunol.* **2020**, *122*, 80–88. [CrossRef] [PubMed]
13. Gross, O.; Poeck, H.; Bscheider, M.; Dostert, C.; Hannesschlager, N.; Endres, S.; Hartmann, G.; Tardivel, A.; Schweighoffer, E.; Tybulewicz, V.; et al. Syk kinase signalling couples to the Nlrp3 inflammasome for anti-fungal host defence. *Nature* **2009**, *459*, 433–436. [CrossRef] [PubMed]
14. Allen, I.C.; Scull, M.A.; Moore, C.B.; Holl, E.K.; McElvania-TeKippe, E.; Taxman, D.J.; Guthrie, E.H.; Pickles, R.J.; Ting, J.P. The NLRP3 inflammasome mediates in vivo innate immunity to influenza A virus through recognition of viral RNA. *Immunity* **2009**, *30*, 556–565. [CrossRef] [PubMed]
15. Kanneganti, T.D.; Body-Malapel, M.; Amer, A.; Park, J.H.; Whitfield, J.; Franchi, L.; Taraporewala, Z.F.; Miller, D.; Patton, J.T.; Inohara, N.; et al. Critical role for Cryopyrin/Nalp3 in activation of caspase-1 in response to viral infection and double-stranded RNA. *J. Biol. Chem.* **2006**, *281*, 36560–36568. [CrossRef] [PubMed]
16. Broz, P.; Monack, D.M. Molecular mechanisms of inflammasome activation during microbial infections. *Immunol. Rev.* **2011**, *243*, 174–190. [CrossRef]
17. Bulgaru, C.V.; Marin, D.E.; Pistol, G.C.; Taranu, I. Zearalenone and the Immune Response. *Toxins* **2021**, *13*, 248. [CrossRef] [PubMed]
18. Pierron, A.; Alassane-Kpembi, I.; Oswald, I.P. Impact of mycotoxin on immune response and consequences for pig health. *Anim. Nutr.* **2016**, *2*, 63–68. [CrossRef]
19. Dahiya, Y.; Pandey, R.K.; Bhatt, K.H.; Sodhi, A. Role of prostaglandin E2 in peptidoglycan mediated iNOS expression in mouse peritoneal macrophages in vitro. *FEBS Lett.* **2010**, *584*, 4227–4232. [CrossRef]
20. Cuzzocrea, S.; Salvemini, D. Molecular mechanisms involved in the reciprocal regulation of cyclooxygenase and nitric oxide synthase enzymes. *Kidney Int.* **2007**, *71*, 290–297. [CrossRef] [PubMed]
21. Paduch, R.; Kandefer-Szerszen, M. Nitric Oxide (NO) and Cyclooxygenase-2 (COX-2) Cross-Talk in Co-Cultures of Tumor Spheroids with Normal Cells. *Cancer Microenviron.* **2011**, *4*, 187–198. [CrossRef]
22. Albrecht, L.J.; Tauber, S.C.; Merres, J.; Kress, E.; Stope, M.B.; Jansen, S.; Pufe, T.; Brandenburg, L.O. Lack of Proinflammatory Cytokine Interleukin-6 or Tumor Necrosis Factor Receptor-1 Results in a Failure of the Innate Immune Response after Bacterial Meningitis. *Mediators Inflamm.* **2016**, *2016*, 7678542. [CrossRef]
23. Wellmer, A.; Gerber, J.; Ragheb, J.; Zysk, G.; Kunst, T.; Smirnov, A.; Bruck, W.; Nau, R. Effect of deficiency of tumor necrosis factor alpha or both of its receptors on Streptococcus pneumoniae central nervous system infection and peritonitis. *Infect. Immun.* **2001**, *69*, 6881–6886. [CrossRef]
24. Lane, K.; Andres-Terre, M.; Kudo, T.; Monack, D.M.; Covert, M.W. Escalating Threat Levels of Bacterial Infection Can Be Discriminated by Distinct MAPK and NF-kappaB Signaling Dynamics in Single Host Cells. *Cell Syst.* **2019**, *8*, 183–196.e4. [CrossRef] [PubMed]
25. Anand, P.K.; Malireddi, R.K.; Kanneganti, T.D. Role of the nlrp3 inflammasome in microbial infection. *Front. Microbiol.* **2011**, *2*, 12. [CrossRef]

26. Mosser, D.M.; Hamidzadeh, K.; Goncalves, R. Macrophages and the maintenance of homeostasis. *Cell. Mol. Immunol.* **2021**, *18*, 579–587. [CrossRef]
27. Katona, P.; Katona-Apte, J. The interaction between nutrition and infection. *Clin. Infect. Dis.* **2008**, *46*, 1582–1588. [CrossRef]
28. Zinedine, A.; Soriano, J.M.; Molto, J.C.; Manes, J. Review on the toxicity, occurrence, metabolism, detoxification, regulations and intake of zearalenone: An oestrogenic mycotoxin. *Food Chem. Toxicol.* **2007**, *45*, 1–18. [CrossRef]
29. Lee, H.J.; Park, J.H.; Oh, S.Y.; Cho, D.H.; Kim, S.; Jo, I. Zearalenone-Induced Interaction between PXR and Sp1 Increases Binding of Sp1 to a Promoter Site of the eNOS, Decreasing Its Transcription and NO Production in BAECs. *Toxins* **2020**, *12*, 421. [CrossRef]
30. Marin, D.E.; Pistol, G.C.; Bulgaru, C.V.; Taranu, I. Cytotoxic and inflammatory effects of individual and combined exposure of HepG2 cells to zearalenone and its metabolites. *Naunyn Schmiedebergs Arch. Pharmacol.* **2019**, *392*, 937–947. [CrossRef]
31. Islam, M.R.; Kim, J.W.; Roh, Y.S.; Kim, J.H.; Han, K.M.; Kwon, H.J.; Lim, C.W.; Kim, B. Evaluation of immunomodulatory effects of zearalenone in mice. *J. Immunotoxicol.* **2017**, *14*, 125–136. [CrossRef]
32. Pistol, G.C.; Braicu, C.; Motiu, M.; Gras, M.A.; Marin, D.E.; Stancu, M.; Calin, L.; Israel-Roming, F.; Berindan-Neagoe, I.; Taranu, I. Zearalenone mycotoxin affects immune mediators, MAPK signalling molecules, nuclear receptors and genome-wide gene expression in pig spleen. *PLoS ONE* **2015**, *10*, e0127503. [CrossRef]
33. Pistol, G.C.; Gras, M.A.; Marin, D.E.; Israel-Roming, F.; Stancu, M.; Taranu, I. Natural feed contaminant zearalenone decreases the expressions of important pro- and anti-inflammatory mediators and mitogen-activated protein kinase/NF-kappaB signalling molecules in pigs. *Br. J. Nutr.* **2014**, *111*, 452–464. [CrossRef] [PubMed]
34. Hung, Y.L.; Wang, S.C.; Suzuki, K.; Fang, S.H.; Chen, C.S.; Cheng, W.C.; Su, C.C.; Yeh, H.C.; Tu, H.P.; Liu, P.L.; et al. Bavachin attenuates LPS-induced inflammatory response and inhibits the activation of NLRP3 inflammasome in macrophages. *Phytomedicine* **2019**, *59*, 152785. [CrossRef]
35. Liu, X.; Quan, N. Immune Cell Isolation from Mouse Femur Bone Marrow. *Bio Protoc.* **2015**, *5*, e1631. [CrossRef]
36. Tang, R.; Zhang, G.; Chen, S.Y. Response gene to complement 32 protein promotes macrophage phagocytosis via activation of protein kinase C pathway. *J. Biol. Chem.* **2014**, *289*, 22715–22722. [CrossRef]
37. Trouplin, V.; Boucherit, N.; Gorvel, L.; Conti, F.; Mottola, G.; Ghigo, E. Bone marrow-derived macrophage production. *J. Vis. Exp.* **2013**, *81*, e50966. [CrossRef]

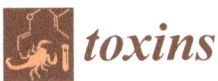

Article

The Reduction of the Combined Effects of Aflatoxin and Ochratoxin A in Piglet Livers and Kidneys by Dietary Antioxidants

Roua Gabriela Popescu [1], Sorin Avramescu [2], Daniela Eliza Marin [3], Ionelia Țăranu [3], Sergiu Emil Georgescu [1,*] and Anca Dinischiotu [1]

[1] Department of Biochemistry and Molecular Biology, Faculty of Biology, University of Bucharest, Splaiul Independentei, No. 91-95, 050095 Bucharest, Romania; roua.popescu@drd.unibuc.ro (R.G.P.); anca.dinischiotu@bio.unibuc.ro (A.D.)

[2] Department of Organic Chemistry, Biochemistry and Catalysis, Faculty of Chemistry, University of Bucharest, Soseaua Panduri, No. 90-92, 050663 Bucharest, Romania; sorin.avramescu@g.unibuc.ro

[3] Laboratory of Animal Biology, National Institute for Research and Development for Biology and Animal Nutrition, Calea Bucuresti, No. 1, 077015 Balotesti, Romania; daniela.marin@ibna.ro (D.E.M.); ionelia.taranu@ibna.ro (I.T.)

* Correspondence: sergiu.georgescu@bio.unibuc.ro

Citation: Popescu, R.G.; Avramescu, S.; Marin, D.E.; Țăranu, I.; Georgescu, S.E.; Dinischiotu, A. The Reduction of the Combined Effects of Aflatoxin and Ochratoxin A in Piglet Livers and Kidneys by Dietary Antioxidants. *Toxins* **2021**, *13*, 648. https://doi.org/10.3390/toxins13090648

Received: 18 August 2021
Accepted: 10 September 2021
Published: 13 September 2021

Publisher's Note: MDPI stays neutral with regard to jurisdictional claims in published maps and institutional affiliations.

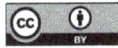

Copyright: © 2021 by the authors. Licensee MDPI, Basel, Switzerland. This article is an open access article distributed under the terms and conditions of the Creative Commons Attribution (CC BY) license (https://creativecommons.org/licenses/by/4.0/).

Abstract: The purpose of this study was to investigate the combined effects of aflatoxin B1 and ochratoxin A on protein expression and catalytic activities of CYP1A2, CYP2E1, CYP3A29 and GSTA1 and the preventive effect of dietary byproduct antioxidants administration against these mycotoxin damage. Three experimental groups (E1, E2, E3) and one control group (C) of piglets after weaning (TOPIGS-40 hybrid) were fed with experimental diets for 30 days. A basal diet containing normal compound feed for starter piglets was used as a control treatment and free of mycotoxin. The experimental groups were fed as follows: E1—basal diet plus a mixture (1:1) of two byproducts (grapeseed and sea buckthorn meal), E2—the basal diet experimentally contaminated with mycotoxins (479 ppb OTA and 62ppb AFB1) and E3—basal diet containing 5% of the mixture (1:1) of grapeseed and sea buckthorn meal and contaminated with the mix of OTA and AFB1. After 4 weeks, the animals were slaughtered, and tissue samples were taken from liver and kidney in order to perform microsomal fraction isolation, followed by protein expression and enzymatic analyses. The protein expressions of CYP2E1 and CYP3A29 were up-regulated in an insignificant manner in liver, whereas in kidney, those of CYP1A2, CYP2E1 and CYP3A29 were down-regulated. The enzymatic activities of CYP1A2, CYP2E1 and CYP3A29 decreased in liver, in a significant manner, whereas in kidney, these increased significantly. The co-presence of the two mycotoxins and the mixture of grape seed and sea buckthorn meal generated a tendency to return to the control values, which suggest that grapeseed and sea buckthorn meal waste represent a promising source in counteracting the harmful effect of ochratoxin A and aflatoxin B.

Keywords: piglets; mycotoxins; CYPs protein expression; CYPs enzyme activity; feed additives; antioxidant effect

Key Contribution: Understanding the combined effects of aflatoxin B1 and ochratoxin A in feed could be a better solution to diminish the deleterious effects of mycotoxins on piglets after weaning.

1. Introduction

Mycotoxin contamination is a major concern with great impact on human and animal health [1], as mycotoxin may be tumorigenic, mutagenic, estrogen mimetic and immunosuppressive. They are absorbed through the gastrointestinal tract [2–5], distributed to different body parts and metabolized especially at the hepatic and renal level [6]. Humans and animals are exposed to these natural contaminants due to consumption of contaminated food and feed components, such as cereals, cereal products, fruits for direct consumption or their derived products [7,8]. Additionally, humans can be exposed to mycotoxin contaminated animal foodstuffs such as milk, eggs and meat, even fish meat [9,10]. One of the main difficulties encountered in controlling mycotoxins incidence and prevalence is that more than one type of mycotoxin is present in a batch of feed or cereal at the same time. Thus, ingestion of contaminated feed with several types of mycotoxins, even if they are at minimum concentrations, can cause numerous negative effects due to their additive, synergic or antagonist effects [11,12].

In general, the metabolism of xenobiotics, respectively the biotransformation process of toxic compounds, into compounds suitable for excretion depends on the structure and physical-chemical properties of parental compound and enzymes available in the exposed tissue [13,14]. Therefore, reactions of xenobiotic metabolism take place in three phases: phase I—modification, by adding a functional group, phase II—conjugation of the functional group with a compound in order to increase the hydrophily of the conjugate and phase III—excretion of the phase II metabolites [15]. As a result of these, changes in protein expression, ROS production and oxidative stress in affected cells or tissues [16–19] could occur. During the biotransformation process, beyond the increased hydrophilicity of xenobiotics, reactive intermediates could be formed, increasing toxicity [20].

Cytochrome P450s play an important role in Phase I of biotransformation of xenobiotics, especially those of the CYP1, CYP2, CYP3 and CYP4 families, which mainly catalyze the reactions of oxidation, reduction or hydrolysis [19]. Phase II metabolism involves glutathione S-transferase, sulfotransferases, N-acetyltransferases and uridine 5′-diphospho-(UDP)-glucuronosyltransferases [21–23]. In the end, Phase III transporters from liver, kidney and intestine remove the produced metabolites in the cells in an active manner. In pigs, such transporters involved in the elimination of mycotoxins' metabolites conjugated with glucuronic acid, reduced glutathione and sulfate are represented by members of transporter family located in the basement membrane of polarized cells, such as MRP2, MRP4, Bcrp, Oat and Oct [19,23–28].

Studies regarding the mycotoxin toxicity in swine are numerous, but solutions for the reduction of these adverse effects are few. For example, the most used method to counteract the negative impact of mycotoxins in animals is adding "mycotoxin binders" or "mycotoxin modifiers", which are very effective for aflatoxins [29] but have limited efficiency against other types of mycotoxins [30] and could bind also vitamins and trace elements [31], generating deficiencies. Adding different plant derived antioxidants in feed could be a better solution to diminish the deleterious effects of mycotoxins on animal health.

To our knowledge, studies regarding cytochromes P450 protein expressions corelated with enzyme activities have not been performed up to now. Previous studies demonstrated that for humans and pigs CYP1A protein expression of liver were decreased whereas CYP3A increased in mycotoxicosis [32,33]. Moreover, in pigs, after a 14-day exposure to T-2 mycotoxin, an inhibition of hepatic CYP3A activity was observed [34].

A number of studies have shown that plant compounds can modulate cytochrome P450s protein expressions and activities [35,36]. For example, in a group of pigs fed for 16 days with a basal diet supplemented with 10% dried chicory root, an important upregulation of CYP1A2 and CYP2A19 mRNA and a small increase in CYP2E1 mRNA increase was noticed, followed by a subsequent increase in the CYP1A2 and 2A19 protein expressions and activities [37]. Therefore, examining the tissue-specific patterns of cytochrome P450s protein expression levels and specific activities provides valuable information toward understanding mycotoxins metabolism and benefits of therapeutic compounds from plants to mitigate the harmful damage produced by the co-presence of mycotoxin in feed.

The aim of our study was to investigate the combined effects of aflatoxin B1 and ochratoxin A in the piglet's liver and kidney on protein expression and catalytic activities of CYP1A2, CYP2E1, CYP3A29 and GSTA1 and the preventive effect of dietary byproduct antioxidants administration against these mycotoxins.

2. Results

2.1. Relative Protein Expression

In liver, the relative protein expression for CYP1A2 increased by 58% in the E1 group, fed with a basal diet supplemented with a mixture of grape seeds and sea buckthorn meal and decreased by 7% for the E2 group. The addition of a mixture of grape seed and sea buckthorn meal to weaned piglets diet contaminated with the mix of AFB1 and OTA (E3 group) has determined an upregulation by 30% of the expression of CYP1A2, compared to control group. At renal level, the CYP1A2 relative protein expression decreased by 18% for the E1 group and 36% for the E2 group, respectively, and increased by 28% for the E3 group compared to control one. These results were basically consistent with our previous data regarding to the relative mRNA expression for *CYP1A2* [38].

As for the protein expression of CYP2E1 in liver, it was practically unchanged in E1 group, and an up-regulation of 22% in E2 group and a significant one of 40% in E3 group ($p < 0.001$) compared to the control group were noticed. In contrast, in the kidney samples, protein expression of CYP2E1 decreased in E2 ($p < 0.01$) and E3 ($p < 0.05$) groups compared to liver ones. In the case of group E3, it was increased by 15% compared to the E2 group and significantly decreased by 39% compared to the E1 group (Figure 1), while for the E2 group, CYP2E1 expression level decreased significantly by 35%, compared to the control one.

For CYP3A29 protein expression, in the case of liver, administration of the basal diet enriched with a mixture of grape seed and sea buckthorn meal (group E1) increased the relative protein expression by 29% for the E1 group, by 47% for the E2 group and by 52% for the E3 group, compared to the control group level. Relative protein expression for CYP3A29 in the kidney increased by 27% for the E1 group and decreased by 20% for E2 and by 1.6% for E3 compared to the control group (Figure 1).

Interestingly, in liver samples, GSTA1 relative protein expression showed a decrease of 3.2% for the E1 group, 23% for the E2 group and 17% for the E3 group, compared to the control group. In kidney, the relative protein expression for GSTA1 showed increases of 19% and 11% for the E1 and E2 groups, respectively, and a decrease of 2.5% for the E3 group compared to the control one.

2.2. Enzymatic Activities

In liver, introduction in the diet of a mixture of grape seed and sea buckthorn meal diminished the activities of CYP1A2, CYP3A29 and GSTA1 in a significant (CYP1A2 and CYP3A29) or insignificant way (GSTA1), whereas CYP2E1 one increased insignificantly. The presence of OTA and AFB1 diminished significantly the CYP1A2, CYP2E1 and CYP3A29 specific activities and insignificantly the GSTA1 one. The concomitant administration of mixture of grape seed and sea buckthorn meal and AFB1 and OTA generated a decrease of all CYPs specific activities except the GSTA1 one compared to control.

In kidney, the mixture of grape seed and sea buckthorn meal added to feed determined an increase of enzymatic activities of CYP1A2, CYP2E1 and GSTA1 and a very significant decrease of CYP3A29 one compared to control ($p < 0.001$). The presence of AFB1 and OTA in piglets' feed increased all four enzymatic activities, whereas the co-presence of the two mycotoxins and the mixture of grape seed and sea buckthorn meal generated a tendency to decrease in all enzymatic activities toward the control values.

The hepatic CYP1A2 activity decreased significantly ($p < 0.001$) by 85% for the E2 group (1.88 U/mg) compared to control (12.35 U/mg) (Figure 2). In the kidney samples, CYP1A2 activity increased significantly ($p < 0.001$) by 2.7 times in the case of the E2 group (0.98 U/mg) compared to the control one (0.36 U/mg).

The specific activity of hepatic CYP2E1 decreased by 27% and 36% for the E2 group and E3 group ($p < 0.001$), respectively, compared to the E1 group. In contrast, the administration of basal diet supplemented with a mixture of AFB1 and OTA resulted in an increase of 56% in the specific activity of renal CYP2E1 compared to the E1 group level.

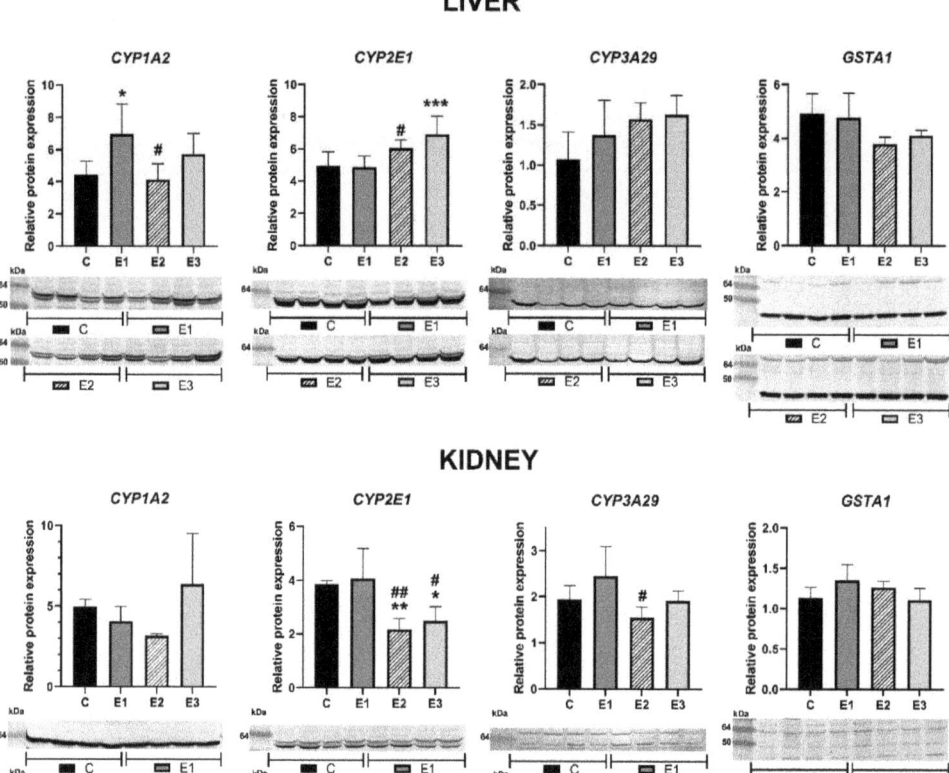

Figure 1. Relative protein expression and the corresponding quantification of Western blot images for CYP1A2, CYP2E1, CYP3A4 and GSTA1 in the hepatic and renal microsomal fractions of weaned piglets subjected to experimental diets. Calnexin band (70 kDa) was used as reference protein. The control group (C) were fed a basal diet. The experimental groups were fed as follows: the basal diet plus a mixture (1:1) of two byproducts (grapeseed and sea buckthorn meal) (E1 group), the basal diet artificially contaminated with AFB1 and OTA (E2 group), and the basal diet containing the mixture (1:1) of grapeseed and sea buckthorn meal and contaminated with the mix of AFB1 and OTA (E3 group). The data are illustrated as average values of the groups ($n = 4$) ± standard deviation of the mean (SE) and statistical significance related to the control group level. * E1/E2/E3 vs. C; # E2/E3 vs. E1; *, # $p < 0.05$; **, ## $p < 0.01$; *** $p < 0.001$.

The administration of basal diet enriched with a mixture of grape seed and sea buckthorn meal (E1 group) increased significantly ($p < 0.001$) the CYP3A29 specific activity in the liver by 15% compared to the E2 group level. Another contrast was observed in the renal CYP3A29 specific activity with a significant decrease of 57% ($p < 0.001$) in the E1 group and 31% in the E3 group ($p < 0.001$), compared to the E2 group level (Figure 2).

In the case of hepatic GSTA1, the specific activity showed decreases of 6% and 23% for the E1 and E2 groups, respectively, and an increase of 7% in the E3 group, compared to the control level. The renal GSTA1 specific activity showed an increase in experimental groups, compared to the control level.

Analyzing Figure 2, it can be noticed that mixture of grape seed and sea buckthorn meal decreased the CYP1A2 and CYP3A29 specific activities at hepatic level in a significant way, whereas at renal level, the CYP1A2 specific activity was significantly increased ($p < 0.01$). Moreover, the presence of OTA and AFB1 in piglet's feed decreased significantly the hepatic CYP1A2, CYP2E1 and CYP3A29 specific activities ($p < 0.001$), whereas in the kidney, the CYP1A2, CYP2E1 and CYP3A29 specific activities were increased significantly ($p < 0.01$). The concomitant administration of the mixture of grape seed and sea buckthorn meal and OTA and AFB1 determined the restauration of specific activity levels to control ones only in the kidney samples.

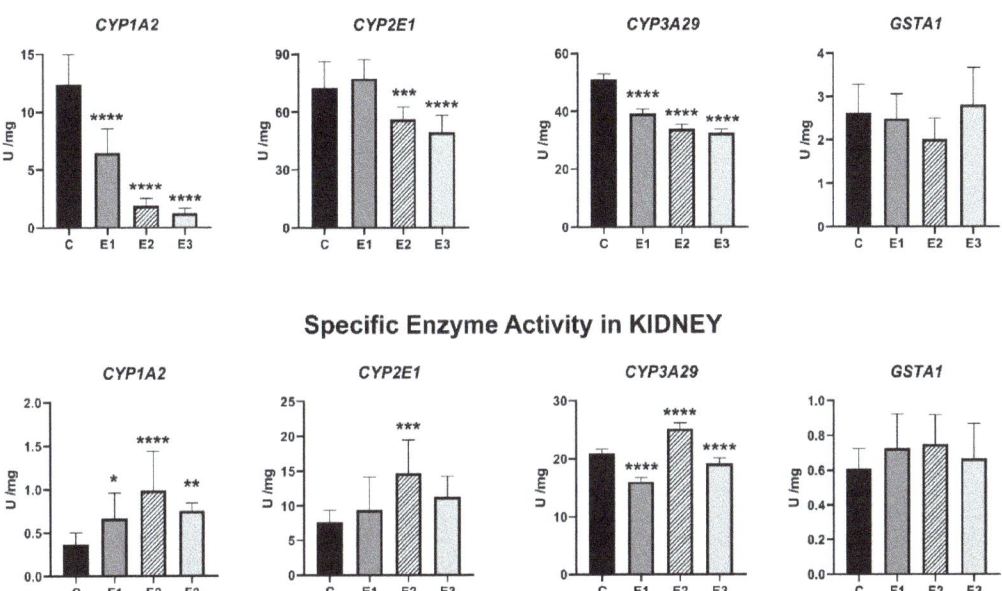

Figure 2. Enzymatic specific activity in the hepatic and renal microsomal fractions for CYP1A2, CYP2E1, CYP3A29 and GSTA1 of weaned piglets subjected to experimental diets. The control group (C) were fed a basal diet. The experimental groups were fed as follows: the basal diet plus a mixture (1:1) of two byproducts (grapeseed and sea buckthorn meal) (E1 group), the basal diet artificially contaminated with AFB1 and OTA (E2 group) and the basal diet containing the mixture (1:1) of grapeseed and sea buckthorn meal and contaminated with the mix of AFB1 and OTA (E3 group). The data are illustrated as average values of the groups ($n = 4$) ± standard deviation of the mean (SE) and statistical significance related to the control group level. * $p < 0.05$; ** $p < 0.01$; *** $p < 0.001$; **** $p < 0.0001$.

3. Discussion

Pigs are important non- rodent models in toxicology as well as in biomedical research [39] due to the fact that they have genetic and physiological traits similar to humans [40]. Pigs' liver presents the highest constitutive protein expressions and enzymatic activities of CYP1A1, CYP 1A2, CYP2E1 and CYP3A compared to other organs such as muscle, adipose tissue and intestine. Their kidney is also metabolically active. The metabolizing enzymes are primarily CYPs and are presented at the highest level in the renal proximal convoluted tubules. In pigs, they have not been studied extensively [39].

The CYP450 enzyme expressions and activities can be regulated by many different factors, including genetic polymorphism, epigenetic influences on xenobiotic metabolism, non-genetic host factors and depend on gene expression, mRNA translation, post-translational processes, protein expression level and inhibition or activation process of the catalytic activity of enzymes [41].

Regulation of porcine CYP450s expression in renal tissue has received less attention. In our study, changes in the renal tissue, compared to the liver samples in the expression level of cytochromes P450 can be observed.

The use of phenolic antioxidants as a feed supplement to pigs has recently attracted considerable attention because of their positive impact on meat quality, particularly by the reduction of skatole levels, which together with androsterone contributes to the development of boar taint [42]. However, there are a number of bioactive secondary metabolites in vegetal by-products, such as sesquiterpene lactones [43], one of these being artemisinin (a sesquiterpene lactone from *Artemisia* sp.) that has been shown to up-regulate CYP3A4 and CYP2B6 expression in humans and mice by binding to the nuclear receptors PXR and CAR [44]. A study of our group has demonstrated that feeding grapeseed and sea buckthorn meal, containing ferulic acid, p-coumaric acid, caffeic acid, vanillic acid, luteolin, quercetin, rutin, epicatechin, catechin in the diet of OTA and AFB1-intoxicated pigs decreased the *CYP1A2, CYP1A19, CYP2E1, CYP3A29* and *CYP4A24* gene expression, suggesting the decrease of bioactivation of these mycotoxins, probably resulting in a diminished toxicity in both organs, as the histological studies have revealed [38].

Previously, direct effects of phytochemicals on CYP450 dependent activity have been shown [45–47]. Scott et al. [48] demonstrated that CYP3A4, CYP19 and CYP2C19 activities in vitro could be modified by various plant constituents, and the magnitude of inhibition is dependent on concentration of the bioactive constituents in extract. Thus, to further investigate the impact of grapeseed and sea buckthorn meal on CYP450s activity, the direct effect of by-products in the diet of pigs was investigated.

In humans, CYP1A2 enzyme plays an important role in the metabolism of several clinically used drugs. It is one of the major P450 enzymes and accounts for approximately 13% of the total content of this enzyme group in the human liver [49]. CYP1A2 mRNA content shows an up to 40-fold variability between individuals [50] and corresponding variability of enzyme activity and drug metabolism [51,52]. The genetic variation in CYP1A2 activity is estimated to be up to 75% depending on environmental factors [53]. According to Klein et al. [54], the genetic variation of CYP1A2 activity might only account for 42%, 38% and 33% of the catalytic activity, protein expression and mRNA levels, respectively, in human liver samples. Taking into account the predominant role of CYP1A2 in activation of toxic xenobiotics compared to its metabolism of prescription drugs, there are many epidemiological reports examining the role of CYP1A2 variants, metabolism of procarcinogens and cancer risk.

In liver, both AFB1 and OTA are metabolized in reactions catalyzed by CYP1A2 and CYP3A4 [55,56]. AFB1 metabolization requires oxidation of the 8,9 double bond to yield the biologically active AFB1-8,9-epoxide that can react with DNA. At high concentrations of AFB1, the major producer of this metabolite is CYP3A4 [55], whereas at lower concentrations, the main enzymatic player is CYP1A2 [57]. Recent studies revealed that, a high dose of OTA, i.e., 3 mg per kg body weight given to ICR-type mice, diminished the protein expression of CYP1A2 [56]. This could be the reason for which CYP1A2 protein expression decreased slightly in the E2 group compared to the control one. AFB1 is also metabolized into a number of hydroxylation products, such as aflatoxin Q1 (AFQ1), aflatoxin P1 (AFP1), aflatoxin B2a (AFB2a), aflatoxin M1 (AFM1), aflatoxicol (AFL) and aflatoxicol H1 (AFH1). These could exert an inhibition of CYP1A2 activity as previously it was proved for other natural compounds [58]. The lower protein expression together with the inhibitory action of hydroxylated compounds could cooperate for the decrease of CYP1A2 specific activity in E2 group. The addition of several flavonoids and phenolic acids present in the byproducts mixed in feed [38] could explain the lower specific activity of CYP1A2 in the liver of the E3 group.

Taking into account that the kidney is implicated in the removal of metabolic wastes and xenobiotics from the circulatory system, a relatively high level of toxic substances can be formed during the urine concentration process [59]. In our experiment, probably the concentration of AFB1 and OTA increased in kidney and induced CYP1A2 biosynthesis. This enzyme catalyzes the oxidation of the xenobiotics and generates superoxide and hydrogen peroxide. Recent data revealed that exposure to OTA and AFB1 increased ROS level in HK-2 human proximal tubule epithelial cells [59] in chickens' kidneys [60].

If these overwhelmed the capacity of antioxidant system [61], hydrogen peroxide could accumulate and operate as a negative feedback loop for CYP1A transcription [62]. On the other hand, advanced oxidation protein products that formed due to the ROS attack on proteins down-regulated the expression of CYP1A2 and CYP3A4 in the kidneys of rats' models for chronic kidney disease [63]. Moreover, probably, antioxidants present in the by-products diminished ROS level, and the protein expression of CYP1A2 was up-regulated in the kidneys of E3 group individuals.

In our opinion, in the kidneys of the E1 group, the increase of CYP1A2 activity might be due to the influence of oleic and linoleic acids, beyond other unsaturated fatty acids and polyphenols present in the byproducts added to piglets' feed [38]. Taking in account that CYP1A2 is located in the endoplasmic reticulum (ER) membrane, its activity could be dependent on this membrane's fluidity. The ER membrane contains high quantities of phosphatidylcholines, phosphatidylethanolamines and phosphatidylinositol and low ones of sphingolipids and cholesterol, and as a result, the lipid packing is tight and ordered [64]. The *cis*-unsaturated fatty acids such as oleic and linoleic ones supplied by diet could be used for de novo synthesis of these phospholipids in ER, and once existing, could decrease the packing compactness of acyl chains, rising membrane fluidity [65]. Furthermore, flavonoids and iso-flavonoids might enter the hydrophobic core of membrane, causing an important decrease of lipid fluidity [66].

The active site of CYPs is present on the cytosolic side of ER membrane, is buried in the enzyme structure and contains the hem cofactor. It could adopt several conformations, and the substrates would bind to its most suitable conformation [67]. The increased fluidity of ER membrane could facilitate adopting such a suitable conformation, and the catalytic activity would be increased in E3 kidneys compared to control. For the E2 group, the high concentration of AFB1 and OTA due to the urine concentration process could increase specific activities of CYP1A2 and CYP3A4, compared to the control one. Moreover, it appears that the co-administration of by-products and mycotoxins (E3 group) decreased these two specific activities compared to those of the E2 group, still remaining higher in comparison with E1 and control groups.

CYP2E1 is an enzyme responsible for the metabolism of a large number of xenobiotics, such as aliphatic, aromatic and halogenated hydrocarbons, many of which are solvents and industrial monomers, mycotoxins and other drugs [68,69]. CYP2E1 is localized in the centrilobular region of the liver, but has also been detected in lung, bronchial tissue, kidneys, nasal mucosa, intestine and lymphocytes [70]. The regulation of CYP2E1 expression depends on transcriptional, post-transcriptional and post-translational factors. Increased hepatic CYP2E1 protein expression for the E2 group might be due to mycotoxins binding to CYP2E1 that stabilize the protein and thus increase CYP2E1 content [70,71]. As shown in Figure 1, renal CYP2E1 protein expression was down-regulated in E2 group. However, inclusion of by-products in mycotoxins contaminated diet effectively restored this decrease in E3 group.

In contrast, the decrease in enzyme activity in liver could be due to poorer transcription or stability of *CYP2E1* gene product rather than a functional change in the enzyme [72], which is in agreement with those reported in our previous study by Popescu et al. [38], when comparing *CYP2E1* mRNA levels to the levels of enzyme activities found for all experimental groups. Moreover, in the liver of E2 group individuals, possibly as response to the increased oxidative stress caused by induction of CYP2E1 activity in hepatocytes, glutathione S-transferase activity was found to be up-regulated, in agreement with the study of Mari and Cederbaum, [73]. The catalytic activity of CYP2E1 has been associated with susceptibility to toxicity under industrial exposure to chemicals such as benzene [68]. Therefore, probably, in the present study, renal CYP2E1 activity increased for the E2 group and was restored for the E3 group, compared to the control level.

It should be noted that our study did not fully cover the entire CYP450s enzyme families with respect to mRNA expression and that this may partially explain the discrepancies between mRNA expression, protein expression and activity measurements.

The discrepancies between mRNA expression and activity between experimental groups and the contradictory results on CYP2E1 need to be addressed in further studies.

In general, the studies regarding porcine CYP450s enzymes have focused on the impact of xenobiotics or antioxidant compounds only at molecular level and for a single type of tissue [38,74–78], while investigations regarding correlation between enzyme activity, protein level and mRNA transcript are few.

The pig is a relevant animal model for xenobiotics metabolic studies due to similarity to humans [79], therefore, studies on porcine CYP3A29 are important for a better understanding of mycotoxins co-exposure in vivo and metabolism studies [80].

Previous works have demonstrated that CYP3A constitutive expression is regulated by nuclear transcription factor Y; specificity protein 1 [81,82]; hepatocyte nuclear factors 1α, 3γ and 4 [83–85]; upstream stimulatory factor 1 [86]; activator protein 1 [87] and CCAAT/enhancer-binding proteins α and β [85,86]. In the presence of xenobiotics, induced expression of CYP3A is mediated by Pregnane X Receptor [80], constitutive androstane receptor (CAR), glucocorticoid receptor (GR) and vitamin D receptor (VDR) [81,88,89].

We demonstrated that by-products addition increased CYP3A29 protein expression in liver and kidney, while CYP3A29 activity was decreased, and only in kidneys, the tendency was opposite in the case of AFB1 and OTA co-contamination of the feed. The restoration of CYP3A29 relative protein expression level in kidney for the E3 group compared to the control one showed that the addition of a mixture of grapeseed and sea buckthorn meal by-products in mycotoxins contaminated diets favored the elimination processes and generated an adaptive response to the perturbation of hepatic and renal metabolism. The results for renal CYP3A29 activity were according with those reported in our previous study by Popescu et al. [38], when comparing *CYP3A29* mRNA levels to the levels of enzyme activities found for the E1 and E2 groups. Although, correlation of enzymatic activity from transcriptomic data was observed in a study [90], based on our results, we would argue that the differences between protein expression and specific activity are due to protein ability to bind specifically substrates and the way in which the enzyme is regulated [91].

Phase-I enzymes catalyze the primary reactions of xenobiotic detoxification [92]. Due to their electrophilic nature, phase-I metabolites have a potential to form stable adducts with nucleic acids and proteins, which act as cell-toxic and carcinogenic compounds [93,94]. The cytotoxic intermediates metabolites generated from Phase I are conjugated with hydrophilic moieties to form more readily excreted metabolites [95] by phase II enzymes, such as UDP–glucuronosyltransferases (UGTs), sulfotransferases, glutathione S-transferases, *N*–acetyltransferases, *N*–methyltransferases, phenol and catechol *O*–methyltransferase, Thiol methyltransferase and amino acid *N*–acyltransferase [96,97].

Glutathione *S*-transferases (GSTs) are dimeric enzymes (EC 2.5.1.18) that catalyze the conjugation of the reduced form of glutathione (GSH) to a broad variety of xenobiotic substrates including arene oxides, mycotoxins, lipoperoxidation-derived aldehydes, highly reactive aldehydes and other substrates [97–99]. GSTA1 is a cytosolic isoenzyme containing 222 amino acids from class alpha (A), based on amino acid sequence and substrate specificity of GSTs, with expression in liver and kidney. It is encoded by *GSTA1* gene [100]. The mycotoxins present in the feed and food chain such as AFB1 that are converted to AFB1-8,9-exo-epoxide (AFBO) via P450 metabolism are substrates for GSTs [101]. The ability of AFBO to conjugate with GSH reflects the expected sensitivity to AFB1-induced carcinogenesis since the pig is prone to develop hepatic tumors in vivo in the presence of xenobiotics [102,103].

Due to the lack of data about GSTs protein expression and catalytic activity in hepatic and renal tissue of pigs, we focused in our study on GSTA1 expression level. In the present study, the variation of GSTA1 protein expression and specific activity were decreased in liver and increased in kidney for the E2 group and restored for the E3 group, compared to the control level. The difference between liver and kidney could possibly be due to the physiological features of these pigs' organs [101], which correlates with the antagonist actions by addition of phenolic antioxidants [104] such as a mixture of grapeseed and sea buckthorn meal by-products (E1 group). The restoration of GSTA1 protein expressions and specific activities post-addition of phenolic antioxidants could be due to the counteracting effect on reactive oxygen species generated by mycotoxins metabolism that might decrease the GSH content [104]. Moreover, recent studies revealed that, in rats, phase I metabolites from OTA react with GSH to produce GSH-conjugates. In kidney, OTB-GSH is the major metabolite, and therefore, higher levels of GSH conjugates suggest a greater level of OTA bioactivation and greater sensitivity of the kidney to OTA [105,106]. Moreover, Gekle et al. [107] demonstrated that kidney is the target organ of OTA toxicity, probably because this mycotoxin is actively accumulated in kidney cells, due to unfavorable kinetics of renal elimination [106].

4. Conclusions

As far as we know, this is the first study analyzing the protein expressions of CYP1A2, CYP2E1, CYP3A29 and GSTA1 in comparison with their specific enzymatic activities in piglets' livers and kidney under combined exposure to AFB1 and OTA. A tissue-dependent response was noticed. Taking in account that CYP1A2, CYP2E1 and CYP3A29 activities were raised in the kidney of the E2 group individuals and decreased in those of the E3 group, it appears that the kidney was more affected compared to liver, and addition of by-products in the piglets' feed was beneficial. These findings along with those of gene expression suggest that grapeseed and sea buckthorn meal waste represent a promising source for counteracting the harmful effect of ochratoxin A and aflatoxin B. The discrepancies between protein expression and activity between experimental groups and the mechanisms involved need to be addressed in further studies.

5. Materials and Methods

5.1. Animals, Treatment and Sampling

Three experimental groups (E1, E2, E3) and one control group (C) of piglets after weaning (TOPIGS-40 hybrid, n = 10 per group, housed in pen two replicates of 5 pigs per pen) with an average body weight of 9.11 ± 0.03 kg were fed with experimental diets for 30 days. They fed on a basal diet which was served as a control (control group—C) with normal compound feed for starter piglets (corn 68.46%, soya meal 19%, corn gluten 4%, milk replacer 5%, L-lysine 0.3%, DL-methionine 0.1%, limestone 1.57%, monocalcium phosphate 0.35%, salt 0.1%, choline premixes 0.1% and 1% vitamin-mineral premixes). The feeding treatments for the experimental groups were as follows: group E1 received basal diet including a mixture (1:1) of two meal by-products (grape seed and sea buckthorn) in a percentage of 5% which replace corn and soya bean meal; group E2 received the basal diet artificially contaminated with a mixture of 62 ppb aflatoxin B1- AFB1 and 479 ppb ochratoxin A-OTA (E2 group) and group E3 get the basal diet with 5% by-product meal mixture and contaminated with AFB1 and OTA mycotoxins (62 and 479 ppb respectively). The AFB1 and OTA contaminated material was kindly provided by Dr. Boudra and Dr. Morgavi (I.N.R.A. Clermont Ferrand, Clermont-Ferrand, France) and was produced by the cultivation of Aspergillus flavus and Aspergillus ochraceus, respectively, on wheat as already described by Boudra et al. [108] resulting in a AFB1 concentration of 30 mg/kg and OTA 230 mg/kg. The grape seed meal and sea buckthorn meal were provided by two local commercials S.C. OLEOMET-S.R.L. and BIOCATINA, Bucharest, Romania. The mixture of mycotoxins was kindly provided by I.N.R.A, Centre of Clermont Ferrand. Data regarding diet composition, fatty acid composition of grapeseed and sea buckthorn, flavonoids and phenolic acids composition of byproducts, mineral composition of byproducts, animal performance and biomarkers of liver and kidney function in plasma were published previously by Popescu et al. 2021. Assigned diet and water were provided ad libitum during the experiment. At the end of the experiment (day 30), animals were slaughtered with the approval of the Ethical Committee of the National Research-Development Institute for

Animal Nutrition and Biology, Baloteşti, Romania (Ethical Committee no. 118/2 December 2019) and in accordance with the Romanian Law 206/2004 and the EU Council Directive 98/58/EC for handling and protection of animals used for experimental purposes. From four animals per group, the liver and kidney were collected and perfused with ice-cold saline solution to remove blood. Right liver lobe and renal cortex samples were collected on ice from all animals and were stored at −80 °C until the microsomal fraction isolation.

5.2. Isolation of the Microsome Fraction

The microsome fraction was isolated according to Rasmussen et al., [37], with slight modifications. Briefly, 6 g liver/kidney tissue were minced with sharp scissors and placed into a pre-chilled Dounce glass tube and added 4–5 volumes (4–5 mL of buffer per g of tissue) of ice-cold Tris–sucrose buffer (10 mM Tris–HCl, 250 mM sucrose, pH 7.4) and homogenized on ice using a thigh-fitting Teflon pestle attached to a Glas-Col Tissue Homogenizing System (Cole-Parmer, setting 70) for 3 min with a 30 s break at each 1 min. After 10 min centrifugation at 10,000× g, 4 °C, the supernatant (crude homogenate) was used for microsome isolation. Therefore, crude homogenate was diluted in Tris–sucrose buffer to a final volume of approximately 18 mL and centrifuged (Beckman Coulter Optima™L-80 XP Ultracentrifuge) with a fixed-angle rotor (Beckman 90 Ti) in OptiSeal tubes (Beckman, Ref 361623) at 100,000× g for 60 min at 4 °C. After ultracentrifugation, the supernatant obtained was collected as cytosolic fractions and the microsomal pellet were suspended in a buffer containing 50 mM Tris–HCl, 10 mM KH_2PO_4, 0.1 mM EDTA, 20% glycerol (pH 7.4) and stored at −80 °C in aliquots of 200 µL for later western blot and enzymatic assays. The purity of the microsomal and cytosolic fractions obtained after ultracentrifugation was assessed by immunoblotting for CYP1A2, CYP2E1, CYP3A29 and GSTA1. All steps were carried out on ice.

5.3. Western Blot Analysis

The obtained microsomes were used to evaluate protein expression for CYP1A2. CYP2E1, CYP3A29 and GSTA1 with Western blotting technique. Quantities of 30 µg microsomal protein from each sample were denatured by heating in the presence of a 5× Laemmlli buffer for 5 min at 95 °C. After cooling, the denatured proteins samples were separated by sodium dodecyl sulphate-polyacrylamide gel electrophoresis (SDS-PAGE, 10% separating gel) under reducing conditions in TRIS-glycine-SDS buffer at 90 V for 2 h. Proteins were transferred onto 0.4 µm poly-(vinylidene difluoride) membrane (Millipore, Billerica, MA, USA) in a wet transfer system (Bio-Rad, Hercules, CA, USA). Membrane blocking, and the incubations of primary and secondary antibodies were performed using the Western Breeze Chromogenic kit (Invitrogen, Themo Fischer Scientific, Waltham, MA, USA), and the membranes were processed according to manufacturer's instructions. Primary antibodies used were rabbit polyclonal antibodies anti-CYP1A2 (MyBioSource, San Diego, CA, USA, MBS9605022, 1:750), anti-CYP2E1 (MyBioSource, San Diego, CA, USA, MBS9605034, 1:750), anti-Cytochrome P450 Enzyme CYP3A4 (Merck, Temecula, CA, USA, AB1254, 1:1000) and anti-GSTA1 (NovusBiologicals, NBP1-33586, Centennial, CO, USA, 1:1000). The obtained bands were visualized with the ChemiDoc MP system (Bio-Rad, Hercules, CA, USA) and quantified using ImageLab software 5.1 (Bio-Rad, Hercules, CA, USA). Each sample analyzed was normalized to the expression corresponding to the calnexin band (Merck, Temecula, CA, USA, AB2301, 1:750) used as a control of protein loading.

5.4. Enzymatic Activity Assays

In accordance with protein expression evaluation from microsome fraction, enzymatic activity was also evaluated for: CYP1A2, CYP2E1, CYP3A29 and GSTA1.

5.4.1. CYP1A2

The activity of CYP1A2 was measured according to Hanioka et al. [109], with modifications. Therefore, a quantity of 200 µg microsomal protein was preincubated with 2 µM methoxy resorufin (MROD) (Sigma, Saint Louis, MO, USA, M1544-1MG) in 50 mM K_2HPO_4/KH_2PO_4 buffer (pH 7.4) in a final volume of 425 µL at 37 °C for 1 min. After preincubation, the reaction was started by adding 75 µL of 6.666 mM NADPH (final concentration of NADPH: 1 mM), incubated at 37 °C for 5 min and stopped with 500 µL of 100% ice-cold methanol with vortexing. After cooling on ice for 5 min, the samples were centrifuged at 10,000× g for 10 min at 4 °C, and the supernatant was collected and added into amber vials for HPLC analysis. The production of resorufin was analyzed by a HPLC method according to Wanwimolruk et al. [110] using a Varian HPLC system, Prostar 410 solvent delivery pumps, Prostar 350 autosampler, and column oven, equipped with a Pack Pro C18 150 × 4.6 mm I.D. S-3 µm, 12 nm column (YMC). The column was kept at 40 °C. A volume of 20 µL of sample was injected, and the metabolite resorufin was eluted isocratically with 20 mM K_2HPO_4/KH_2PO_4 buffer (pH 6.8), methanol and acetonitrile (30:35:35 v/v) at a flow rate of 0.5 mL/min (Supplementary Materials Figure S1B). The eluent was monitored by a fluorescence detector ProStar 363 with excitation and emission wavelengths of 560 and 586 nm, respectively. The obtained data were analyzed using Varian Workstation 6.3 software (Santa Clara, CA, USA). For quantification of resorufin, a standard calibration curve of resorufin (Sigma, Saint Louis, MO, USA, 73144-20MG) from 1 to 200 nM was prepared (Supplementary Materials Figure S1A). The enzyme activity was calculated by relating the amount of produced resorufin to blank incubations and was expressed as specific activity (units per mg of protein). One unit of activity represented the amount of enzyme that released one pmole of resorufin in one minute at 37 °C.

5.4.2. CYP2E1

The activity of CYP2E1 was measured according to Zamaratskaia et al. [111], with slight modifications. Briefly, 500 µg microsomal protein was preincubated with 0.2 mM p-nitrophenol (Sigma, Bellefonte, PA, USA, 48549) in 100 mM K_2HPO_4/KH_2PO_4 buffer (pH 6.8) in a final volume of 475 µL at 37 °C for 5 min. The reaction was started by adding 25 µL of 20 mM NADPH (final concentration of NADPH: 1 mM), incubated at 37 °C for 120 min, and immediately, a volume of 20 µL was injected into the HPLC system. The production of p-nitrocathechol was analyzed by High-Performance Liquid Chromatography with Diode-Array Detection (HPLC-DAD), using a High-Performance Liquid Chromatography Systems L-3000 from RIGOL Technologies, Inc. (Beijing, China), equipped with a Kinetex EVO C18 column (150 × 4.6 mm, 5 µm). The mobile phase consisted of 0.1% trifluoroacetic acid in water as solvent A and 0.1% trifluoroacetic acid in acetonitrile as solvent B. The gradient profile was as follows: 0–10 min 85% solvent A; 10–12 min 85% solvent B; 12–15 min 100% solvent A. The flow rate of the mobile phase was 1 mL/min, and the UV detector was set to 345 nm (Supplementary Materials Figure S2B). For quantification of produced metabolite, p-nitrocatechol, a standard calibration curve of p-nitrocatechol (Sigma, Saint Louis, MO, USA, N15553-1G) from 5 to 400 µM was prepared (Supplementary Materials Figure S2A). One unit of CYP2E1 activity represented the amount of enzyme that produces one pmole of p-nitrocatechol in one minute at 37 °C. The Enzyme activity was calculated by relating the amount of produced p-nitrocatechol/minute/mg protein to blank incubations and was expressed as specific activity (units per mg of protein).

5.4.3. CYP3A29

The activity of CYP3A29 was measured using the specific substrate nifedipine, as previously described by Sohl et al. [112] and Cheng et al. [113], with the following modifications: 500 µg microsomal protein and 200 µM nifedipine were preincubated in 100 mM K_2HPO_4/KH_2PO_4 buffer (pH 7.85) in a final volume of 425 µL at 37 °C for 3–5 min. The enzymatic reactions were initiated by addition of the 75 µL NADPH-generating system (50 parts 100 mM glucose 6-phosphate with 25 parts of NADP+ 10 mg/mL and with

1 part of glucose 6-phosphate dehydrogenase from *Leuconostoc mesenteriodes* at 1 mg/mL). After incubation at 37 °C for 10 min, the reaction was terminated by addition of 1.5 mL of ice-cold acetonitrile, followed by centrifugation for 10 min at $15,000\times g$ to precipitate the proteins. The supernatants were collected in amber vials and subjected to HPLC analysis, using a High-Performance Liquid Chromatography Systems L-3000 from RIGOL Technologies, Inc. (Beijing, China). The column was Kinetex EVO C18 column (150 × 4.6 mm, 5 μm) with the isocratic mobile phase of 0.1% trifluoroacetic acid in water/acetonitrile/methanol (40:30:30) at a flow rate of 1 mL/min at 30 °C. The consumption of nifedipine in the reaction mixture for each of the samples was determined based on calibration curves (Supplementary Materials Figure S3B) constructed from a series of standards of 2.5–250 μM nifedipine (Sigma, Saint Louis, MO, USA, N7634-1G). The remaining substrate was detected as the absorbance at 235 nm (Supplementary Materials Figure S3A). One unit of CYP3A29 activity represented the amount of enzyme that consumes one nmole of nifedipine in one minute at 37 °C. The enzyme activity was calculated by relating the amount of consumed nifedipine/minute/mg protein to blank incubations and was expressed as specific.

5.4.4. GSTA1

Glutathione S-transferase (GST; EC 2.5.1.18) activity was determined by measuring the conjugation rate of GSH with 1-chloro-2,4-dinitrobenzene (CDNB) substrate at 340 nm, according to the method described by Habig et al. [114] and adapted for 96 well plates with a 200 μL final volume per well. One unit of GSTA1 represented the amount of enzyme that releases one μmole of GS-CDNB product in one minute at 25 °C. Enzyme activity was expressed as specific activity (units per mg of protein).

5.4.5. Protein Determination

Each time after thawing a sample aliquot of microsomal fraction for Western blot and enzymatic activity assays, the protein concentration was determined by Bradford method [115] using bovine serum albumin as standard.

5.5. Statistical Analysis

Statistical analyses to identify differences in protein expression and enzyme activities were evaluated by one-way ANOVA method performed with GraphPad Prism 3.03 software (GraphPad Software, La Jolla, CA, USA). Post hoc comparisons between all groups were run using the Bonferroni test. The statistical significance (p value) was presented for all groups in contrast to the Control group (C). For each analysis, each of biological replicate was run in three technical replicates.

Supplementary Materials: The following are available online at https://www.mdpi.com/article/10.3390/toxins13090648/s1, Figure S1: Quantification and separation of resorufin using reversed-phase HPLC (C18). Figure S2: Quantification and separation of 4-nitrocatechol using reversed-phase HPLC (C18), Figure S3: Quantification and separation of nifedipine using reversed-phase HPLC (C18).

Author Contributions: Conceptualization, A.D. and S.E.G.; methodology, R.G.P., S.A., D.E.M. and I.Ț.; software, R.G.P.; validation, R.G.P. and S.A.; formal analysis, R.G.P. and S.A.; investigation, R.G.P.; resources, R.G.P., I.Ț., S.A. and A.D.; data curation, R.G.P. and I.Ț.; writing—original draft preparation, R.G.P.; writing—review and editing, A.D., I.Ț. and S.E.G.; visualization, A.D.; supervision, A.D. and S.E.G.; project administration I.Ț. and S.E.G.; funding acquisition, R.G.P. and S.E.G. All authors have read and agreed to the published version of the manuscript.

Funding: This research was funded by a grant of the Romanian Ministry of Research and Innovation, CCCDI—UEFISCDI, project number PN-III-P1-1.2-PCCDI-2017-0473/ "From classical animal nutrition to precision animal nutrition, scientific foundation for food security", within PNCDI.

Institutional Review Board Statement: The study was conducted according to the guidelines of the Declaration of Helsinki, and approved by the Ethical Committee of the National Research-Development Institute for Animal Nutrition and Biology, Baloteşti, Romania (Ethical Committee no. 118/2 December 2019) and in accordance with the Romanian Law 206/2004 and the EU Council Directive 98/58/EC for handling and protection of animals used for experimental purposes.

Informed Consent Statement: Not applicable.

Data Availability Statement: The data presented in this study are available on request from the corresponding author. The data are not publicly available due to privacy reason.

Acknowledgments: This work was supported by a grant of the Romanian Ministry of Research and Innovation, CCCDI—UEFISCDI, project number PN-III-P1-1.2-PCCDI-2017-0473/"From classical animal nutrition to precision animal nutrition, scientific foundation for food security", within PNCDI I "Use of agro-food residues by feeding solutions which to control the feed contaminants".

Conflicts of Interest: The authors declare no conflict of interest.

References

1. Omotayo, O.P.; Omotayo, A.O.; Mwanza, M.; Babalola, O.O. Prevalence of Mycotoxins and Their Consequences on Human Health. *Toxicol. Res.* **2019**, *35*, 1–7. [CrossRef]
2. Khan, A.; Aalim, M.M.; Khan, M.Z.; Saleemi, M.K.; He, C.; Khatoon, A.; Gul, S.T. Amelioration of immunosuppressive effects of aflatoxin and ochratoxin A in White Leghorn layers with distillery yeast sludge. *Toxin Rev.* **2017**, *36*, 275–281. [CrossRef]
3. Liu, Y.; Yang, Y.; Dong, R.; Zhang, Z.; Jia, F.; Yu, H.; Wang, Y. Protective effect of selenomethionine on intestinal injury induced by T-2 toxin. *Res. Veter. Sci.* **2020**, *132*, 439–447. [CrossRef]
4. Peltomaa, R.; Mickert, M.J.; Brandmeier, J.C.; Hlav, A.; Moreno-bondi, M.C.; Gorris, H.H.; Benito-pe, E. Competitive upconversion-linked immunoassay using peptide mimetics for the detection of the mycotoxin zearalenone. *Biosens. Bioelectron.* **2020**, *170*, 112683. [CrossRef] [PubMed]
5. Koletsi, P.; Schrama, J.; Graat, E.; Wiegertjes, G.; Lyons, P.; Pietsch, C. The Occurrence of Mycotoxins in Raw Materials and Fish Feeds in Europe and the Potential Effects of Deoxynivalenol (DON) on the Health and Growth of Farmed Fish Species—A Review. *Toxins* **2021**, *13*, 403. [CrossRef] [PubMed]
6. Rai, A.; Das, M.; Tripathi, A. Occurrence and toxicity of a fusarium mycotoxin, zearalenone. *Crit. Rev. Food Sci. Nutr.* **2020**, *60*, 2710–2729. [CrossRef]
7. Gonçalves, B.L.; Coppa, C.C.; De Neeff, D.V.; Corassin, C.H.; Oliveira, C. Mycotoxins in fruits and fruit-based products: Occurrence and methods for decontamination. *Toxin Rev.* **2019**, *38*, 263–272. [CrossRef]
8. Abdolmaleki, K.; Khedri, S.; Alizadeh, L.; Javanmardi, F.; Oliveira, C.A.; Khaneghah, A.M. The mycotoxins in edible oils: An overview of prevalence, concentration, toxicity, detection and decontamination techniques. *Trends Food Sci. Technol.* **2021**, *115*, 500–511. [CrossRef]
9. Carballo, D.; Moltó, J.; Berrada, H.; Ferrer, E. Presence of mycotoxins in ready-to-eat food and subsequent risk assessment. *Food Chem. Toxicol.* **2018**, *121*, 558–565. [CrossRef]
10. Adegbeye, M.J.; Reddy, P.R.K.; Chilaka, C.A.; Balogun, O.B.; Elghandour, M.M.; Rivas-Caceres, R.R.; Salem, A.Z. Mycotoxin toxicity and residue in animal products: Prevalence, consumer exposure and reduction strategies—A review. *Toxicon* **2020**, *177*, 96–108. [CrossRef]
11. Heussner, A.; Dietrich, D.; O'Brien, E. In vitro investigation of individual and combined cytotoxic effects of ochratoxin A and other selected mycotoxins on renal cells. *Toxicol. Vitr.* **2006**, *20*, 332–341. [CrossRef]
12. Smith, M.-C.; Madec, S.; Coton, E.; Hymery, N. Natural Co-Occurrence of Mycotoxins in Foods and Feeds and Their in vitro Combined Toxicological Effects. *Toxins* **2016**, *8*, 94. [CrossRef] [PubMed]
13. Park, Y.-C.; Lee, S.; Cho, M.-H. The Simplest Flowchart Stating the Mechanisms for Organic Xenobiotics-induced Toxicity: Can it Possibly be Accepted as a "Central Dogma" for Toxic Mechanisms? *Toxicol. Res.* **2014**, *30*, 179–184. [CrossRef] [PubMed]
14. Pelkonen, O.; Raunio, H. Metabolic activation of toxins: Tissue-specific expression and metabolism in target organs. *Environ. Health Perspect.* **1997**, *105*, 767–774. [CrossRef] [PubMed]
15. Caldwell, J.; Gardner, I.; Swales, N. An Introduction to Drug Disposition: The Basic Principles of Absorption, Distribution, Metabolism, and Excretion. *Toxicol. Pathol.* **1995**, *23*, 102–114. [CrossRef]
16. Mulero, J.; Martínez, G.; Oliva, J.; Cermeño, S.; Cayuela, J.M.; Zafrilla, P.; Martínez-Cachá, A.; Barba, A. Phenolic compounds and antioxidant activity of red wine made from grapes treated with different fungicides. *Food Chem.* **2015**, *180*, 25–31. [CrossRef]
17. Jarolim, K.; Del Favero, G.; Pahlke, G.; Dostal, V.; Zimmermann, K.; Heiss, E.; Ellmer, D.; Stark, T.D.; Hofmann, T.; Marko, D. Activation of the Nrf2-ARE pathway by the *Alternaria alternata* mycotoxins altertoxin I and II. *Arch. Toxicol.* **2016**, *91*, 203–216. [CrossRef]
18. Wen, J.; Mu, P.; Deng, Y. Mycotoxins: Cytotoxicity and biotransformation in animal cells. *Toxicol. Res.* **2016**, *5*, 377–387. [CrossRef]
19. Antonissen, G.; Devreese, M.; De Baere, S.; Martel, A.; Van Immerseel, F.; Croubels, S. Impact of Fusarium mycotoxins on hepatic and intestinal mRNA expression of cytochrome P450 enzymes and drug transporters, and on the pharmacokinetics of oral enrofloxacin in broiler chickens. *Food Chem. Toxicol.* **2017**, *101*, 75–83. [CrossRef]
20. Gu, X.; Manautou, J.E. Molecular mechanisms underlying chemical liver injury. *Expert Rev. Mol. Med.* **2013**, *14*, e4. [CrossRef]

21. Mathur, S.; Constable, P.D.; Eppley, R.M.; Waggoner, A.L.; Tumbleson, M.E.; Haschek, W.M. Fumonisin B1 Is Hepatotoxic and Nephrotoxic in Milk-Fed Calves. *Toxicol. Sci.* **2001**, *60*, 385–396. [CrossRef]
22. Kojima, M.; Degawa, M. Biochemical and Biophysical Research Communications Serum androgen level is determined by autosomal dominant inheritance and regulates sex-related CYP genes in pigs. *Biochem. Biophys. Res. Commun.* **2013**, *430*, 833–838. [CrossRef] [PubMed]
23. Lehman-McKeeman, L.D.; Ruepp, S.U. Chapter 2—Biochemical and Molecular Basis of Toxicity. In *Fundamentals of Toxicologic Pathology*, 3rd ed.; Academic Press: Waltham, MA, USA, 2018; pp. 15–33.
24. Anzai, N.; Jutabha, P.; Endou, H. Molecular Mechanism of Ochratoxin a Transport in the Kidney. *Toxins* **2010**, *2*, 1381–1398. [CrossRef]
25. Kok-Yong, S.; Lawrence, L. *Drug Distribution and Drug Elimination, Basic Pharmacokinetic Concepts and Some Clinical Applications*; Ahmed, T.A., Ed.; IntechOpen: London, UK, 2015; Available online: https://www.intechopen.com/chapters/48275 (accessed on 18 August 2021). [CrossRef]
26. Arana, M.R.; Tocchetti, G.N.; Rigalli, J.P.; Mottino, A.D.; García, F.; Villanueva, S.S. Hepatic and Intestinal Multidrug Resistance-Associated Protein 2: Transcriptional and Post-transcriptional Regulation by Xenobiotics. In *Toxicology New Aspects to This Scientific Conundrum*; Soloneski, S., Larramendy, M.L., Eds.; IntechOpen: London, UK, 2016; Available online: https://www.intechopen.com/chapters/51996, (accessed on 18 August 2021).
27. Kőszegi, T.; Poór, M. Ochratoxin A: Molecular Interactions, Mechanisms of Toxicity and Prevention at the Molecular Level. *Toxins* **2016**, *8*, 111. [CrossRef]
28. Szilagyi, J.T.; Gorczyca, L.; Brinker, A.; Buckley, B.; Laskin, J.D.; Aleksunes, L.M. Placental BCRP/ABCG2Transporter Prevents Fetal Exposure to the Estrogenic Mycotoxin Zearalenone. *Toxicol. Sci.* **2019**, *168*, 394–404. [CrossRef]
29. Ullah, H.A.; Durrani, A.Z.; Ijaz, M.; Javeed, A.; Sadique, U.; Hassan, Z.U.; Rahman, A.U.; Shah, M.; Khattak, I. Dietary mycotoxins binders: A strategy to reduce aflatoxin m1 residues and improve milk quality of lactating Beetal goats. *J. Consum. Prot. Food Saf.* **2016**, *11*, 305–309. [CrossRef]
30. Huwig, A.; Freimund, S.; Käppeli, O.; Dutler, H. Mycotoxin detoxication of animal feed by different adsorbents. *Toxicol. Lett.* **2001**, *122*, 179–188. [CrossRef]
31. Elliott, C.T.; Connolly, L.; Kolawole, O. Potential adverse effects on animal health and performance caused by the addition of mineral adsorbents to feeds to reduce mycotoxin exposure. *Mycotoxin Res.* **2020**, *36*, 115–126. [CrossRef] [PubMed]
32. Meissonnier, G.; Laffitte, J.; Raymond, I.; Benoit, E.; Cossalter, A.-M.; Pinton, P.; Bertin, G.; Oswald, I.; Galtier, P. Subclinical doses of T-2 toxin impair acquired immune response and liver cytochrome P450 in pigs. *Toxicology* **2008**, *247*, 46–54. [CrossRef] [PubMed]
33. Sun, L.-H.; Zhang, N.-Y.; Zhu, M.-K.; Zhao, L.; Zhou, J.-C.; Qi, D.-S. Prevention of Aflatoxin B1 Hepatoxicity by Dietary Selenium Is Associated with Inhibition of Cytochrome P450 Isozymes and Up-Regulation of 6 Selenoprotein Genes in Chick Liver. *J. Nutr.* **2015**, *146*, 655–661. [CrossRef]
34. Goossens, J.; De Bock, L.; Osselaere, A.; Verbrugghe, E.; Devreese, M.; Boussery, K.; Van Bocxlaer, J.; De Backer, P.; Croubels, S. The mycotoxin T-2 inhibits hepatic cytochrome P4503A activity in pigs. *Food Chem. Toxicol.* **2013**, *57*, 54–56. [CrossRef]
35. Shang, Y.; Huang, S. Engineering Plant Cytochrome P450s for Enhanced Synthesis of Natural Products: Past Achievements and Future Perspectives. *Plant Commun.* **2020**, *1*, 100012. [CrossRef] [PubMed]
36. Chang, T.K.H.; Crespi, C.L.; Waxman, D.J.; Ian, P.R.; Elizabeth, S.A. Spectrophotometric Analysis of Human CYP2E1-Catalyzed p-Nitrophenol Hydroxylation. *Methods Mol. Biol.* **2006**, *320*, 127–132. [CrossRef]
37. Rasmussen, M.K.; Ekstrand, B.; Zamaratskaia, G. Comparison of cytochrome P450 concentrations and metabolic activities in porcine hepatic microsomes prepared with two different methods. *Toxicol. Vitr.* **2011**, *25*, 343–346. [CrossRef]
38. Popescu, R.; Bulgaru, C.; Untea, A.; Vlassa, M.; Filip, M.; Hermenean, A.; Marin, D.; Țăranu, I.; Georgescu, S.; Dinischiotu, A. The Effectiveness of Dietary Byproduct Antioxidants on Induced CYP Genes Expression and Histological Alteration in Piglets Liver and Kidney Fed with Aflatoxin B1 and Ochratoxin A. *Toxins* **2021**, *13*, 148. [CrossRef]
39. Helke, K.L.; Nelson, K.N.; Sargeant, A.M.; Jacob, B.; McKeag, S.; Haruna, J.; Vemireddi, V.; Greeley, M.; Brocksmith, D.; Navratil, N.; et al. Pigs in Toxicology: Breed Differences in Metabolism and Background Findings. *Toxicol. Pathol.* **2016**, *44*, 575–590. [CrossRef] [PubMed]
40. Schook, L.B.; Collares, T.; Darfour-Oduro, K.A.; De, A.K.; Rund, L.A.; Schachtschneider, K.; Seixas, F.K. Unraveling the Swine Genome: Implications for Human Health. *Annu. Rev. Anim. Biosci.* **2015**, *3*, 219–244. [CrossRef] [PubMed]
41. Zanger, U.M.; Schwab, M. Pharmacology and Therapeutics Cytochrome P450 enzymes in drug metabolism: Regulation of gene expression, enzyme activities, and impact of genetic variation. *Pharmacol. Ther.* **2013**, *138*, 103–141. [CrossRef]
42. Zamaratskaia, G.; Žlábek, V.; Chen, G.; Madej, A. Modulation of porcine cytochrome P450 enzyme activities by surgical castration and immunocastration. *Animal* **2009**, *3*, 1124–1132. [CrossRef] [PubMed]
43. Bais, H.P.; Ravishankar, G.A. *Cichorium intybus* L.—Cultivation, processing, utility, value addition and biotechnology, with an emphasis on current status and future prospects. *J. Sci. Food Agric.* **2001**, *81*, 467–484. [CrossRef]
44. Burk, O.; Arnold, K.A.; Geick, A.; Tegude, H.; Eichelbaum, M. A role for constitutive androstane receptor in the regulation of human intestinal MDR1 expression. *Biol. Chem.* **2005**, *386*, 503–513. [CrossRef]
45. Doehmer, J.; Weiss, G.; McGregor, G.P.; Appel, K. Assessment of a dry extract from milk thistle (*Silybum marianum*) for interference with human liver cytochrome-P450 activities. *Toxicol. Vitr.* **2011**, *25*, 21–27. [CrossRef]

46. Slaughter, R.L.; Edwards, D.J. Recent Advances: The Cytochrome P450 Enzymes. *Ann. Pharmacother.* **1995**, *29*, 619–624. [CrossRef]
47. Teel, R.W.; Huynh, H. Modulation by phytochemicals of cytochrome P450-linked enzyme activity. *Cancer Lett.* **1998**, *133*, 135–141. [CrossRef]
48. Obach, R.S.; Walsky, R.L.; Venkatakrishnan, K.; Gaman, E.A.; Houston, J.B.; Tremaine, L.M. The Utility of in Vitro Cytochrome P450 Inhibition Data in the Prediction of Drug-Drug Interactions. *J. Pharmacol. Exp. Ther.* **2006**, *316*, 336–348. [CrossRef] [PubMed]
49. Shimada, T.; Yamazaki, H.; Mimura, M.; Inui, Y.; Guengerich, F.P. Interindividual variations in human liver cytochrome P-450 enzymes involved in the oxidation of drugs, carcinogens and toxic chemicals: Studies with liver microsomes of 30 Japanese and 30 Caucasians. *J. Pharmacol. Exp. Ther.* **1994**, *270*, 414–423. [PubMed]
50. Zhou, S.-F.; Liu, J.-P.; Chowbay, B. Polymorphism of human cytochrome P450 enzymes and its clinical impact. *Drug Metab. Rev.* **2009**, *41*, 89–295. [CrossRef] [PubMed]
51. Potkin, S.G.; Bera, R.; Gulasekaram, B.; Costa, J.; Hayes, S.; Jin, Y.; Richmond, G.; Carreon, D.; Sitanggan, K.; Gerber, B. Plasma clozapine concentrations predict clinical response in treatment-resistant schizophrenia. *J. Clin. Psychiatry* **1994**, *55*, 133–136. [PubMed]
52. Faber, M.; Jetter, A.; Fuhr, U. Assessment of CYP1A2 Activity in Clinical Practice: Why, How, and When? *Basic Clin. Pharmacol. Toxicol.* **2005**, *97*, 125–134. [CrossRef]
53. Rasmussen, B.B.; Brix, T.H.; Kyvik, K.O.; Brøsen, K. The interindividual differences in the 3-demthylation of caffeine alias CYP1A2 is determined by both genetic and environmental factors. *Pharmacogenetics* **2002**, *12*, 473–478. [CrossRef] [PubMed]
54. Klein, K.; Winter, S.; Turpeinen, M.; Schwab, M.; Zanger, U.M. Pathway-Targeted Pharmacogenomics of CYP1A2 in Human Liver. *Front. Pharmacol.* **2010**, *1*, 129. [CrossRef] [PubMed]
55. Ueng, Y.-F.; Shimada, T.; Yamazaki, H.; Guengerich, F.P. Oxidation of Aflatoxin B1 by Bacterial Recombinant Human Cytochrome P450 Enzymes. *Chem. Res. Toxicol.* **1995**, *8*, 218–225. [CrossRef]
56. Shin, H.S.; Lee, H.J.; Pyo, M.C.; Ryu, D.; Lee, K.-W. Ochratoxin A-Induced Hepatotoxicity through Phase I and Phase II Reactions Regulated by AhR in Liver Cells. *Toxins* **2019**, *11*, 377. [CrossRef] [PubMed]
57. Gallagher, E.P.; Kunze, K.L.; Stapleton, P.L.; Eaton, D.L. The Kinetics of Aflatoxin B1Oxidation by Human cDNA-Expressed and Human Liver Microsomal Cytochromes P450 1A2 and 3A4. *Toxicol. Appl. Pharmacol.* **1996**, *141*, 595–606. [CrossRef] [PubMed]
58. Bojić, M.; Kondža, M.; Rimac, H.; Benković, G.; Maleš, Ž. The Effect of Flavonoid Aglycones on the CYP1A2, CYP2A6, CYP2C8 and CYP2D6 Enzymes Activity. *Molecules* **2019**, *24*, 3174. [CrossRef]
59. Pyo, M.C.; Shin, H.S.; Jeon, G.Y.; Lee, K.-W. Synergistic Interaction of Ochratoxin A and Acrylamide Toxins in Human Kidney and Liver Cells. *Biol. Pharm. Bull.* **2020**, *43*, 1346–1355. [CrossRef] [PubMed]
60. Longobardi, C.; Andretta, E.; Romano, V.; Lauritano, C.; Avantaggiato, G.; Schiavone, A.; Jarriyawattanachaikul, W.; Florio, S.; Ciarcia, R.; Damiano, S. Effects of Some New Antioxidants on Apoptosis and ROS Production in AFB1 Treated Chickens. *Med. Sci. Forums* **2020**, *2*, 12. [CrossRef]
61. Zangar, R.C. Mechanisms that regulate production of reactive oxygen species by cytochrome P450. *Toxicol. Appl. Pharmacol.* **2004**, *199*, 316–331. [CrossRef]
62. Moorthy, B. *The CYP1A Subfamily. Issues in Toxicology of Cytochromes P450*; Royal Society of Chemistry: Cambridge, UK, 2008; pp. 97–135.
63. Xun, T.; Lin, Z.; Wang, X.; Zhan, X.; Feng, H.; Gan, D.; Yang, X. Advanced oxidation protein products downregulate CYP1A2 and CYP3A4 expression and activity via the NF-κB-mediated signaling pathway in vitro and in vivo. *Lab. Investig.* **2021**, *101*, 1197–1209. [CrossRef]
64. Jacquemyn, J.; Cascalho, A.C.C.; Goodchild, R.E. The ins and outs of endoplasmic reticulum-controlled lipid biosynthesis. *EMBO Rep.* **2017**, *18*, 1905–1921. [CrossRef] [PubMed]
65. Casares, D.; Escribá, P.V.; Rosselló, C.A. Membrane Lipid Composition: Effect on Membrane and Organelle Structure, Function and Compartmentalization and Therapeutic Avenues. *Int. J. Mol. Sci.* **2019**, *20*, 2167. [CrossRef] [PubMed]
66. Arora, A.; Byrem, T.M.; Nair, M.G.; Strasburg, G.M. Modulation of Liposomal Membrane Fluidity by Flavonoids and Isoflavonoids. *Arch. Biochem. Biophys.* **2000**, *373*, 102–109. [CrossRef]
67. Hlavica, P. Challenges in assignment of allosteric effects in cytochrome P450-catalyzed substrate oxidations to structural dynamics in the hemoprotein architecture. *J. Inorg. Biochem.* **2017**, *167*, 100–115. [CrossRef]
68. Caro, A.A.; Cederbaum, A.I. Oxidativestress, Toxicology, Andpharmacology of CYP2E1. *Annu. Rev. Pharmacol. Toxicol.* **2004**, *44*, 27–42. [CrossRef] [PubMed]
69. Gonzalez, F.J. Role of cytochromes P450 in chemical toxicity and oxidative stress: Studies with CYP2E1. *Mutat. Res. Mol. Mech. Mutagen.* **2005**, *569*, 101–110. [CrossRef]
70. Neafsey, P.; Ginsberg, G.; Hattis, D.; Johns, D.O.; Guyton, K.Z.; Sonawane, B. Genetic Polymorphism in CYP2E1: Population Distribution of CYP2E1 Activity. *J. Toxicol. Environ. Health Part B* **2009**, *12*, 362–388. [CrossRef] [PubMed]
71. Bolt, H.M.; Roos, P.H.; Thier, R. The cytochrome P-450 isoenzyme CYP2E1 in the biological processing of industrial chemicals: Consequences for occupational and environmental medicine. *Int. Arch. Occup. Environ. Health* **2003**, *76*, 174–185. [CrossRef] [PubMed]
72. Hu, Y.; Oscarson, M.; Johansson, I.; Yue, Q.Y.; Dahl, M.L.; Tabone, M.; Arincò, S.; Albano, E.; Ingelman-Sundberg, M. Genetic polymorphism of human CYP2E1: Characterization of two variant alleles. *Mol. Pharmacol.* **1997**, *51*, 370–376.

73. Marí, M.; Cederbaum, A.I. CYP2E1 Overexpression in HepG2 Cells Induces Glutathione Synthesis by Transcriptional Activation of γ-Glutamylcysteine Synthetase. *J. Biol. Chem.* **2000**, *275*, 15563–15571. [CrossRef]
74. Rasmussen, M.K.; Zamaratskaia, G. Regulation of Porcine Hepatic Cytochrome P450—Implication for Boar Taint. *Comput. Struct. Biotechnol. J.* **2014**, *11*, 106–112. [CrossRef]
75. Willard, R.R.; Shappell, N.W.; Meekin, J.H.; Talbot, N.C.; Caperna, T.J. Cytochrome P450 expression profile of the PICM-19H pig liver cell line: Potential application to rapid liver toxicity assays. *Vitr. Cell. Dev. Biol. Anim.* **2009**, *46*, 11–19. [CrossRef]
76. Howard, J.T.; O'Nan, A.T.; Maltecca, C.; Baynes, R.E.; Ashwell, M. Differential Gene Expression across Breed and Sex in Commercial Pigs Administered Fenbendazole and Flunixin Meglumine. *PLoS ONE* **2015**, *10*, e0137830. [CrossRef] [PubMed]
77. Bee, G.; Silacci, P.; Ampuero-Kragten, S.; Čandek-Potokar, M.; Wealleans, A.; Litten-Brown, J.; Salminen, J.-P.; Mueller-Harvey, I. Hydrolysable tannin-based diet rich in gallotannins has a minimal impact on pig performance but significantly reduces salivary and bulbourethral gland size. *Animal* **2017**, *11*, 1617–1625. [CrossRef]
78. Zhou, X.; Li, X.; Wang, X.; Jin, X.; Shi, D.; Wang, J.; Bi, D. Cecropin B Represses CYP3A29 Expression through Activation of the TLR2/4-NF-κB/PXR Signaling Pathway. *Sci. Rep.* **2016**, *6*, 27876. [CrossRef] [PubMed]
79. Li, X.; Jin, X.; Zhou, X.; Wang, X.; Shi, D.; Xiao, Y.; Bi, D. Pregnane X receptor is required for IFN-α-mediated CYP3A29 expression in pigs. *Biochem. Biophys. Res. Commun.* **2014**, *445*, 469–474. [CrossRef]
80. Yao, M.; Dai, M.; Liu, Z.; Huang, L.; Chen, D.; Wang, Y.; Peng, D.; Wang, X.; Liu, Z.; Yuan, Z. Comparison of the substrate kinetics of pig CYP3A29 with pig liver microsomes and human CYP3A4. *Biosci. Rep.* **2011**, *31*, 211–220. [CrossRef] [PubMed]
81. Taneja, G.; Maity, S.; Jiang, W.; Moorthy, B.; Coarfa, C.; Ghose, R. Transcriptomic profiling identifies novel mechanisms of transcriptional regulation of the cytochrome P450 (Cyp)3a11 gene. *Sci. Rep.* **2019**, *9*, 6663. [CrossRef]
82. Chen, R.; Jiang, J.; Hu, Z.; Ye, W.; Yuan, Q.; Li, M.; Wen, J.; Deng, Y.; Jun, J. Coordinated Transcriptional Regulation of Cytochrome P450 3As by Nuclear Transcription Factor Y and Specificity Protein 1. *Mol. Pharmacol.* **2019**, *95*, 507–518. [CrossRef] [PubMed]
83. Dong, L.; Chen, Q.; Liu, X.; Wen, J.; Jiang, J.; Deng, Y. Role of Specificity Protein 1, Hepatocyte Nuclear Factor 1α, and Pregnane X Receptor in the Basal and Rifampicin-Induced Transcriptional Regulation of Porcine Cytochrome P450 3A46. *Drug Metab. Dispos.* **2015**, *43*, 1458–1467. [CrossRef] [PubMed]
84. Qin, X.; Wang, X. Role of vitamin D receptor in the regulation of CYP3A gene expression. *Acta Pharm. Sin. B* **2019**, *9*, 1087–1098. [CrossRef] [PubMed]
85. Jover, R.; Bort, R.; Gomez-Lechon, M.J.; Castell, J.V. Cytochrome P450 regulation by hepatocyte nuclear factor 4 in human hepatocytes: A study using adenovirus-mediated antisense targeting. *Hepatology* **2001**, *33*, 668–675. [CrossRef]
86. Saito, T.; Takahashi, Y.; Hashimoto, H.; Kamataki, T. Novel Transcriptional Regulation of the Human CYP3A7Gene by Sp1 and Sp3 through Nuclear Factor κB-like Element. *J. Biol. Chem.* **2001**, *276*, 38010–38022. [CrossRef]
87. Kuban, W.; Daniel, W.A. Cytochrome P450 expression and regulation in the brain. *Drug Metab. Rev.* **2021**, *53*, 1–29. [CrossRef] [PubMed]
88. Rodrigues, E.; Vilarem, M.-J.; Ribeiro, V.; Maurel, P.; Lechner, M.C. Two CCAAT/enhancer binding protein sites in the cytochrome P4503A1 locus. Potencial role in the glucocorticoid response. *JBIC J. Biol. Inorg. Chem.* **2003**, *270*, 556–564. [CrossRef] [PubMed]
89. Luo, G.; Guenthner, T.; Gan, L.-S.; Humphreys, W. CYP3A4 Induction by Xenobiotics: Biochemistry, Experimental Methods and Impact on Drug Discovery and Development. *Curr. Drug Metab.* **2004**, *5*, 483–505. [CrossRef] [PubMed]
90. Glanemann, C.; Loos, A.; Gorret, N.; Willis, L.B.; O'Brien, X.M.; Lessard, P.A.; Sinskey, A.J. Disparity between changes in mRNA abundance and enzyme activity in Corynebacterium glutamicum: Implications for DNA microarray analysis. *Appl. Microbiol. Biotechnol.* **2003**, *61*, 61–68. [CrossRef]
91. Lodish, H.; Berk, A.; Zipursky, S.L.; Matsudaira, P.; Baltimore, D.; Darnell, J. *Molecular Cell Biology*, 4th ed.; W. H. Freeman: New York, NY, USA, 2000; Section 3.3, Functional Design of Proteins. Available online: https://www.ncbi.nlm.nih.gov/books/NBK21733/ (accessed on 18 August 2021).
92. Hassan, I.; Jabir, N.R.; Ahmad, S.; Shah, A.; Tabrez, S. Certain Phase I and II Enzymes as Toxicity Biomarker: An Overview. *Water Air Soil Pollut.* **2015**, *226*, 1–8. [CrossRef]
93. Yagishita, Y.; Uruno, A.; Yamamoto, M. *NRF2-Mediated Gene Regulation and Glucose Homeostasis*; Elsevier: Amsterdam, The Netherlands, 2016; ISBN 9780128015858.
94. Hakkola, J.; Hukkanen, J.; Turpeinen, M.; Pelkonen, O. Inhibition and induction of CYP enzymes in humans: An update. *Arch. Toxicol.* **2020**, *94*, 3671–3722. [CrossRef]
95. Kedderis, G. Biotransformation of Toxicants. *Compr. Toxicol.* **2010**, *1–14*, 137–151.
96. Jančová, P.; Siller, P.J.A.M. *Phase II Drug Metabolism*; Paxton, J., Ed.; IntechOpen: London, UK, 2012; Available online: https://www.intechopen.com/chapters/29241 (accessed on 18 August 2021). [CrossRef]
97. Singh, R.R.; Reindl, K.M. Glutathione S-Transferases in Cancer. *Antioxidants* **2021**, *10*, 701. [CrossRef]
98. Strange, R.C.; Jones, P.W.; Fryer, A.A. Strange bedfellows in the personal computer industry: Technology alliances between ibm and apple. *Toxicol. Lett.* **2000**, *113*, 357–363. [CrossRef]
99. Allocati, N.; Masulli, M.; Di Ilio, C.; Federici, L. Glutathione transferases: Substrates, inihibitors and pro-drugs in cancer and neurodegenerative diseases. *Oncogenesis* **2018**, *7*, 1–15. [CrossRef] [PubMed]
100. Chatterjee, A.; Gupta, S. The multifaceted role of glutathione S-transferases in cancer. *Cancer Lett.* **2018**, *433*, 33–42. [CrossRef] [PubMed]

101. Murcia, H.W.; Diaz, G.J. Protective effect of glutathione S-transferase enzyme activity against aflatoxin B1 in poultry species: Relationship between glutathione S-transferase enzyme kinetic parameters, and resistance to aflatoxin B1. *Poult. Sci.* **2021**, *100*, 101235. [CrossRef] [PubMed]
102. Zain, M.E. Impact of mycotoxins on humans and animals. *J. Saudi Chem. Soc.* **2011**, *15*, 129–144. [CrossRef]
103. Mitchell, J.; Tinkey, P.T.; Avritscher, R.; Van Pelt, C.; Eskandari, G.; George, S.K.; Xiao, L.; Cressman, E.; Morris, J.S.; Rashid, A.; et al. Validation of a Preclinical Model of Diethylnitrosamine-Induced Hepatic Neoplasia in Yucatan Miniature Pigs. *Oncology* **2016**, *91*, 90–100. [CrossRef]
104. Surai, P.F. Antioxidants in Poultry Nutrition and Reproduction: An Update. *Antioxidants* **2020**, *9*, 105. [CrossRef] [PubMed]
105. Tozlovanu, M.; Canadas, D.; Pfohl-Leszkowicz, A.; Frenette, C.; Paugh, R.J.; Manderville, R.A. Glutathione Conjugates of Ochratoxin a as Biomarkers of Exposure / Glutationski Konjugati Okratoksina a Kao Biomarkeri Izloženosti. *Arch. Ind. Hyg. Toxicol.* **2012**, *63*, 417–427. [CrossRef] [PubMed]
106. Sorrenti, V.; Di Giacomo, C.; Acquaviva, R.; Barbagallo, I.; Bognanno, M.; Galvano, F. Toxicity of Ochratoxin and Its Modulation by Antioxidants: A Review. *Toxins* **2013**, *5*, 1742–1766. [CrossRef]
107. Gekle, M.; Sauvant, C.; Schwerdt, G. Ochratoxin A at nanomolar concentrations: A signal modulator in renal cells. *Mol. Nutr. Food Res.* **2005**, *49*, 118–130. [CrossRef]
108. Boudra, H.; Saivin, S.; Buffiere, C.; Morgavi, D. Short communication: Toxicokinetics of ochratoxin A in dairy ewes and carryover to milk following a single or long-term ingestion of contaminated feed. *J. Dairy Sci.* **2013**, *96*, 6690–6696. [CrossRef]
109. Hanioka, N.; Tatarazako, N.; Jinno, H.; Arizono, K.; Ando, M. Determination of cytochrome P450 1A activities in mammalian liver microsomes by high-performance liquid chromatography with fluorescence detection. *J. Chromatogr. B Biomed. Sci. Appl.* **2000**, *744*, 399–406. [CrossRef]
110. Wanwimolruk, S.; Wanwimolruk, P. Characterization of CYP1A enzyme in Adélie penguin liver. *Comp. Biochem. Physiol. Part C Toxicol. Pharmacol.* **2006**, *144*, 148–154. [CrossRef] [PubMed]
111. Zamaratskaia, G.; Chen, G.; Lundström, K. Effects of sex, weight, diet and hCG administration on levels of skatole and indole in the liver and hepatic activities of cytochromes P4502E1 and P4502A6 in pigs. *Meat Sci.* **2006**, *72*, 331–338. [CrossRef] [PubMed]
112. Sohl, C.D.; Cheng, Q.; Guengerich, F.P. Chromatographic assays of drug oxidation by human cytochrome P450 3A4. *Nat. Protoc.* **2009**, *4*, 1252–1257. [CrossRef] [PubMed]
113. Cheng, G.; Liu, C.; Wang, X.; Ma, H.; Pan, Y.; Huang, L.; Hao, H.; Dai, M.; Yuan, Z. Structure-Function Analysis of Porcine Cytochrome P450 3A29 in the Hydroxylation of T-2 Toxin as Revealed by Docking and Mutagenesis Studies. *PLoS ONE* **2014**, *9*, e106769. [CrossRef] [PubMed]
114. Habig, W.H.; Pabst, M.J.; Jakoby, W.B. Glutathione S-transferases. The first enzymatic step in mercapturic acid formation. *J. Biol. Chem.* **1974**, *249*, 7130–7139. [CrossRef]
115. Bradford, M.M. A rapid and sensitive for the quantitation of microgram quantities of protein utilizing the principle of protein-dye binding. *Anal. Biochem.* **1976**, *72*, 248–254. [CrossRef]

MDPI
St. Alban-Anlage 66
4052 Basel
Switzerland
Tel. +41 61 683 77 34
Fax +41 61 302 89 18
www.mdpi.com

Toxins Editorial Office
E-mail: toxins@mdpi.com
www.mdpi.com/journal/toxins

www.ingramcontent.com/pod-product-compliance
Lightning Source LLC
LaVergne TN
LVHW070616100526
838202LV00012B/658